YOGA BODY

Praise for
Yoga Body: The Origins of Modern Posture Practice
Mark Singleton

"Mark Singleton's *Yoga Body: The Origins of Modern Posture Practice* is an outstanding scholarly work which brings so much insight and clarity to the historic and cultural background of modern haṭha yoga. I highly recommend this book, especially for all sincere students of yoga."—John Friend, founder of Anusara Yoga

"From the moment I started reading Mark Singleton's *Yoga Body* I couldn't put it down. It is beautifully written, extensively researched, and full of fascinating information. It stands alone in its depth of insight into a subject which has intrigued me for forty years."—David Williams, the first non-Indian to learn the complete Ashtanga Yoga syllabus

"Mark Singleton's book *Yoga Body* traces the evolution of the ever-expanding practice of āsana world-wide. His work offers a much needed historical perspective that will help correct much of the mythology and group-think that is emerging in the modern āsana based 'yoga world.' Any serious āsana practitioner who wishes to understand the place of āsana in the greater tradition of yoga will do well to read it carefully."—Gary Krafstow, founder of the American Viniyoga Institute, author of *Yoga for Wellness and Yoga for Transformation*

"Mark Singleton has written a sweeping and nuanced account of the origins and development of modern postural yoga in early twentieth-century India and the West, arguing convincingly that yoga as we know it today does not flow directly from the *Yoga Sūtras* or India's medieval *haṭha* yoga traditions, but rather emerged out of a confluence of practices, movements and ideologies, ranging from contortionist acts in carnival sideshows, British Army calisthenics and women's stretching exercises to social Darwinism, eugenics, and the Indian nationalist movement. The richly illustrated story he tells is an especially welcome contribution to the history of yoga, demonstrating the ways in which an ancient tradition was reinvented against the backdrop of India's colonial experience."—David Gordon White, professor of Religious Studies, University of California, Santa Barbara.

YOGA BODY

THE ORIGINS OF MODERN POSTURE PRACTICE

MARK SINGLETON

OXFORD
UNIVERSITY PRESS

2010

OXFORD
UNIVERSITY PRESS

Oxford University Press, Inc., publishes works that further
Oxford University's objective of excellence
in research, scholarship, and education.

Oxford New York
Auckland Cape Town Dar es Salaam Hong Kong Karachi
Kuala Lumpur Madrid Melbourne Mexico City Nairobi
New Delhi Shanghai Taipei Toronto

With offices in
Argentina Austria Brazil Chile Czech Republic France Greece
Guatemala Hungary Italy Japan Poland Portugal Singapore
South Korea Switzerland Thailand Turkey Ukraine Vietnam

Published by Oxford University Press, Inc.
198 Madison Avenue, New York, NY 10016

www.oup.com

Library of Congress Cataloging-in-Publication Data
Singleton, Mark, 1972–
Yoga body : the origins of modern posture practice / Mark Singleton.
p. cm.
Includes bibliographical references and index.
ISBN 978-0-19-539535-8; ISBN 978-0-19-539534-1 (pbk.)
1. Hatha yoga. 2. Posture. I. Title.
RA781.7.S568 2010
613.7'046—dc22
2009014275

7 9 8
Printed in the United States of America
on acid-free paper

contents

acknowledgments

Many people have contributed to the development of the ideas in this book. I would like to thank Peter Schreiner for his thorough and insightful comments on an earlier version; James Mallinson for helping to clarify certain issues regarding contemporary Indian *haṭha* yoga practitioners, and for sharing his images of the murals of the Nātha Mahāmandir in Jodhpur; Gudrun Bühnemann for spotting some egregious errors in my Sanskrit diacritics; and Dagmar and Dominik Wujastyk for the discussions on the topic of modern yoga over the last five years. Thanks also to Felicia M. Tomasko, editor of *LA Yoga Magazine*, for her continued insights into current developments in yoga. I'm grateful to Gavin Flood and David Smith, who gave valuable feedback at the Ph.D stage of this project; and to Joseph S. Alter and Kenneth Liberman for their extensive comments and suggestions as OUP readers. Thanks also to Eivind Kahrs of Queen's College, Cambridge, for reading and commenting on early drafts, and to Julius Lipner for his guidance on the research process throughout my time at the Faculty of Divinity in Cambridge.

I am grateful to the participants at the Modern Yoga Graduate Workshop, organized by Elizabeth De Michelis, Suzanne Newcombe, and me at the Divinity Faculty, University of Cambridge, in April 2006. Ongoing interaction with several of the participants has been invaluable in refining the ideas in this book, and in particular, I thank Elliott Goldberg, who was generous in sharing his reflections on physical culture and yoga both prior to and during this workshop. Thanks are also due to Vivienne Lo and Ronit Yoeli-Tlalim of University College, London, for supporting me through the task of editing a special yoga issue of *Asian Medicine, Tradition and Modernity* in 2007, and to Jean Marie Byrne of

Queensland University, Australia, for her collaboration on our collection of yoga scholarship, *Yoga in the Modern World* (2008). Editorial work on these projects has given me the opportunity to engage in sustained dialogue with many international scholars currently working in the field of modern yoga and has contributed greatly to the shape of this book.

I am much obliged to Laura Cooley of the Meem Library, St. John's College, Santa Fe, for obtaining the many, sometimes obscure, interlibrary loan requests I made during the final stages of this book, and to Paige Roberts of the Babson Library, Springfield College, Massachusetts, for going out of her way to provide material on YMCA physical culture programs in India. Thanks also to senior staff member and scholar of yoga at the YMCA College of Physical Education in Bangalore, Śrī Vasudeva Bhāt, who was extremely helpful in directing my research in Karnataka in 2005.

I am indebted to Śrī M. A. Narasimhan and Dr. M. A. Jayashree of Mysore, India, for their good-humored support in reading Sanskrit yoga texts during 2005, and to Professor Lakṣmī Tattācarya for his guidance in my reading of the *Yogasūtrabhāṣya*. Thanks to Dr. K. V. Karna of Bangalore for sharing his memories of his father, K. V. Iyer and for providing otherwise unavailable textual and photographic material; and to Professor T. R. S. Sharma, who was so generous with his records and his memories of Mysore in the 1930s and 1940s. Thanks also to Śrī K. Pattabhi Jois, Shankara Narayan Jois, Anant Rao and A. G. Mohan for the interviews they granted, and to B. K. S. Iyengar, for the free use of his library in Pune.

Thanks to all my teachers of *āsana*, in particular, Śrī K. Pattabhi Jois, Sharat Rangaswami, B. N. S. Iyengar, Rudra Ḍev, Hamish Hendry, Barbara Harding, and Sasha Perryman; and to all those friends who have helped to sustain and inspire my practice, especially Louie Ettling, Norman Blair, Emma Owen-Smith, Nigel Jones, Tara Fraser, Romola Davenport, Louise Palmer, and Jennifer Morrison. Thanks also to Lorin Parrish, who never fails to see the funny side.

This project was funded by a Domestic Research Scholarship from the University of Cambridge and by various travel scholarships made available by the Faculty of Divinity and Sidney Sussex College, Cambridge. I am grateful for the opportunity that these scholarships provided. Finally, I owe an enormous debt of gratitude to Dr. Elizabeth De Michelis, for her unflagging support and friendship over the last six years.

abbreviations

GŚ:	*Gorakṣa Śataka*	HR:	*Haṭharatnāvalī*
ŚS:	*Śiva Saṃhitā*	GhS:	*Gheraṇḍa Saṃhitā*
HYP:	*Haṭhayogapradīpikā*		

YOGA BODY

Introduction

An Outline of the Project

This book investigates the rise to prominence of *āsana* (posture) in modern, transnational yoga. Today yoga is virtually synonymous in the West with the practice of *āsana*, and postural yoga classes can be found in great number in virtually every city in the Western world, as well as, increasingly, in the Middle East, Asia, South and Central America, and Australasia. "Health club" types of yoga are even seeing renewed popularity among affluent urban populations in India. While exact practitioner statistics are hard to come by, it is clear that postural yoga is booming.[1] Since the 1990s, yoga has become a multimillion dollar business, and high-profile legal battles have even been fought over who owns *āsana*. Styles, sequences, and postures themselves have been franchised, copyrighted, and patented by individuals, companies, and government,[2] and yoga postures are used to sell a wide range of products, from mobile phones to yoghurt. In 2008, it was estimated that U.S. yoga practitioners were spending 5.7 billion dollars on yoga classes, vacation, and products per year (*Yoga Journal* 2008), a figure approximately equal to half the gross domestic product of Nepal (CIA 2008).

However, in spite of the immense popularity of postural yoga worldwide, there is little or no evidence that *āsana* (excepting certain seated postures of meditation) has ever been the primary aspect of any Indian yoga practice tradition—including the medieval, body-oriented *haṭha* yoga—in spite of the self-authenticating claims of many modern yoga schools (see chapter 1). The primacy of *āsana* performance in transnational yoga today is a new phenomenon that has no parallel in premodern times.

In the late 1800s, a mainly anglophone yoga revival began in India, and new syntheses of practical techniques and theory began to emerge, most notably with the teachings of Vivekananda (1863–1902). But even in these new forms the kind of *āsana* practice so visible today was missing. Indeed, *āsana*, as well as other techniques associated with *haṭha* yoga, were explicitly shunned as being unsuitable or distasteful by Vivekananda and many of those who followed his lead. As a result, they remained largely absent from initial expressions of practical anglophone yoga. In this study I set out to examine the reasons *āsana* was initially excluded from most modern yogas and what changes it underwent as it was assimilated into them.[3] With such unpromising beginnings, how did *āsana* attain the standing it enjoys today as the foundation stone of transnational yoga? What were the conditions that contributed to its exclusion from the vision of early modern yoga teachers, and on what grounds was it able to make its return?

At the time of Vivekananda's synthesis of yoga in the 1890s, postural practice was primarily associated with the *yogin* (or, more popularly, "yogi"). This term designated in particular the *haṭha* yogins of the Nāth lineage, but was employed more loosely to refer to a variety of ascetics, magicians, and street performers. Often confused with the Mohammedan "fakir," the yogi came to symbolize all that was wrong in certain tributaries of the Hindu religion. The postural contortions of *haṭha* yoga were associated with backwardness and superstition, and many people considered them to have no place in the *scientific* and *modern* yoga enterprise. In the first half of this study I investigate the figure of the yogin as he appears in travel writing, scholarship, popular culture, and the literature of popular practical yoga, with a view to understanding the particular status of *haṭha* yoga at this time. This provides the necessary context for the second half of the study, which focuses on the particular modifications that *haṭha* yoga had to undergo to avoid being perceived as a blight on the Indian religious and social landscape.

The book targets an essential, but hitherto largely ignored, aspect of yoga's development. Studies of modern yoga have tended to elide the passage from Vivekananda's *āsana*-free manifestos of yoga in the mid-1890s to the well-known posture-oriented forms that began to emerge in the 1920s. The two main studies in this area to date, by De Michelis (2004) and Alter (2004a), have focused on both these moments in the history of transnational yoga, but they have not offered a good explanation of why *āsana* was initially excluded and the ways in which it was eventually reclaimed.[4] The present work aims to identify the factors that initially contributed to the shape that transnational yoga has taken today, and constitutes in some ways a "prehistory" of the international *āsana* revolution that got into full swing with B. K. S. Iyengar and others from the 1950s onward.

That prehistory involves an examination of the international physical culture movement and the ways that it made an impact on the consciousness of Indian youth at the turn of the nineteenth century and into the twentieth. Quasi-religious forms of physical culture swept Europe during the nineteenth century and found their way to India, where they informed and infiltrated popular new interpretations of nationalist Hinduism. Experiments to define the particular nature of *Indian* physical culture led to the reinvention of *āsana* as the timeless expression of Hindu exercise. Western physical culture–oriented *āsana* practices, developed in India, subsequently found their way (back) to the West, where they became identified and merged with forms of "esoteric gymnastics," which had grown popular in Europe and America from the mid-nineteenth century (independent of any contact with yoga traditions). Posture-based yoga as we know it today is the result of a dialogical exchange between para-religious, modern body culture techniques developed in the West and the various discourses of "modern" Hindu yoga that emerged from the time of Vivekananda onward. Although it routinely appeals to the tradition of Indian *haṭha* yoga, contemporary posture-based yoga cannot really be considered a direct successor of this tradition.

Sources, Methods, and Demarcations

The initial primary sources for this study were popular English-language yoga manuals from the late 1800s to about 1935. De Michelis (2004) has proposed that "Modern Yoga" begins with Vivekananda's *Raja Yoga* of 1896, and while there are a few exceptions—such as the Theosophical Society–sponsored works of M. N. Dvivedi (1885, 1890) and Ram Prasad (1890)—it is largely true that the practice-oriented anglophone yoga manual begins to emerge as a genre only after this date. Indeed, J. Gordon Melton credits Ram Prasad's book with being the *first* "to explain and advocate the practice of yoga" (Melton 1990: 502). A literature survey of the holdings of the Cambridge University Library and the India Office of the British Library in London revealed that prior to the 1920s the subjects of *āsana* and *haṭha* yoga tended to be absent in popular primers. Subsequent examinations of the collections at Stanford University's Green Library and the library of the University of California, Berkeley, helped to confirm this impression with regard to American-based yoga authors. These surveys enabled me to consult the majority of available practical, anglophone, book-form yoga primers published in India, Britain, and the United States prior to the 1930s. In the post–World War II years, there was an explosion of interest in yoga and in titles dedicated to the subject, and although I have some familiarity with many of these, they fall outside the period under question and I lay no claim to authoritative or comprehensive knowledge of them. However, it is easy to see that after World War II, popular English-language yoga manuals tend to give far greater primacy to the *postures* of yoga than they did before.[5]

The research questions that arose from these literature surveys were the following: why is *āsana*, and *haṭha* yoga more generally, absent from early popular instruction manuals of yoga? What were the conditions whereby postural practice could, by the mid-twentieth century, rise to prominence as the single most important feature of transnational yoga, to become, in certain non-Asian contexts, a virtual synonym for yoga itself? Can the modes of practice of postural yoga today, and the belief frameworks that inform them, be considered "modern" in a typological sense? And, if so, how do these modern forms mediate their supposed relationship with the medieval *haṭha* yoga traditions of which they often claim to be heir?

It is well known that the work of Bombay-based gurus Sri Yogendra (1897–1989) and Swami Kuvalayananda (1883–1966), along with the teachings of T. Krishnamacharya (1888–1989) and his now famous Mysore disciples, were instrumental in bringing *haṭha* yogic *āsanas* into the public eye. It was largely due to their efforts, and those of their disciples, indeed, that postural practice is now so prominent in transnational yoga circles, and these men's publications do serve as significant primary sources for my investigations of modern expressions of *āsana* (chapters 6 through 9). However, these sources alone do not explain why there was a three-decade gap between Vivekananda's exposition of yoga for the modern practitioner, and the arrival of *haṭha* yoga as a significant component of yoga practice. What were the conditions that allowed Kuvalayananda and others to bring *āsana* into the field of popular yoga? And conversely, how could Vivekananda see fit to omit treatment of it in his new synthesis?

These questions led me to examine representations of *haṭha* yoga, and yogins themselves, in European travel writing, scholarship, and popular media from the seventeenth to the early twentieth century. Richard Schmidt's 1908 study of *haṭha* yogic "fakirism" first alerted me to early accounts of yogins by Bernier (1670), Tavernier (1676), J. de Thevenot (1684), and Fryer (1698). These editions furnished further references to the accounts of Mundy (1628–1634), Ovington (1696), Heber (1828), and the compilation of Bernard (ed. 1733–36). What is clear in these works is that the yogin, and the postural austerities he undertakes, are objects of moral and judicial censure, disgust, and morbid fascination. Nineteenth-century scholarship, both by Europeans and English-educated Indians, tends to show similar attitudes to the practitioner of *haṭha* yoga. My sources here include E. W. Hopkins, W. J. Wilkins, M. Monier-Williams, and Max Müller. Also vital to my understanding of the status of the yogin in the last quarter of the nineteenth century are the early *haṭha* yoga translations by

S.C. Vasu (from 1884 on) and, to a lesser extent, those of C. R. S. Ayangar (1893), B. N. Banerjee (1894), and Pancham Sinh (1915). Vasu's translations in particular were instrumental in bringing a modern interpretation of *haṭha* yoga to a widespread public and in creating the conditions whereby "medicalized" *haṭha* yoga could begin to emerge from the 1920s onward as legitimate mode of practice. Once again, scholars have hitherto neglected this crucial stage in the development of modern anglophone yoga.

Sources for the representation of the yogin in popular media include British illustrated periodicals of the nineteenth century, like *The Strand, Pearson's Magazine*, and *Scribner's Magazine*; turn-of-the-century, popular esoteric works which treat the "fakir-yogi" and his methods; later popular ethnographies of India; and some early films featuring fictional Indian yogins.[6] Eighteenth-century newspaper advertisements for performances by "Posture Masters," a European precursor to the "vaudeville yogin" of the late 1800s, were initially found via references in secondary sources and then obtained in either Cambridge or London. These visions of the yogin, from the European travelogues of Bernier onward, through nineteenth-century Orientalist scholarship and popular media representations, show clearly the status of the yogin in early formulations of popular anglophone yoga and go a long way to explaining the absence of *haṭha* teachings in the early practical manuals. The works of Swami Vivekananda and Mme. H. P. Blavatsky, the two most significant arbiters of taste in early modern yoga, have been particularly important sources here, insofar as their writings reflect and reinforce prevailing attitudes to *haṭha* yoga. It is also important to note, however, that the *haṭha* yogin had always been an agent of ritual pollution for caste Hindus, well prior to the kind of European interpretations I consider here. This status is a key factor in the exclusion of the yogin from the Indian yoga renaissance.

The above sources helped to explain the initial exclusion of *haṭha* practice from popular anglophone yoga but did not offer any evidence as to how it eventually made its comeback. Where to look was, once again, suggested by early popular yoga manuals. My initial survey showed that the *āsanas* of *haṭha* yoga were commonly, indeed routinely, compared with gymnastics in these manuals. These interpretations of postural yoga were significantly divergent from those given by "classical" *haṭha* yoga texts, such as those translated by Vasu. Indeed, the whole somatic and philosophical framework of this new English-language yoga appeared to have been replaced by a modern discourse of health and fitness. An examination of the eighteenth- to early twentieth-century European gymnastics manuals in the British Library and Cambridge University Library showed without much doubt that anglophone yoga authors had grafted elements of modern physical culture onto *haṭha* yoga orthopraxy and seemingly excised those parts that were difficult to reconcile with the emerging health and fitness discourse.

Of especial relevance here are Scandinavian systems stemming from Ling, the teachings of Sandow, and the methods of the YMCA. These three were the major foreign players in the shaping of modern physical culture in India and thereby also helped to determine the shape of the new *haṭha* yoga syntheses. My primary sources for YMCA physical culture programs in India come from several places: the archives and special collections of the Babson Library of Springfield College (Massachusetts) where Luther Halsey Gulick pioneered the Y's first Department of Physical Education in 1887; books and records at India's pioneer YMCA College of Physical Education in Chennai; and material found at the YMCA College of Physical Education in Bangalore as well as interviews conducted there. Other primary sources for the exploration of modern physical culture in India include the Maharastrian periodical *Vyāyam, the Bodybuilder* and the works of Indian physical culture authors like P. K. Gupta, P. K. Ghose, and, most important, K. Ramamurthy. I also draw substantially on British physical culture periodicals of the early twentieth century, such as *Health and Strength* and *The Superman*, for evidence of the dialogue between yoga and fitness in the milieu of international physical culture.

Some of the material for chapters 6 and 9, regarding the practices of yoga and physical culture in the Mysore and Bangalore area during the 1930s, was derived from interviews with informants who had either studied or taught these disciplines at the time or who had close relatives who had. All were conducted during a three-month fieldwork visit to the region in 2005. These men were often in their eighties or nineties (one was over a hundred years old) and represent living links between the historical past, which is the subject of this study, and the evolving present of modern transnational yoga. My aim in tracking them down and interviewing them was, on the one hand, to obtain firsthand accounts of what it was like to practice yoga or physical culture during this period and, on the other, to garner specific details concerning key figures in these respective fields (particularly T. Krishnamacharya and the "bodybuilding yogins" associated with K. V. Iyer).

The period in question is still—though only just—within living memory, and often these memories are hazy. Indeed, my interviews brought into sharp relief the limits of this method of enquiry: here were old men, struggling to recall the particulars of over half a century ago, when they were themselves mere children, and it is probably inevitable that some details should have faded or been lost. Furthermore, factionalism and vested interests in the management of memory are still alive and well in the realm of modern yoga. In particular, the legacy of T. Krishnamacharya has been, and remains, the locus of power struggles within and among the several schools of postural yoga that stem from his teaching (see chapter 9). Orthopraxy (i.e., what counts as the true and authentic way to practice) is hotly contested in contemporary, transnational yoga, and authority is often established by means of hagiography and the editorializing of memory. This needed to be taken into account in the interpretation of interview transcriptions. In spite of these caveats, however, the interviews provided invaluable and otherwise inaccessible insights into the experiences of those practicing yoga and physical culture in 1930s Karnataka, as well as access to some rare textual sources.

Key informants include three original Mysore students of Krishnamacharya: the internationally famous, and recently deceased, guru Śrī K. Pattabhi Jois; the less well-known Mysore *āsana* teacher B. N. S. Iyengar; and Professor T. R. S. Sharma, who was kind enough to share at length and on several occasions his memories and mementos of his time at the Mysore *yogaśālā*. Another ex-student, the illustrious pioneer of international postural yoga, B. K. S. Iyengar, refused my repeated requests for an interview on these topics but did allow me to make use of his personal library at his institute in Pune. A fifth ex-student whom I interviewed was the well-known teacher A. G. Mohan, who studied under Krishnamcharya during his later years in Chennai but who had no direct experience of the Mysore period.

Mention should also be made of Śrī M. G. Narasimhan, custodian of the administrative records of the Jaganmohan Palace in Mysore, who generously provided me with annual reports from the 1930s and 1940s concerning Krishnamacharya's *yogaśālā* there. His wife, Dr. M. A. Jayashree, and brother-in-law Śrī M. A. Narasimhan, were also helpful in developing my understanding of *haṭha* yoga theory, guiding me through a close reading of the Sanskrit text of Brahmānanada's *Jyotsnā* commentary to the *Haṭhayogapradīpikā*. On my return from Mysore, I edited Śrī Narasimhan's translation from the Kannada of Krishnamacharya's hitherto untranslated and unpublished *Yoga Makaranda* of 1935. Although the text has quasi-legendary status among contemporary students of Pattabhi Jois, very few have actually seen it. Plans for the publication of the complete text have been temporarily postponed, but part of Śrī Narasimhan's translation, with a discussion of the contexts in which it was written, will appear in Singleton 2009b. This seminal, though unknown work has been, along with Śrī Narasimhan's translation of Krishnamacharya's *āsana* manual *Yogāsanagalu* of c.1941, a key source for my understanding of Krishnamacharya's teaching in Mysore in the thirties and forties. The partial translation of *Yogāsanagalu* by Autumn Jacobsen and R.V.S. Sundaram has also been helpful in cross-checking translations.

"Transnational Anglophone Yoga"

Modern, transnational yoga was and is a predominantly anglophone phenomenon, and therefore the majority of my sources are in English (or sometimes in another European language). My quarry is the forms of yoga that were formulated and transmitted in *a dialogical relationship between India and the West through the medium of English*, and this is why I refer to it as "transnational anglophone yoga," rather than simply "modern yoga." I take "transnational" in this context to indicate a flow of ideas, beliefs, and practices that extends or operates across national boundaries. On this basis, I have not found it necessary or relevant to engage in any substantial Sanskritic exegesis nor to attempt a sustained consideration of modern yoga texts in Indian vernacular languages (although there are exceptions) since, by definition, such work falls for the most part outside the parameters of the field under examination.

Primary and Secondary Sources

I treat all material of the period that claims to present the nature of yoga (and in particular *haṭha* yoga) as *primary* sources, whether it be popular yoga primers or academic translations and studies of "classical" texts. Both contributed to the processes of production that shaped the idea of yoga in the modern period: they do not stand outside this production as descriptions of a priori phenomena, although of course both commonly claim precisely this as legitimation for their interpretations. Scholarship structured and informed practical modern yoga by obliquely sanctioning its choice of texts and endowing "classical" status to certain methods and belief frameworks. In this sense scholarship is not a meta-discourse that reveals the truth about yoga (though, of course, it may) but a constituent part of its historical production in the modern age. For example, I treat the translations and commentaries of S. C. Vasu as key moments in the construction and legitimation of a particular, historically situated, *rendition* of *haṭha* yoga rather than as documents revealing its true substance. This is not to say that Vasu's work could not contribute to this end (were one seeking to define the true substance of *haṭha* yoga), nor do I thereby intend to lessen Vasu's achievements as a translator and commentator or to impugn his scholarly integrity. My purpose is simply to foreground those emphases, innovations, and omissions that colored the interpretation and implementation of *haṭha* yoga in modern times, not to determine how reliable they are in terms of their fidelity to tradition.

Orientalism

The same is true for my approach to "Orientalist" scholarship more generally. By "Orientalist" here I mean the self-designation of mainly nineteenth-century British and German scholars studying the languages and the texts of Asia.

I emphatically do not intend the connotations that the term has acquired since the publication of Edward Said's *Orientalism* (1978). Said extended the semantic range of the term *Orientalist* to include all those Europeans who wrote about the East and not just the linguists and philologists that it originally referred to. These writers, according to him, were part of a larger, imperial enterprise to project an image of the Orient as Europe's subordinate "Other," to the ends of political, economic, and cultural subjugation. David Smith contends that the conflation of Said's Orientalist with the European scholar of India represents a "perverse sleight-of-hand [which] magics away into thin air the editions, translations, and dictionaries of the true and original Orientalists who devoted their lives to understanding the meaning of instances of Oriental culture and civilization" (2003: 46). Smith attacks, in particular, Ronald Inden's development of Said's project in his (Inden's) *Imagining India* (1992), a book that, Smith claims, belittles the accomplishments of Sanskrit scholars such as Louis Renou by implicating their work in the project of empire building: an implication for which, he insists, there is no evidence whatever (2003: 46).

I draw attention to Smith's critique in order to clarify my own position with regard to theses such as Inden's and, to a lesser extent, Richard King's (1999). The fact that I seek out evidence of pervasive attitudes and opinions regarding yoga among scholars does not imply a denigration of these scholars' achievements nor an attempt to "magic away" their significance for the field of Indology. The "true and original Orientalists," in Smith's phrase, most certainly devoted their lives to their scholarship, but this does not mean that they did not also hold certain current, negative views concerning what was good and bad yoga. It is these attitudes that have the greatest import for this study, rather than the relative strengths of each man's Sanskrit philology, because they directly reflect and contribute to the climate of opinion regarding the function, status, and desirability of yoga as philosophical system and as practice.

Often, editions by Orientalists and anglophone *paṇḍitas* were the only "classical" yoga texts available to those wishing to learn more about the subject, and as such the personal pronouncements inscribed in their introductions, commentaries, addenda, and footnotes(on, for example, the moral standards of the yogin)take on considerable significance for our understanding of modern yoga's development. There is little to be gained from the kind of accusation and recrimination that Smith discerns in Inden's work, and it is not my intention to adopt such colonial discourse theories and apply them to modern yoga. Orientalist-bashing aside, it is simply a fact that there were certain prevalent attitudes regarding yoga among these men (though not without significant variation between them); this requires no lamentation nor recrimination on my part and is not employed in this study to tarnish their worth as scholars. Nor do I believe that my position in this regard is indicative of any intellectual "perversity," such as that discerned by Smith in Inden's work.

Similarly, while I have found it necessary to highlight the Orientalists' almost complete reliance on textual material, as well as the neglect of ethnography and oral data, my aim is not to use this as a stick to beat them with. This reliance is particularly evident in scholarship on yoga, which tended to limit itself almost exclusively to a handful of "classical" texts, themselves often endowed with that status during the very period in question (Singleton 2008a), and to ignore oral tradition and the actual, current practices of yoga in India. There are several exceptions to this trend, such as the on-the-ground analysis of mid-nineteenth-century yoga in India by N. C. Paul, via his British informant (the "gone native" deserter and would-be yogin, Captain Seymour), but by and large the kind of modern, English-language yoga that is the focus of this study is greatly informed by the textual vision of Orientalist and anglo-Indian scholarship of the late nineteenth century.

While it is vital, then, to document how the specific aspects of this textualization process influenced modern understandings of the nature of yoga, it is *not* necessary to decry the attendant lack of ethnographic fieldwork that was its corollary. There were good reasons that scholars stuck to classical texts. One is that they usually had deep intellectual roots in the classical scholastic traditions of Europe, which relied primarily on the *textual* sources of Greece and Rome. They quite naturally sought analogous *classical* sources for India and were just not interested in the activities of contemporary yogins, particularly of the *haṭha* variety. Indeed, they tended to be downright suspicious of such figures and their activities, and it is these views (held perhaps, in some cases, with good reason) that concern me, *insofar as they mediate the modern development of yoga*. By pointing to such attitudes, I am not suggesting that these scholars took the wrong path nor that they would have been better employed (or modern yoga better served) by taking their notebooks into "the field." Lines between disciplines were clearer then, and the kind of ethnography undertaken by researchers today was simply not what a philologist or cultural historian was expected to do at the time.

It is important, however, to see that this resulted in a heavy reliance on textual material in scholastic attempts to understand yoga, and that the intellectual structure of modern, anglophone yogas reflects this emphasis to a significant extent. That is to say, despite a prevailing anti-intellectualism among teachers and practitioners of yoga—and a concomitant distaste for "practical yoga" among some scholars—scholarly editions nevertheless often provided the former with access to the traditions from which their practices claimed to stem.

Representations of Yoga: Methodological Considerations

In the first part of this book, I set out examples of yoga and the yogin as they appear in popular media and academia during the late nineteenth and early twentieth centuries. My focus is on perceptions and representations of yoga and on the particular forms of modern practice and theory that emerged from, or in reaction to, these perceptions. Beyond a short summary of *haṭha* yoga as it is known to us through a handful of medieval texts, I do not seek to define or describe what *haṭha* yoga "really" is (or was).

Two elucidations are necessary here. First, I have no intention of suggesting that the Orientalists and the early pioneers of international anglophone yoga dreamed up their notions about yoga and yogins as a component of some overarching ideological plot (the "imagining India" thesis). There is little doubt that the bad reputation of so-called yogins among colonial administrators, Orientalist scholars, and certain sectors of Indian society was not without basis in fact: yogins could indeed be sinister, dangerous people. But more significant than the relative truth of their much publicized malfeasances, however, is the influence that their reputation had on the constitution of modern anglophone yogas.

Second, I have sought to avoid a methodological approach that negatively contrasts "modern yoga" against presumably more authentic, older forms of yoga. Of course, this is an appealing way to structure a study of modern yogas because it provides a ready-made framework for comparison and contrast: we hold up aspects of "modern yoga" against the template of "classical" forms and determine to what extent they converge with or diverge from the latter. For example, we might easily and convincingly demonstrate the discontinuities of logic, method, and soteriology between modern, international "hatha" yoga and the "classical" texts from which it claims to derive, such as *Haṭhayogapradīpikā*, *Gheraṇḍasaṃhitā*, and *Śivasaṃhitā*. Implicit in this approach, however, is the sense that such divergences are errors and that modern yoga is flawed precisely to the extent that it departs from the perceived tradition. In its more extreme formulations, this method seems to be a remnant of the kind of textual essentialism that shaped the attitudes of the Orientalist scholars themselves. But more than this, it gives insufficient recognition to the plurality and mutability of (chronologically) premodern forms of yoga and to the fact that "Indian tradition" has itself been subject to fragmentation, accretion, and innovation in much the same way as "modern yoga." It also tends to place the writer on the scholastic moral high ground. By foregrounding a firsthand familiarity with the primary classical sources, that is, he or she is able to give the impression of "knowing better" what constitutes authentic yoga than those unversed in this learning, but who nevertheless make truth claims about the nature of yoga. This obviously functions to endow the scholar with an authority that the nonscholastic modern yoga practitioner is seen to lack, and it provides the moral authority for the kind of "debunking" approach that, intentionally or otherwise, is a fairly common feature of writing about modern yoga.[7] In this model, premodern yoga as represented in "the classical texts" is the touchstone of authenticity for modern forms.

Let me be clear that to reject this "gold standard" approach to yoga is not to embrace the kind of relativism that regards all truth claims about yoga in the modern period as "true," in the sense of being accurate historical statements about tradition. The problem is that in spite of the sincerity with which such claims are made, they often simply do not stand up to the slightest critical scrutiny. To adopt an artificial naivety in this regard as a scholar is to ignore (or defer) one's own awareness of the history of ideas. As Joseph Alter has recently argued, a key methodological issue is therefore "how to exercise ethnographic relativism, historical perspectivity and intellectual skepticism all at the same time" (Alter 2008). This means critically examining modern yoga's truth claims while seeking to understand under what circumstances and to what ends such claims are made. In terms of the present study, this requires an analysis of the merger of *haṭha* yoga with the international physical culture movement, not with a view to demonstrating that popular modern yoga has become "mere" gymnastics but to understand the development of postural modern yoga in the world today. This certainly includes a critical awareness of the unreliability of truth claims made about the product of this merger but is in no way meant to unmask international *haṭha* yoga's imposture. This is a vital distinction.

For example, the claim that specific gymnastic *āsana* sequences taught by certain postural schools popular in the West today are enumerated in the *Yajur* and *Ṛg* Vedas is simply untenable from a historical or philological point of view. This claim is made by K. Pattabhi Jois about the *sūryanamaskār* sequences in his Ashtanga Vinyasa system (see note 4 in chapter 9).[8] Assertions such as this are made with some frequency in popular yoga discourse, and there is no question of accepting them as statements of historical or philological fact. However, the practices themselves cannot be written off as lacking interest or validity merely on the grounds of their late accession to the postural vocabulary of yoga or because of their divergence from the "traditional yoga" invoked on their behalf. Geoffrey Samuel has recently insisted that "modern yoga has become a significant part of contemporary western practices of bodily cultivation, and it should be judged in its own terms, not in terms of its closeness to some presumably more authentic Indian practice" (Samuel 2007: 178). I largely agree with Samuel here: an approach aiming solely to identify the dislocations from "tradition" inherent in today's global yoga forms is sterile and limited insofar as it fails to give serious consideration to the substance of these modern forms. It is for these reasons that I do not base this study on a comparison of modern "hatha" yoga with its purported medieval forebears. In the first chapter, I nevertheless offer a brief outline of some older forms of yoga and provide references for readers wishing to find out more concerning the theory, practice, and history of these forms, in particular *haṭha* yoga.

I am well aware—on the basis of several years of presentations and informal discussions on the material presented here—that my work will elicit some very specific reactions in certain quarters. For those who prefer hagiography to history, such as some Western apologists of "traditional" systems of postural modern yoga, this work is easily dismissed as either irrelevant or malign in intent, and its author as an academic trespasser on hallowed ground. Others, who situate themselves in an antagonistic relationship to the authority of modern traditions (or who are angry about what "has been done" to yoga), revel in what they see as a much needed exposure of convenient but specious myths. Both these responses are based on the assumption that my intention is to "demolish" the validity of modern yoga or to show that the postural forms that abound today are "bastardized," "compromised," "watered down," "confected" (and so on) with regard to the true meaning and authentic practice of yoga. Both responses, however, aside from misrepresenting my position, are inadequate and undesirable as they stifle genuine and sustained thinking about the substance of modern yoga. While there seems little point in protesting that this material is not presented through love of controversy or iconoclasm on my part, it *is* worth suggesting that there may be more profitable ways to view this book than as a hostile but ultimately irrelevant academic exercise on the one hand, or a righteous destruction of false idols on the other.

A more valid and helpful way of thinking beyond such unproductive positions might be to consider the term *yoga* as it refers to modern postural practice as a *homonym*, and not a synonym, of the "yoga" associated with the philosophical system of Patañjali, or the "yoga" that forms an integral component of the Śaiva Tantras, or the "yoga" of the *Bhagavad Gītā*, and so on. In other words, although the word "yoga" as it is used popularly today is identical in spelling and pronunciation in each of these instances, it has quite different meanings and origins. It is, in short, a homonym, and it should therefore not be assumed that it refers to the same body of beliefs and practices as these other, homonymous terms. If this is admitted as the basis for further discussion, we are free to consider postural modern yoga on its own terms instead of in negative comparison to other traditions called "yoga." The apologist might then concede, with no sense of self-betrayal, that his or her practices and belief systems have indeed changed and adapted, and that there is real value in investigating the historical course of these changes insofar as they relate to their own tradition. And the iconoclast might stop flogging a dead horse.

This is not to say that I take popular yoga today to be necessarily divorced and isolated from other, prior traditions of yoga. The relationship is rather one of dialectical homology, wherein structural similarities can still obtain (to a greater or lesser degree), but where the composition of practical and theoretical elements, and the overall orientation of the system, proceed in markedly divergent fashion. There are often, in short, far more plausible historical explanations for the way yoga is practiced today than the claim of direct, wholesale, genealogical affiliation to a tradition with the same or similar sounding name. As the next section shows, recent studies have made it amply clear that yoga, in its dissemination in the Western world, has undergone radical transformation in response to the differing worldviews, logical predispositions, and aspirations of modern audiences. These modern forms, it is also evident, were the result of a reframing of practices and belief frameworks within India itself over the last 150 years, in response to encounters with modernity and the West. Modern, popular yogas in and out of India bear the clear traces of this dialectic exchange. In this study I endeavor to present some of these reasons as they relate to modern postural practice. If they prove at all compelling, I hope that this will encourage further careful, intelligent discussion of modern forms of postural yoga and not merely their dismissal or jingoistic defense.

The Academic Study of Modern Yoga

It is only since the 1990s that modern forms of yoga have begun to be examined within the humanities and social sciences. Among the first studies were Christian Fuchs's history of yoga's reception in Germany (1990); Norman Sjoman's study of the Mysore Palace yoga tradition (1996); Karl Baier's analysis of yoga's passage to the West (1998); and Sylvie Ceccomori's detailed overview of the history of yoga in France (2001). Two major works on modern forms of yoga appeared in 2004: Joseph Alter's *Yoga in Modern India: The Body between Philosophy and Science*, and Elizabeth De Michelis's *A History of Modern Yoga: Patañjali and Western Esotericism*. Alter's book is anthropological in approach and is substantially concerned with the medical and scientific experiments carried out by Swami Kuvalayananda from the 1920s onward in the Bombay area (see Singleton 2006 for my review of this book). De Michelis (2004), who styles herself in this book as a historian of religious ideas (6), examines the Western esoteric influences at play in Swami Vivekananda's popular yoga synthesis of 1896, and traces these to the later teachings of the postural yoga guru B. K. S. Iyengar. On the basis of her analysis of Vivekananda, De Michelis devises a typology of "Modern Yoga" that has since become influential in scholarly thinking on this topic. In 2005, Sarah Strauss published her study of the "transnational" yoga teachings of Swami Sivananda of Rishikesh. Like Alter, Strauss is an anthropologist by training, and her work is based on periods of fieldwork in India. She tends to be less critically aware in this book of modern yoga's dialectical relationship with tradition than either Alter or De Michelis.

Since then, there has been a swell of interest in this area, and a substantial increase in the number of scholars and students researching modern yoga. Two recent doctoral studies, hopefully soon to be published, by Suzanne Newcombe (2007a, on yoga in Britain) and Klas Nevrin (forthcoming, on yoga in Sweden) are particularly worthy of attention in this regard; also noteworthy is the new collection of modern yoga scholarship edited by me and Jean Byrne (2008), which brings together established scholars like Alter, De Michelis, and Strauss, as well as important new voices in the field. The recently completed three-year "Modern Yoga" consultation at the American Academy of Religions annual meetings (2006–2008) is another indication of increased scholarly interest in this area. De Michelis (2007) offers a convenient and detailed summary of scholarship in this field, which I will not endeavor to duplicate here.

Of all these studies, perhaps the closest to mine thematically is Norman Sjoman's *The Yoga Tradition of the Mysore Palace* (1996). Sjoman suggests that the "godfather" of today's global *āsana* boom, T. Krishnamacharya, evolved his influential postural forms out of an extant royal gymnastics tradition of the Mysore Palace. He attempts to trace the poses made famous by this latter's disciples (esp. B. K. S. Iyengar and K. Pattabhi Jois) back to an exercise manual from the palace library. It is unfortunate that Sjoman's principal work has received less attention than it deserves. There are at least two reasons for this: first, the book is often dismissed or greeted with hostility by apologists of modern postural systems like Ashtanga Vinyasa because it undermines orthodox accounts of that system's origins. And it has been sometimes overlooked by scholars because it is published in a way that makes it seem unacademic. Now, while my subject matter is proximate to Sjoman's (especially in chapter 9), it is worth making explicit that I have no intention of offering a genealogy of *āsana* in the modern period. My aim is to examine the cultural contexts of modern *haṭha* yoga's emergence, not to trace the derivation of individual postures.

In conjunction with Sjoman, I should also mention the as-yet unpublished writing of Elliott Goldberg. Goldberg has done substantial work on the famous Indian bodybuilder and yoga synthesist K.V. Iyer, who is treated in my chapter 6. Building on Sjoman's work, as well as Alter's, Goldberg attempts to push further the thesis that the postures and techniques of modern postural yoga can be directly derived from modern gymnastics and bodybuilding. Goldberg was generous in sharing with me his reflections on physical culture and yoga in the form of undeveloped notes and a workshop paper on *sūryanamaskār* (sun salutations) delivered in Cambridge in 2005. While his approach and material have not been a significant influence in this book (except where acknowledged), it should be noted that his extensive knowledge of K.V. Iyer, and his disciple Anant Rao, predates and exceeds mine. Goldberg's forthcoming study on physical culture and yoga is currently still in preparation, but it should provide a useful complement to, and amplification of, some of the bare details in the current study concerning Iyer and his coterie.

This book is informed by the orientations and conceptual understandings made explicit by recent scholarship, as well as by its lacunae. It was conceived while I was a research assistant to Elizabeth De Michelis at the Dharam Hinduja Institute of Indic Research in Cambridge in 2003–2004 and developed as a Ph.D. thesis under her supervision. Since it is inevitably influenced to some degree by her way of thinking about modern yoga, I should point out where this study departs from her work.

Primarily, I am skeptical of the typological application of the term *Modern Yoga* (capitalized) and its subdivisions—conceptual entities that did not exist prior to De Michelis's work but that have already become the predominant nomenclature among scholars of contemporary, transnational yoga. While they have proven invaluable in delineating a field of enquiry, it seems to me that they have quickly exceeded their mandate as provisional and workable constructs with a finite heuristic value. That is to say, as a "way in" to thinking about expressions of yoga in the modern age, these are extremely useful categorizations. But typology is not a good starting point for history insofar as it subsumes detail, variation, and exception. Can we really refer to an entity called Modern Yoga and assume that we are talking about a discrete and identifiable category of beliefs and practices? Does Modern Yoga, as some seem to assume, differ in ontological status (and hence intrinsic value) from "traditional yoga"? Does it represent a rupture in terms of tradition rather than a continuity? And in the plethora of experiments, adaptations, and innovations that make up the field of transnational yoga today, should we be thinking of all these manifestations as belonging to Modern Yoga in any typological sense? Can Modern Yoga really be viewed as an enterprise with a unitary agenda?

One result of answering "yes" to these questions has been that Modern Yoga is sometimes subject to deconstructive attack in a way that "Classical" yoga is not. Another is that it is viewed as a mission initiated by Vivekananda and continued to this day, in various guises but fundamentally of a piece, conceptually and ideologically. Though such readings should not be attributed to

De Michelis herself, who explicitly acknowledges her typology's provisional, heuristic status, they are a common consequence of adopting it as if it were more than a working construct. I have therefore sought to avoid using the term Modern Yoga (or "modern yoga") in any rigidly typological sense. When I do refer to "modern yoga" it is intended to designate yoga in the modern age (or, more often than not, transnational anglophone yogas of the period) rather than De Michelis's 2004 interpretive framework.

It should also be noted that De Michelis's study bypasses a full seventy-year period between the milestones of *Raja Yoga* (1896) and Iyengar's *Light on Yoga* (1966). In many ways, it is in this gap that the present study begins. The vast paradigmatic divide that separates Vivekananda's teaching from the heavily postural forms of Iyengar Yoga simply cannot be explained by the typology of Modern Yoga. While De Michelis's analysis of Iyengar's permeability to the New Age is convincing, it does not engage with *why* his teaching is so overwhelmingly concerned with *āsana*, nor point to the radical departure from Vivekananda's teaching that this represents (nor, indeed, this latter's distinct antipathy toward *āsana*). Given the ascendancy of *āsana* in transnational anglophone yoga, these omissions weaken the case for the primary dominance of Vivekananda's yoga within Modern Yoga. That is not to say that Vivekananda is not a figure of monumental importance here nor that his teachings were not an inspiration to later *āsana* pioneers like Shri Yogendra, but they were not the direct practical source for the emergent postural yoga revival. So while it is clear from De Michelis's account that Iyengar was receptive to Vivekananda's message and to later New Age influence, this does little to account for the primacy of postural practices in his teaching. That is to say, the postural tenor that defines Iyengar yoga in form and practice, like a majority of postural yoga forms today, simply cannot be extrapolated from Vivekananda.

Postwar Developments in Transnational Yoga

This is a study of the conditions that gave rise to the practical and semantic hegemony of *āsana* within modern yoga. It does not concern itself in any detail with post–World War II developments of postural yoga: this would be another, substantial study. However, it may be useful to provide a brief synopsis of transnational yoga's development in the decades following the experiments under examination here to convey how these experiments shaped today's popular postural yoga forms. It is a necessarily schematic picture and omits many important details concerning yoga's development. More detailed accounts can be found in my overview of Modern Yoga in Singleton 2007m, in chapter 6 of De Michelis 2004, and in Newcombe 2007a.

The second half of the twentieth century saw a phenomenal growth of popular interest in yoga in the West and the rise to prominence of several posture-oriented systems. During the 1950s, a proliferation of practical manuals, such as those of Krishnamacharya disciple Indra Devi, promised unassailable health and youthfulness through a radically secularized and medicalized version of yoga. American physical culturists like former Mr. America Walt Baptiste also helped to further align yoga with Western notions of sport and exercise. Also influential was the work of Theos Bernard, whose participant/observer account of a *haṭha* yoga *sādhana* (*Hatha Yoga: The Report of a Personal Experience*, 1950) was an important forerunner of the encyclopedic *āsana* guides of Vishnudevananda (*The Complete Book of Yoga*, 960) and Iyengar (*Light on Yoga*, 1966).

In the 1960s, the rise of "flower power" brought yoga to the attention of a generation of young Americans and Europeans. The wholesale embrace of Indian metaphysics and yoga by many countercultural icons (such as The Beatles' spiritual romance with the Maharishi Mahesh Yogi) reinforced the position of yoga in the popular psyche and inspired many to join the "hippy trail" to India in pursuit of alternative philosophies and lifestyles. Increased media attention brought yoga closer to the mainstream, and printed primers and television series throughout the 1960s and 1970s, such as Richard Hittleman's *Yoga for Health* (first broadcast in 1961), encouraged many to take up posture-based yoga in the comfort of their own homes. The 1970s and 1980s were a period of consolidation for yoga in the West with the establishment and expansion of a significant number of dedicated schools and institutes. The period also saw a further, and enduring, rapprochement of yoga with the burgeoning New Age movement, which in many ways represents a new manifestation of yoga's century-old association with currents of esotericism. By the mid-1990s posture-based yoga had become thoroughly acculturated in many urban centers in the West. The 1990s "boom" turned yoga into an important commercial enterprise, with increasing levels of merchandising and commodification.

It is clear that the majority of popular *āsana*-based forms of transnational yoga today are profoundly influenced by the postural revivals that are the topic of this book. In some cases, such as the Ashtanga Vinyasa system—and its "Power Yoga" spin-offs—a direct line can be traced from modern urban health clubs and yoga studios to educational gymnastics institutions in India during the early twentieth century (the subject of chapter 9). The lucrative Bikram Yoga system, similarly, can be traced directly to the physical culture syntheses developed during the 1930s by the bodybuilder B.C. Ghosh (chapter 6). But alongside cases such as these are the innumerable new forms of postural yoga that, I contend, ultimately grow out of the early context of physical culture and esoteric body movement that are the subject of this book.

This is by no means an obvious assertion, nor can this study in any way be characterized as a simple re-description of previously delineated, or self-evident, historical processes. While scholarship has certainly noticed transnational practitioners' infatuation with *āsana*, as yet there has been no thorough investigation of the genesis of the postural forms we see today. Moreover, among outsiders and practitioners alike, there is often little awareness that these modes of practice have no precedent (prior to the early twentieth century, that is) in Indian yoga traditions. This study focuses on a period of approximately forty years during which the foundations of today's popular postural yoga forms were laid. Obviously, it cannot provide an exhaustive account of yoga's development up to the present day, nor does it claim that these early developments fully determined the way yoga is practiced in the twenty-first century. In other words, just as postural forms cannot be extrapolated from Vivekananda's work, the systems examined here are not the last word on transnational postural yoga. Experimentation did not stop at World War II, and *āsana* forms continue to mutate and grow today. However, I believe it is clear, based on the evidence I have gathered, that the forms and belief frameworks underlying postural yoga practice in the world today are, at their root, the result of the singularly creative period treated here.

Chapter Summary

Chapter 1 presents a very brief overview of yoga in the Indian tradition, with particular reference to *haṭha* yoga, as we know it through medieval texts and modern historical scholarship. What is clear from such a summary is that modern postural orthopraxis does not really resemble the yoga forms from which it claims to derive.

Chapter 2 considers some of the earliest European encounters with yogins during the seventeenth century and goes on to analyze their increasingly inferior status during colonial rule. Nineteenth-century Orientalist scholarship, it is suggested, consolidated the position of the yogin, and the first English translations of *haṭha* texts evidence a deep-seated hostility to the very practices they present. I also consider here the nineteenth-century roots of modern medical yoga, one of the conduits by which "*haṭha*" practices could eventually be reclaimed by twentieth-century pioneers like Kuvalayananda.

In chapter 3 I look to the topos of the performing yogin. As a result of economic and political repression in the late eighteenth century, many *haṭha* yogins resorted to street performance as a means of livelihood. This, combined with new technologies of photojournalism, made the postural contortions of the yogin a familiar component of the "exotic East." The late nineteenth-century yoga syntheses of Vivekananda, Blavatsky and others betray a profound distaste for the posture-practicing yogin, and their writings tend to denigrate the value of such practices. It is for this reason that *āsana* was initially absent from transnational anglophone yogas.

The first three chapters examine the reasons for the exclusion of *haṭha* yogic practices, particularly *āsana*, from the modern yoga renaissance. In the remaining chapters, I analyze how *āsana* was reclaimed, and thereby refashioned, as a key component of transnational yoga practice, through interaction with the worldwide physical culture movement.

In chapter 4 I offer a brief account of modern nationalist physical culture. This provides the context for an examination of several of the most important forms of (Western) physical culture present in India during the late nineteenth and early twentieth centuries. These forms were Scandinavian gymnastics on the model of Ling, the bodybuilding techniques and ethos of Sandow, and the various methods promoted by the Indian YMCA, headed by H. C. Buck. Each of these, I argue, has had a profound effect on the shape of transnational yoga, both in terms of formal praxis and belief.

Chapter 5 considers more closely the Indian physical culture scene of the period. Colonial educators tended to present Hindu Indians as a weakling race who deserved to be dominated. The British physical culture regimes, however, were adopted by Indians and used as components of nationalist programs of regeneration and resistance to colonial rule. It is in this context that *āsana* began to be combined with modern physical culture and reworked as an "indigenous" technique of man-building. Considered here are what are probably the earliest experiments in the synthesis of yoga and physical culture.

Chapters 6 and 7 consider early twentieth-century developments of these first experiments. *Āsana* remains largely absent from the practical, anglophone yoga primer in the first decades of the twentieth century. Here, I analyze the ways in which it progressively became the most prominent practice component of mainstream modern yoga. As I hope to make clear, the new yogic body is one that is thoroughly shaped by the practices and discourses of modern physical culture, "healthism," and Western esotericism. Chapter 6 examines formulations of yoga as a species of gymnastics and bodybuilding, often linked to the kind of nationalist man-building projects examined in chapter 5. Chapter 7 takes another facet of modern postural yoga's relationship with physical culture: the "harmonial gymnastic" tradition. Largely practiced by women, such "spiritualized" methods of movement and dance became firmly associated at the end of the nineteenth century with Hindu yoga. Here I make the claim that "hatha yoga" classes, as practiced in many twenty-first-century urban settings, recapitulate the philosophical, practical, and demographic circumstances of women's physical culture classes of the early twentieth century.

In Chapter 8, I argue that modern postural practice cannot be understood without an examination of the technologies of visual reproduction. Advances in photography and print distribution created the conditions for a popular yoga of the body and dictated to a large extent the features of that body. The result of modern yoga's overwhelming reliance on photographic realism has elided the body of "traditional" *haṭha* yoga.

Chapter 9, finally, considers the vastly influential postural forms developed by T. Krishnamacharya during his tenure as yoga teacher in Mysore during the 1930s and 1940s. The preceding chapters force us to see these radically innovative forms, which are at the root of several of today's preeminent postural systems, as stemming from a modern preoccupation with physical culture. I demonstrate that Krishnamacharya's distinctive style of yoga practice is not as unique as one might assume but is a powerful synthesis of Western and Indian modes of physical culture, contextualized within "traditional" *haṭha* yoga.

1

A Brief Overview of Yoga in the Indian Tradition

Yoga in Traditional Hinduism

Some scholars have found evidence of early yogic practice in the archaeological artifacts from the Indus Valley civilization in Sind, which developed from about 2500 BCE. Sir John Marshall, director general of the Archaeological Survey of India, began excavating two sites, Mohenjo-Daro and Harappa, in 1921 and discovered the remains of a highly developed urban culture. Among the artifacts unearthed was the "Paśupati Seal," so-called because Marshall believed that the horned figure surrounded by animals which it depicts was a prototype of Śiva, the "Lord of the Beasts" (*paśupati*), seated in a yoga posture. As Eliade notes, this would make it by far "the earliest plastic representation of a yogin" (1969: 355). Although the links of this (and other seals) with *yogāsana* are highly speculative, they have continued to be cited as an instantiation of postural yoga's ancient roots. Thomas McEvilley (1981), for example, has suggested that one of the "proto-Śiva" seals represents a "shamanic" posture of *haṭha* yoga, later referred to as *utkaṭāsana* by the *Gheraṇḍa Saṃhitā* (2.23) and as *mūlabandhāsana* in the modern Iyengar system (Iyengar 1966). Doris Srinivasan (1984), on the other hand, has convincingly argued that these seals cannot be taken as proofs of the Indus origins of Śiva, and therefore that the interpretation of the seals as evidence of proto-yogic forms is misplaced. Geoffrey Samuel has recently summarized the Indus Valley controversy by noting that little or nothing can be known of the *religious* practices of these peoples via archaeological findings and that any evidence for the existence of yogic practices at this time is "so dependent on reading later practices into the material that it is of little or no use for constructing any kind of history of practices" (2008: 8).

Textual evidence of yoga practice begins to emerge only at a much later stage. While there are references to *tapas*-practicing ascetics (called *muni, keśin,* or *vrātya*) as early as the vedic Brāhmaṇas, the first occurrence of the word "yoga" itself is in the *Kaṭha Upaniṣad* (third century BCE?), where it is revealed to the boy Naciketas by Yama, god of death, as a means to leave behind joy and sorrow and overcome death itself (2.12 ff). The *Śvetāśvatara Upaniṣad* (third century BCE?) outlines a procedure in which the body is maintained in an upright posture while the mind is brought under control by the restraint of the breath (2.8–14). The much later *Maitrī Upaniṣad* describes a six-fold yoga method of yoga, namely (1) breath control (*prāṇāyāma*), (2) withdrawal of the senses (*pratyāhāra*), (3) meditation (*dhyāna*), (4) placing of the concentrated mind (*dhāraṇā*), (5) philosophical inquiry (*tarka*), and (6) absorption (*samādhi*). These technical terms will later (with the exception of *tarka*) be used to designate five of the eight elements of Patañjali's *aṣṭāṅgayoga* scheme.[1]

The section of the *Mahābhārata* known as the *Bhagavad Gītā* lays out three paths of yoga by which the aspirant can know the Lord, or supreme person, here known as Kṛṣṇa. The first is the path of action (*karmayoga*), in which one gives up the fruits of one's actions but continues to be an agent in the world, guided by Kṛṣṇa himself.[2] The second is the path of devotion (*bhaktiyoga*), in which one's devotion to Kṛṣṇa swiftly liberates one from worldly suffering, regardless of caste.[3] The third is the path of knowledge (*jñānayoga*), which liberates through discrimination of the true nature of self and universe.[4] The *Gītā* also describes a range of practices undertaken by yogins of the day (such as an internalization of the vedic ritual, as in the sacrifice of the inhalation (*prāṇa*) into the exhalation (*apāna*) (26 [4]: 22–31), as well as instructions for the preparation of a yoga *sādhana* and for the withdrawal of the senses (28 [6]: 1–29).

The *Yogasūtras* (YS, c. 250 CE?) ascribed to Patañjali consist of 195 brief aphorisms (*sūtrāṇi*) outlining diverse methods for the attainment of yoga. It is heavily influenced by Sāṃkhya philosophy (Larson 1989, 1999; Bronkhorst 1981), but also contains distinct elements from Buddhism[5] and a variety of *śramaṇa* (renunciant ascetic) traditions.[6] The *Yogasūtrabhāṣya* attributed to Vyāsa (c. 500–600 CE), is the first and most influential commentary on the text and is sometimes even regarded as a component part of the YS itself (e.g., Bronkhorst 1981). Although the text has received an enormous amount of interest from modern scholars, even coming to be known as the "Classical Yoga," bear in mind that it is one among many texts on yoga and may not necessarily be *the* authoritative source for Indian yoga traditions, as is commonly supposed. It has become the primary text for anglophone yoga practitioners in the twentieth century, largely due to the influence of European scholarship, on the one hand, and early promoters of practical yoga, like Vivekananda and

H. P. Blavatsky, on the other. However, it is common for modern yoga teachers to confine their discussion of the text to the *aṣṭāṅgayoga* section (II.29–III.8) as if this were the sum of Patañjali's message.

In spite of the scarcity of information regarding *āsana* in the *sūtras* themselves and in the traditional commentaries, the text is routinely invoked as the source and authority of modern postural yoga practice (e.g., Iyengar 1993a; Maehle 2006). This is in no small measure due to the authority and prestige that the association with Patañjali confers on modern schools of yoga and their practices. Although I do not deal with it at any length in the present study, it is clear that the refurbishment of Patañjali in the modern era is one of the key loci of transnational yoga's development (see Singleton 2008a).

Śaiva Tantras and other Āgamic compendia often contain detailed descriptions of yoga practice. For example, the *Vijñānabhairava*, an eighth-century CE collection from the Śaivāgama, contains 112 types of yoga aiming at the union of the aspirant with Śiva (cf. Singh 1979). Or we find the yogic teachings from the *Mālinīvijayottaratantra*, a Tantra of the Trika division of Śaivism, which "attempts to integrate a whole plethora of competing yoga systems," the common feature of which is that they all require the yogin "to traverse a 'path' (*adhvan*) towards a 'goal' (*lakṣya*)" (Vasudeva 2004: xi–xii).[7] In all the systems of yoga mentioned here, not much emphasis is placed on the practice of *āsana*. Even early Tantric works such as that examined by Vasudeva teach only a small number of seated postures (Vasudeva 2004: 397–402). Any assertion that transnational postural yoga is of a piece with the dominant orthopraxy of Indian yogic tradition is therefore highly questionable.

Haṭha Yoga

The techniques and philosophical frameworks of the Śaiva Tantras form the basis for the teachings of *haṭha* yoga, which flourished from the thirteenth century CE and which entered its decline in the eighteenth (Gonda 1965: 268; Bouy 1994: 5). The term *haṭha* means "forceful" or "violent," but it is also interpreted to indicate the union of the internal sun (*ha*) and moon (*ṭha*), which symbolically indicates the goal of the system (Eliade 1969: 229). As Mallinson (2005: 113) has noted, the corpus of *haṭha* yoga is not doctrinally whole and does not "belong" to any one single school of Indian thought. It is nevertheless closely associated with Gorakṣanāth and his teacher Matsyendranāth, who is credited with founding the Śaiva Nāth *saṃpradāya* (twelfth century CE?).[8] In practice, however, there was a high level of orthopractical and organizational fluidity between the Nāths (also called Kānphaṭa, or "split eared") and other yoga-practicing groups. The yoga-practicing *tyāgīs* of the Vaiṣṇava Rāmānandīs, for example, were closer to the Nāths in terms of ritual and religious experience than to their devotionally inclined (*rasik*) Rāmānandī brethren (van der Veer 1987: 688); close organizational trade ties obtained between Nāths, Sufi fakirs, and Daśnāmi *saṃnyāsins*, and there was a great deal of interchange between these various groups (Dasgupta 1992: 18; Bouiller 1997: 9; Green 2008); and at least until the late 1800s, Nāth yogins recruited novitiates without regard for caste or religion, attracting many Muslim yogins into their fold (Pinch 2006: 10). This all contributed to a permeability among *haṭha* yoga practicing groups.

The earliest of the well-known texts of *haṭha* yoga is probably *Gorakṣa Śataka* (GŚ), ascribed to Gorakṣanātha, followed by *Śiva Saṃhitā* (ŚS, fifteenth century CE), *Haṭhayogapradīpikā* (HYP, fifteenth–sixteenth century), *Haṭharatnāvalī* (HR, seventeenth century), *Gheraṇḍa Saṃhitā* (GhS, seventeenth–eighteenth century CE), and the *Jogapradīpakā* (JP, eighteenth century).[9] As Bouy (1994) has shown, *haṭha* yoga techniques aroused much interest among the followers of Śaṇkara's *advaita vedānta*, and a number of texts from Nāth literature were assimilated wholesale into the corpus of 108 Upaniṣads compiled in South India during the first half of the eighteenth century.[10] Mallinson (2007: 10) has demonstrated that the orthodox *vedāntin* bias of these compilers resulted in the omission of some key aspects of Nāth *haṭha* yoga, such as the practice of *khecarīmudrā*.[11] As we shall see, a similar process of omission occurred during the modern *haṭha* yoga revival. Since many of the *āsana* systems considered in this study purport to derive from, or to be, *haṭha* yoga, a brief examination of the main features of its doctrines and practices is in order. This account is drawn mainly from HYP, GhS, and ŚS, which are the *haṭha* yoga texts best known to English language readers.

Haṭha yoga is concerned with the transmutation of the human body into a vessel immune from mortal decay. GhS compares the body to an unbaked earthenware pot which must be baked in the fires of yoga to purify it and even refers to this system as the "yoga of the pot" (*ghaṭasthayoga*) rather than *haṭha* yoga.[12] A preliminary stage of the *haṭha* discipline is the six purifications (*ṣaṭkarmas*), which are (with some variation between texts) (1) *dhauti*, or the cleansing of the stomach by means of swallowing a long, narrow strip of cloth; (2) *basti*, or "yogic enema," effected by sucking water into the colon by means of an abdominal vacuum technique (*uḍḍiyāna bandha*); (3) *neti*, or the cleaning of the nasal passages with water and/or cloth; (4) *trāṭaka*, or staring at a small mark or candle until the eyes water; (5) *nauli* or *laulikī*, in which the abdomen is massaged by forcibly moving the rectus abdominus muscles in a circular motion; and (6) *kapālabhāti*, where air is repeatedly and forcefully expelled via the nose by contraction of the abdominal muscles. These six purifications are described at HYP

II and GS I. The texts promise miraculous results for the proper practice of these purifications, such as the indefinite prevention of illness and old age.

The HYP names *āsana* as the first accessory (*aṅga*) of *haṭha* yoga and lists its benefits as the attainment of steadiness (*sthairya*), freedom from disease (*ārogya*), and lightness of body (*aṅgalāghava*) (I.19). The text outlines fifteen *āsanas*, some of which are credited with curative properties, such as destroying poisons (e.g., *mayūrāsana*, I.33). The GhS places the *āsanas* after the purifications, and briefly describes thirty-two of them. The ŚS mentions that there are eighty-four *āsanas*, but describes only four seated postures. The mainstay of *haṭha* practice is *prāṇāyāma* (also called *kumbhaka*, or "retention," in HYP). *Prāṇāyāma* cleanses and balances the subtle channels of the body (*nāḍī*) and in combination with certain bodily "seals," or *mudrās*,[13] forces the *prāṇa* (vital air) into the central channel called *suṣumṇā* or *brahmanāḍī*. This in turn raises the *kuṇḍalinī* energy, which is visualized as a serpent sleeping at the base of the spine.

A little more explication of the "subtle physiology" of *haṭha* yoga may be helpful here. According to these texts, the human body is made up of networks of subtle channels called *nāḍīs*. The ŚS numbers these channels at 300,000 (II.14) and the HYP at 72,000 (IV.8). The entire process of *ṣaṭkarmāṇi, āsana, prāṇāyāma*, and *mūdra* aims at the purification and balancing of the *nāḍīs*. The two principal *nāḍīs, iḍā* and *piṅgala*, are situated respectively on the left and the right sides of the central channel (*suṣumnā*) and are identified with a microcosmic, corporeal moon and sun. Also of vital importance here are the famous *cakras* ("wheels") or *padmas* (lotuses) of *haṭha* yoga and Tantra, which are commonly numbered six or seven and which lie at intervals along the spine (HYP III.2; ŚS V.56–131). They are intersected by *iḍā* and *piṅgala nāḍīs*. The serpent *kuṇḍalinī* (also known as the goddess *Śakti*), lying coiled and sleeping at the base of the spine where all the *nāḍīs* converge (*ādhāra*), is drawn up along the *suṣumnā*, piercing the *cakras* as it goes. The result is that the vital breath (*prāṇa*) becomes absorbed in voidness (*śūnya*) and the practitioner attains the condition of *samādhi* (HYP IV.9–10), which in turn leads to *mokṣa*, or liberation.

Transnational "Hatha" Yoga

What is initially striking about the kind of transnational "hatha" yoga commonly taught today is the degree to which it departs from the model outlined in these texts. The most prominent departure is the primacy accorded to *āsana* as a system of health, fitness, and well-being, and the relegation or elimination of other key aspects such as *ṣaṭkarmas*, *mudrā*, and even (though to a slightly lesser extent)

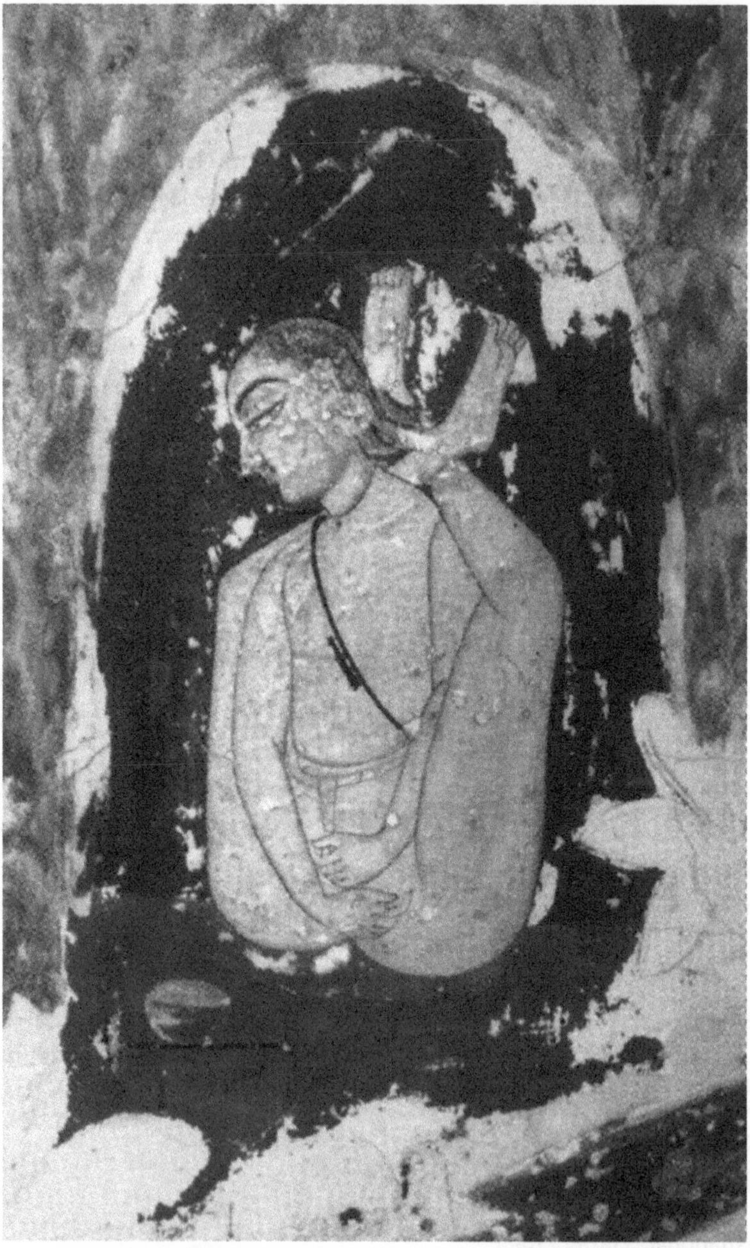

Āsanas from the Nātha Mahāmandir murals (photographs courtesy of James Mallinson)

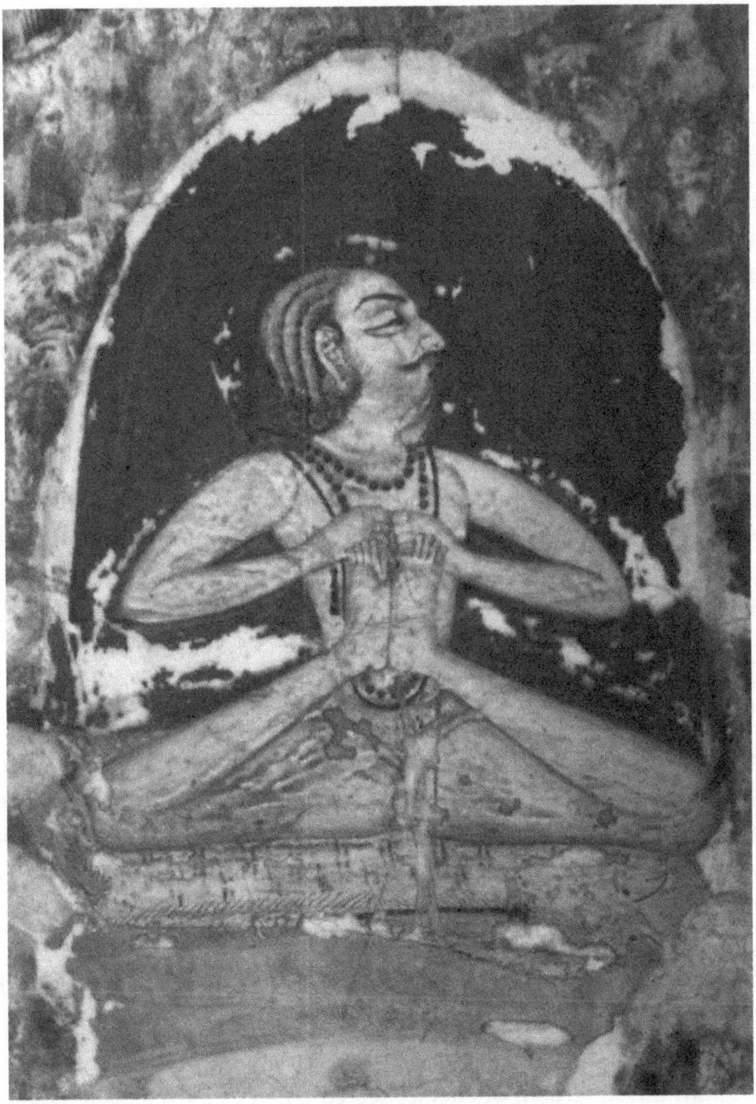

prāṇāyāma. While some schools of modern yoga catering to an international audience do conserve some of these elements,[14] in the main they have become distinctly subordinate to the practice of *āsana*, which is itself rationalized in ways markedly alien to the kind of *haṭha* yoga outlined in GŚ, GhS, ŚS or HYP.

The Tantric physiology that underpins traditional expressions of *haṭha* yoga has also generally played only quite a minor role in popular modern yoga. The international public has long been interested in such topics, as demonstrated by the popularity of Sir John Woodroofe's translation of the *Ṣaṭcakranirūpaṇa* of 1924, which Eliade credits as "the most authoritative treatise on the doctrine of the *cakras*" (1969: 241 n.142). Theosophical explanations of *nāḍīs* and *cakras*, such as C. W. Leadbeater's *The Chakras* of 1927, also helped to disseminate interest in these subjects, albeit in a distinctly Western esoteric format. Modern medical *haṭha* yoga, as initiated by the likes of N. C. Paul, Major D. Basu, and, some decades later, Swami Kuvalayananda (1883–1966) and Shri Yogendra (1897–1989), is deeply concerned with this subtle physiology,[15] and New Age books about the "spiritual anatomy" of the *cakras* (such as the current best-selling works of Caroline Myss) continue to draw readers even today.

But essentially their application to modern forms of yoga is limited to a general recognition of the three principal *nāḍīs*, the *cakras*, and the role that these may play in *kuṇḍalinī*-type experiences. While such references are commonly to be found in popular texts fashionable in yoga circles and in practitioners' *imaginaire*, the larger theories and related practices are usually kept to a minimum, and only occasionally are they encountered in actual yoga teaching and practice. Indeed, the average anglophone yoga class today is far more likely to foreground the sole practice of *āsana* and largely ignore the subtle system of *haṭha* yoga. Student yoga teachers commonly learn something about *nāḍīs* and *cakras* during their training, and many will read a modern commentary and translation of HYP, but it is rare for this theoretical knowledge to be applied as part of a *haṭha* yoga practice such as that outlined in the traditional texts or that described by Theos Bernard during his experience of a traditional *haṭha sādhana* in India (Bernard 1950). Tibetan systems of physical yoga from the Bön and Buddhist Vajrayāna traditions, which have recently begun to be taught in the West and which bear a close affinity to *haṭha* yoga, are far more likely to retain an emphasis on the subtle physiology of the body and on practices that work with this body (Chaoul 2007). These Tibetan techniques highlight the extent to which transnational, Indian "hatha" yoga has become decontextualized from the system it claims to represent.[16] In sum, the Indian tradition shows no evidence for the kind of posture-based practices that dominate transnational anglophone yoga today. We should except from this assertion, of course, seated postures such as *padmāsana* and *siddhāsana*, which have played an enormously important practical and symbolic rôle throughout the history of yoga. And today, largely thanks to modern advertising, cross-legged yoga postures such as these have become powerful and universally recognized signifiers of relaxation, self-control, self-cultivation, a balanced lifestyle, good health, fitness, and spiritual urban cool.

Gudrun Bühnemann's recent work on the tradition of 84 *āsanas* (2007a) has summarized various sets of Indian illustrations of *āsanas* and reproduced several, including an illustrated manuscript of the *Jogapradīpakā* (1737) and selections from the murals of the Nātha Mahāmandir in Jodhpur (c.1810). While these rare illustrations are evidence of *āsana* within *haṭha* yoga prior to the postural yoga revivals of the twentieth century, Bühnemann is of the opinion that (in spite of claims to the contrary) the practices of the many modern schools of yoga are not directly based on any known textual tradition of yoga:

> All traditional systems of Yoga... assign a preparatory and subordinate place to *āsanas* in the pursuit of liberation from the cycle of rebirth. Neither the YS nor the Upaniṣads nor the epic texts on Yoga emphasize *āsanas*. Even most texts of the Nātha or *haṭha* traditions teach a very limited number of *āsanas*.... This view of the subordinate position of *āsanas* clearly differs from that of most modern Yoga schools. (Bühnemann 2007a: 20–21)

The practice of *āsanas* within transnational anglophone yogas is not the outcome of a direct and unbroken lineage of *haṭha* yoga. While it is going too far to say that modern postural yoga has no relationship to *āsana* practice within the Indian tradition, this relationship is one of radical innovation and experimentation. It is the result of adaptation to new discourses of the body that resulted from India's encounter with modernity. The main objective of this book is to trace the emergence of these new expressions of yoga, particularly as it relates to modern physical culture. In the next two chapters, I examine the anti-*haṭha* sentiment that initially kept *āsana* out of the yoga revival and which gave rise to the conditions under which *haṭha* yoga came to be remodeled as physical culture. For those wishing to look more deeply into the theory, practice, and history of tantric and *haṭha* yoga, I have included some suggestions for further reading in footnote 17.[17]

2

Fakirs, Yogins, Europeans

> It sounds like a degradation of the very name of religion to apply it to the wild ravings of Hindu Yogins or the blank blasphemies of Chinese Buddhists. But as we slowly and patiently wend our way through the dreary prisons, our own eyes seem to expand, and we perceive a glimmer of light where all was darkness at first.
>
> (Müller 1881: 16, vol. 2)

In this chapter I briefly consider some early representations of yogins by European visitors to India, before going on to examine their status in European scholarship of the late nineteenth century. I then consider the important early modern *haṭha* yoga translations of S. C. Vasu, particularly as they mediate the figure, and the practices, of the *haṭha* yogin. My aim is to demonstrate the extent to which the practices of the *haṭha* yogins were negatively viewed by scholars during the crucial period leading up to the first reformulations of yoga for modern, anglophone audiences. The new, English-language yogas devised by Vivekananda and others emerged in a climate of opinion that was highly suspicious of the yogin, especially the practitioner of *haṭha* yoga. Yogins were more likely to be identified by their critics (both Indian and European) with black magic, perverse sexuality, and alimentary impurity than with "yoga" in any conventional sense (see White 1996: 8). Scholars of the period tended to admire what they saw as the rational, philosophical, and contemplative aspects of yoga while condemning the obnoxious behavior and queer ascetic practices of the yogins themselves. This situation resulted in the exclusion of *haṭha* yoga from the initial stages of the popular yoga revival.

Early European Encounters

Although the European interest in Indian holy men probably began as far back as the ancient Greeks' encounters with the so-called gymnosophists (Halbfass 1988: 3, 7, 11), we will begin by examining perceptions of the yogin during the period of modern European colonial expansion. *Yogi* (or "jogi"/"ioghee") was the usual shorthand designation for *haṭha* practitioners of the Nāth and Kānphaṭa orders (Lorenzen 1978: 68), but the term acquired a far broader significance in colonial India. European visitors commonly had difficulty distinguishing between the various categories of mendicant orders, and would commonly conflate the (Hindu) yogin and the (Mohammedan) fakir. From the seventeenth century onward, indeed, European travelers to India rarely made much of a "methodological or functional distinction" between them (Siegel 1991: 149). For these visitors, "yogi" tended to signify the social group of itinerant renouncers known for their disreputable (and sometimes violent) behavior, mendicancy, and outlandish austerities. In the eighteenth century, the term *sannyasi*, or "sannyasi fakir," also came into widespread usage among British officials as a catch-all phrase designating the kind of itinerant holy man who would periodically disrupt the East India Company's trade routes (Ghosh 1930: 9–11). The imprecision and interchangeability of these terms among European merchants and observers increased the general confusion as to the actual religious and ethnic identity of the yogin—a confusion that may have been tactically exploited by the yogi-sannyasi-fakirs themselves to ensure anonymity and freedom of movement (Pinch 2006: 6). What is more important for the discussion that follows, however, is that these undifferentiated mendicant marauders tended to be regarded with hostility and suspicion.

François Bernier's letters from India, written between 1659 and 1669, set the tone for the many descriptions of yogins that would follow. Bernier notes that there are those acetics who "enjoy the reputation of being peculiarly enlightened saints, perfect *Jauguis*, and really united to God" (Bernier 1968 [1670]: 318–19). Such yogins spend their lives in contemplation and prayer, much like the European monk, and while Bernier suspects that the "ravissement" of these men may be the result of imagination or illusion, he nonetheless seems to have some respect for their efforts. That said, Bernier was wont to negatively compare the mystical practices of yogins to those of his occult-inclined foes in Europe, such as the astrologers Jean-Baptiste Morin and Girolamo Cardano (Dew 2009, ch.3). Even eighteen years later, just before his death, he was still comparing the French vogue for quietistic prayer to the practices of Indian yogins and suggesting that both partake of the kind of "maladies d"esprit," madness, and extravagances common to men of all cultures (Bernier 1688: 47–52).

Bernier notes another species of yogin: naked, covered in ashes and with long matted hair, often to be found sitting under trees engaging in painful austerities (1968 [1670]: 316). Of this latter group Bernier comments,

> No *Fury* in the infernal regions [mégère d'enfer] can be conceived more horrible than the *Jauguis*, with their naked and black skin, long hair, spindle arms, long twisted nails, and fixed in the posture which I have mentioned [i.e., arms raised overhead]. (316–17)

Some carry heavy chains of the kind usually seen on elephants while others spend hours in handstand position, or in a variety of other postures which are "so difficult and painful that they could not be imitated by our tumblers" (317).[1] Such figures, he opines, are actually "vegetative rather than rational beings" (the terms are borrowed from Aristotle) who have been seduced by a life of lazy vagrancy or by their own vanity (318).

Other European observers of the time had similar reactions. Jean-Baptiste Tavernier, writing in 1676, claims that these "Fakīrs" are imitators of Rāvaṇa, the demon of the *Rāmāyaṇa*, who was forced into a life of mendicancy after Rāma's

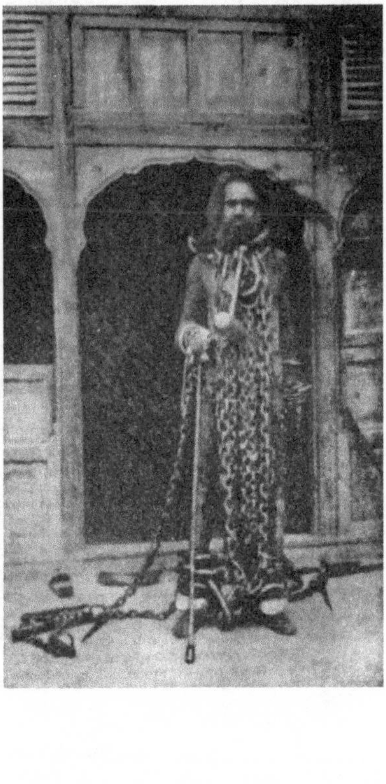

Chain-bearing fakir, Oman 1903

army destroyed his land. He estimates that there are 800,000 Muslim fakirs in India, and 1,200,000 "among the idolators [i.e., Hindus]" (1925 [1676]: 139). His sketches and description of a group of fakirs under a banyan tree at Surat provide a vivid picture of the fakir-yogi's life and recapitulate some of the practices remarked upon by Bernier. There are, notes Tavernier, an "infinity" of penitents, "some of whom assume positions altogether contrary to the natural attitude of the human body" (154).

John Ovington's account of fakirs encountered during his voyage to Surat in 1689 is very similar to Tavernier's, even down to the explanation of Rāvaṇa as "The Original of these Holy Mendicants" (1696: 360). Both Gentiles (Hindus) and Moors (Muslims), he notes, have a "sordid aspect" (362). Being possessed by "the Delusions of Satan," they take solemn vows to remain in "such and such kind of Postures all the days of their life" (363). These "unnatural postures" (367) are much the same as those described by Bernier. Jean de Thevenot's account of 1684 also matches in many details the accounts of Bernier and Ovington. He compares "faquirs" and "Jauges" to the Bohemians of France, suggesting that both originate in "libertinage" (1684: 192). It is probable that the commonalities in these accounts result from all three authors visiting Surat with a few years of each other and that Ovington and de Thevenot had access to the the reports of Tavernier, as well as other European visitors.

As a final example, in his travelogue of East India and Persia of 1698, John Fryer notes that fakirs, operating under a pretense of religious piety, "are Vagabonds, and are the Pest of the Nation they live in" (Fryer 1967 [1698] vol. 1:

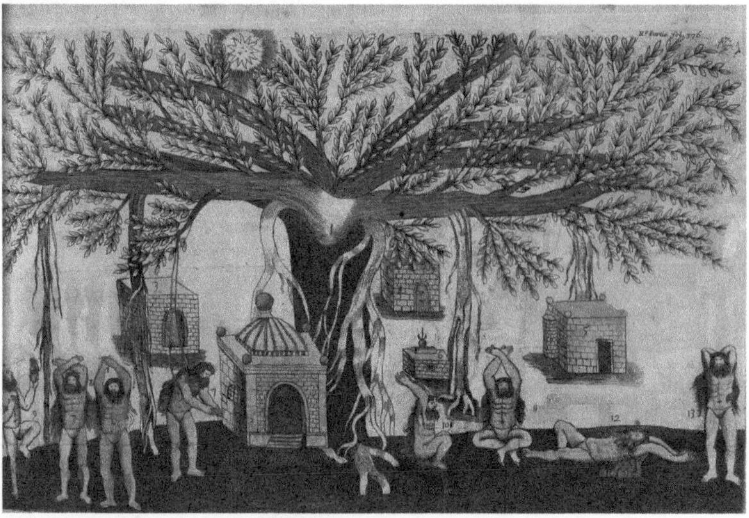

Tavernier's sketch of fakirs at Surat, 1676 (courtesy of Philippe Nicolet)

241). Their aggressive begging has made them feared by the citizens, "nor is the Governour powerful enough to correct their Insolencies" (242). Like Bernier, Tavernier, and Thevenot, Fryer sketches some of the austerities that would fascinate ethnographic writers well into the twentieth century, such as overgrown nails that pierce the flesh of the hand, dislocated arms, and excruciating postures held for so long that the limbs in question become ossified and shriveled. Fryer also mentions one "Jougie" who "as a check to Incontinency, had a Gold Ring fastened to his Viril Member" (vol.2: 35).[2]

Perceived as dissolute, licentious, and profane, these groups were greeted with puzzlement and hostility by early European observers. The performance of yogic postural austerities was the most visible and vaunted emblem of Indian religious folly, and as yogins increasingly took to exhibitionism as a means of livelihood, this association became consolidated in the popular imagination.[3]

Fighting Yogins and Bhakti Ascendancy

As Fryer's account suggests, the European dislike for yogins was not merely due to offended moral sensibilities: yogins were also difficult people to bring to order. From the fifteenth century until the early decades of the nineteenth century, highly organized bands of militarized yogins controlled trade routes across Northern India, becoming so powerful in the eighteenth century as to be able to challenge the economic and political hegemony of the East India Company (Farquhar 1925b; Ghosh 1930; Ghurye 1953; Lorenzen 1978; Dasgupta 1992; Pinch 2006.). As a result of their harassment, notes YMCA literary secretary and historian J. N. Farquhar, "the income of the British Government in Bengal was seriously curtailed... more than once" (1925b: 448). These ascetic mercenaries were from a variety of religious backgrounds and often purposefully masked their allegiance to avoid detection and punishment, even moving between denominations as profit dictated (Ghosh 1930: 11, 12, 20. Pinch 2006). It was in fact the *haṭha* yoga-practicing Nāth yogins themselves (usually simply referred to as *yogīs* or *jogīs*) who were the first major religious group to organize militarily (Lorenzen 1978: 68; Ghurye 1953: 108). Indeed, they became so influential and powerful as the "supernatural power brokers of medieval India" that they were able to make or break kings (White 1996: 7–8). They also continued to be identified as a threat to British economic interests: for employees of the Company, the term *yogi* connoted less the Himālayan hermit than the ascetic marauder. Even though the designation pointed to a confused agglomeration of violent ascetics as seen through British eyes (and not a practitioner of *haṭha* yoga *sensu stricto*), it was nonetheless the *haṭha*-practicing Nāths who were most closely associated with religious trade-soldiering.

The life of the marauding yogin offered a world of opportunity in Moghul and early British India. Militant asceticism furnished trade networks, social opportunities, and equality without caste hindrances. With the arrival of the Pax Britannica, however, such opportunities began to dwindle. In 1773, Warren Hastings enforced a ban on the wandering yogins of Bengal and began to promote the more sedentary, mainly Vaiṣṇava forms of devotional religious practice, which were already in the ascendant in India at the time.[4] The interests of the mainly Vaiṣṇava mercantile and commercial elites, and those of the British, thus intersected in the condemnation of the wandering (Śaiva) yogin.[5]

Although pockets of violent resistance remained and certain "criminal tribes" were kept under surveillance well into the twentieth century, the ever-widening scope of police powers in India meant that yogins were increasingly demilitarized and forced to settle in cities and villages (Briggs 1938: 59). It even became an offense to wander naked or to carry a weapon, the two defining marks of the *nāga* ascetic—a reflection, perhaps, of the double affront they posed to British decency on the one hand and military and economic hegemony on the other (Farquhar 1925b: 449). No longer able to make a living by trade-soldiering, large numbers were forced into lives of yogic showmanship and mendicancy, becoming objects of scorn for many sections of Hindu society, and of voyeuristic fascination or disgust for European visitors (this is the subject of chapter 3). As mercenaries, yogins were feared and reviled. As good-for-nothing social parasites parading their contortions for money or tied up in "nefarious and libidinous intrigues," yogins were "despised rather than honoured" by orthodox Hindus (Bose 1884b: 191–92). In a culture where the "polarity of purity and pollution organizes Hindu social space" (Flood 1998: 57), the caste-less yogin was the embodiment of ritual impurity, as well as the emblem of the savagery and backwardness from which modern Hindus sought to dissociate themselves. Orthodox Hindus despised them, and the British inhabitants of India looked askance at anyone dealing with "those dirty yogi blokes" (Dane 1933: 224). The (*haṭha*) yogin was the common pariah of colonial India.

It should also be noted that militant yogins of all lineages engaged in exercise regimes designed to inure their bodies to the harsh physical conditions of the itinerant life and to prepare them for combat. These regimes were, notes Ghurye, "almost the counterpart of the military drill that a regular [i.e., modern, Westernized] regiment receives as a part of its training to keep it in trim" (1953: 108). Dasgupta argues that the *nāga saṃnyāsins* of the Daśanāmi *akhāṛas* practiced "physical penance and difficult postures" alongside combat techniques and training in the use of arms (Dasgupta 1992: 14). Matthew Clark (2006) has recently shown that these *akhāṛas* owe a great deal to the Sufi martial organizations that had come to dominate northern and central India by the seventeenth century, and Vijay Pinch (2006) has similarly shown the extent to which "Hindu" militant cadres were porous to Sufi institutions. While I have found no hard evidence of any overlap in premodern times between *haṭha* yogic practice per se and elements of military training (Sufi or otherwise), it is clear that the semantic slippage we have seen in the very term *yogi* (from a practitioner of yoga per se to an ascetic mercenary) broadens the term's scope to include those who practice physical culture to non-yogic ends. It is this space of slippage that will later provide an important rationale for the incorporation of physical culture–oriented practice into modern yoga, by the likes of militant physical culturist, Manick Rao (chapter 5). It also helps to explain the apparent discrepancy between postures described in medieval *haṭha* yoga texts and the kind of postural practice ascribed to *haṭha* yoga by modern innovators: in modern times, that is, *āsana* comes to imply both yogic *and* martial practices of the body as well as newer, imported forms of physical culture.

Nineteenth-Century Scholarship

During the decades around Vivekananda's reformulation of yoga it is common to find European scholarship characterizing yogins as dangerous, mendicant tricksters, often in contradistinction to the contemplative, devotional practitioners of "true" yoga. In this sense, scholarship contributed to keeping the *haṭha* yogin and his practices beyond the pale of acceptable religious observance. In his *The Religions of India* of 1885, for example, the American Sanskritist E. W. Hopkins writes that "the Yogi jugglers" of the day share with Islamic fakirs the reputation "of being not only ascetics but knaves" (1970 [1885]: 486 n.1). Two years later, W. J. Wilkins, in *Modern Hinduism*, records that the yogins have become mere "fortune-tellers," "conjurors," and "jugglers" who impose themselves on the ignorance and credulity of the people (87). Neither author presents these yogins as legitimate representatives of Hinduism nor gives any serious consideration to their religious worldview nor to their practices as valid in themselves. It is noteworthy that in his 1901 essay on yoga techniques in the "Great Epic," Hopkins gives "classical" and Vedic precedents for the practice of austerities but has little time for present-day exponents who, he suggests, have no brains in their heads and are "nearly idiotic" (1901: 370 n.1). He insists that it is wrong to consider postural austerities—such as the familiar yoga posture of keeping one leg behind the neck (termed *ekapādaśīrṣāsana* in Iyengar 1966)—as yoga, even though the practitioner may call himself a yogin (Iyengar 1966). *Haṭha* yogic practice, in other words, holds little interest for these scholars.

M. Monier-Williams's 1891 study, *Brahmanism and Hinduism*, shows a distinct preference for Vaiṣṇava forms of belief and praxis over the apparently distasteful religious exhibitions of Śaiva yogins. As Oxford University's Boden Professor of Sanskrit, Monier-Williams was (along with Max Müller) one of the most distinguished and influential scholars of India of his day, and his writing helped to reinforce the negative reputation of the Śaiva yogins. These yogins' "appearance as self-mortifying mendicants" is, he avers, "often revolting to Europeans" (87), a situation only exacerbated by their disreputable moral character and "decidedly dirty habits" (88). The following pronouncement on a Śaiva ritual he has been permitted to witness is typical of his stance:

> I came away sick at heart. No one could be present at such a scene without feeling depressed by the thought that, notwithstanding all our efforts for the extension of education and the diffusion of knowledge, we have as yet done little to loosen the iron grip of idolatry and superstition on the masses of the people. (1891: 93)

His explicit intention in this book is both to convey to English readers the essential features of Hinduism and to reach English-speaking *Indian* readers who, being unable to give a "clear explanation of their own religious creeds or practices," will benefit from the clarity of his exposition (1891: vi). This mission is evident in his assessment of the Śaiva yogins. Monier-Williams was perhaps the single most influential exponent of the doctrine of "fulfillment," in which Indian religious concepts were taken to be underdeveloped truths that could, with the right kind of guidance, pass beyond their limitations and on to the ultimate truth of Christianity (Halbfass 1988: 52). Within this paradigm, Indians (particularly those of the Śaiva persuasion) were considered incapable of interpreting the real significance of their own sacred texts and required the superior intellectual and spiritual counsel of the Christian West. In this interpretation of Indian religious traditions, as well as in Hindu responses to such interpretations, the practices of Śaiva yogins do not have a legitimate place and consistently invite censure and condemnation. Indeed, in his 1879 work, *Modern India and the Indians*, Monier-Williams had noted that the official prohibition of these yogic "self-tortures" was, along with bans on self-immolation and human sacrifices, "among the greatest blessings which India has hitherto received from her English rulers" (1879: 79). Monier-Williams's vision is consistent with the British promotion of devotional forms of Vaiṣṇavism as the paradigm of Indian religious practice.

Max Müller, the first "celebrity academician" and "Captain of the Orientalist enterprise" (Girardot 2002: 215; 221) was similarly ill-disposed toward practitioners of *haṭha* yoga. In his 1899 book on the six orthodox systems of Hindu philosophy, he condemns "all these postures and tortures" of *haṭha* yoga, asserting that he is treating the topic of yoga at all only insofar as it may represent "a useful addition to the Sâṃkhya"—itself subordinate to the supreme philosophical system of the *Vedānta* (1899: 407). He accounts for the presence of such lower yogas by describing an ostensibly historical process of corruption and reformation within the Indian religious sphere. In its "early stages," he claims, yoga "was truly philosophical" (465) but eventually degenerated into practical systems like *haṭha* yoga. Even within Patañjali's *Yogasūtras*, he maintains, "we are able to watch the transition from rational beginnings to irrational exaggerations, the same tendency which led from intellectual to practical Yoga" (465).

Müller is not alone in his negative attitude toward the *practices* of yogins, and his admiration for the "intellectual" schema of *Sāṃkhya* and *Vedānta*. Narratives of "practical yoga" as a symptom of religious degeneration are often related to explain the lowly position of the *haṭha* yogin within the religio-philosophical systems of Hinduism. Hopkins, for example, asserts that during the period of the *Brāhmaṇas*, the wild, unscrupulous yogin began to corrupt Brahminism's admirable aim of attaining oneness with God (1970 [1885]: 351). These "charlatan" yogins, with their reputation for sanctity, easily infiltrated Brahmin society and contributed to religious decline (351). Like Müller, Hopkins has an admiration for *Sāṃkhya* and (especially) *Vedānta* as well as for the yoga of the *Bhagavad Gītā*. Forms such as *haṭha*, however, appear not only inferior but parasitic on other, worthier expressions of yoga.[6] A similar account is given by Max Weber in his *Religions of India* of 1909 in which "the irrational mortification, the *atha Yoga* [*sic*] of pure magical asceticism," is eventually superseded by the "classical Brahmanical holy technique," itself comparable to contemplative Christianity (1958 [1909]: 164). Like Hopkins and Müller, who are probably among his sources here, Weber considers *haṭha* yoga an inferior relative of "classical"—that is, orthodox, and Vaiṣṇava—Indian religion (see also Singleton 2008b).

Girardot argues that such narratives stem from attempts by scholars like Müller and Hopkins to explain "the amalgamation of the religiously (and morally) pure and corrupt in authoritative sacred texts"; in fact, they unconsciously recapitulate a European Protestant narrative of an originally pure religion corrupted by power interests but eventually restored to its former pristine glory (2002: 238). Whatever the degree of historical legitimacy we wish to accord such accounts, the verdicts of Müller and Hopkins are representative of the unfavorable light in which *haṭha* yogins tended to be cast by scholars of the period.

Haṭha Yoga in Translation

Even in modern translations and exegeses of "classical" *haṭha* yoga texts, there is often a marked hostility toward the very practitioners of the doctrines under consideration. A clear example of this is Richard Schmidt's 1908 watercolor-illustrated translation of the *Gheraṇḍa Saṃhitā*, which draws freely on J. C. Oman's 1903 account of the "mystics, ascetics and saints of India" for information regarding yogins (1908: iii). The book contains a collection of European accounts of yogins by authors such as Bernier and Fryer, and so it is not surprising that Schmidt should, like the majority of these authors, regard yogins unfavorably. He is, he declares, "as personally opposed as possible to fakirdom in India and its derivates in Europe and America" (i), and he characterizes yogi-fakirs as nothing but "petty thieves and swindlers" (iv).[7] What is noteworthy here is that the practitioners of the very doctrine Schmidt takes the time to translate and explain are condemned as morally opprobrious. They are, furthermore, confounded, as they always had been, with the Mohammedan fakir. Schmidt's indignation regarding the introduction of yoga to the West is particularly interesting here, insofar as he judges these experiments to be expressions of *haṭha* yoga. As we shall see in the next chapter, the foremost exponents of practical yoga in the West, Swami Vivekananda and Mme. H. P. Blavatsky, were actually themselves pointedly antagonistic to *haṭha* practices and purposefully avoided association with them in their respective formulations (even though such elements are not entirely absent from their teachings). That Schmidt should consider yogic experimentation in the West at this time to represent *haṭha* practice is illustrative of the close ties that yoga in its practical expression had with the figure of the yogi-fakir. It was precisely this association, however, that modern yoga reformers sought to avoid.

S. C. Vasu and the Sacred Books of the Hindus

Other translations of the time reflect a similar ambivalence regarding the teachings of *haṭha* yoga: if the texts themselves merit translation into English, the yogin himself remains a figure of utmost suspicion. Let us consider here the important translations by Rai Bahadur Srisa Chandra Vasu, which were among the first and most popular editions of "classical" *haṭha* yoga available to a wide, English-speaking audience. The first of these translations, *Śiva Saṃhitā*, originally appeared in the *Arya of Lahore* in 1884 and was reprinted in book form under the title *The Esoteric Science and Philosophy of the Tantras* in 1893 as part of Heeralal Dhole's "Vedanta Series." This series included translations of many of the major texts of Vedānta as well as new studies on Hindu religion, medicine, and theosophy. This 1893 edition of the *Śiva Saṃhitā* was published in Calcutta by Dhole himself, in Bombay by Jaishtaram Mookundji, in Madras and London by the Theosophical Society, and in Chicago by Open Court, a company that, according to a full-page advertisement on page 33, published a weekly journal of the same name, edited by Paul Carus and "devoted to the work of conciliating Religion with Science." Vasu's translation should thus be seen as part of the international effort to reconcile (medical) science with religion. This edition is dedicated to the co-founder of the Theosophical Society, Colonel H. S. Olcott, "in recognition of his services for the Revival of Aryan Religion and Ancient Philosophy" (frontispiece).

Two years later in 1895, Vasu's *Gheraṇḍa Saṃhitā, a Treatise on Haṭha Yoga* was published by the Bombay Theosophical Society. In 1914, Vasu's *Śiva Saṃhitā* was republished as a separate volume in the widely available "Sacred Books of the Hindus" series. In 1915 it was combined with the *Gheraṇḍa Saṃhitā* and published as a twin volume in the same series entitled *The Yoga Śāstra*, which included an extensive "Introduction to Yoga Philosophy" and commentary by Vasu. The book is edited by Vasu's brother, Major B. D. Basu (also general editor of the Sacred Books) and published by another family member, Sudhīndranātha Vasu.

Alongside his *haṭha* translations, S. C. Vasu was an energetic and prolific voice in the definition of modern Hinduism, and he wrote and translated widely for the Sacred Books series. His *Catechism of Hindu Dharma* (first edition 1899), for instance, is a credo of unitary Hinduism which, as Major Basu's 1919 preface reads, reflects "a growing tendency to liberal and broad interpretation of the texts and to the need which is becoming felt in certain classes of educated Hindu Society for greater freedom, both of thought and practice" (Vidyārṇava 1919: i).[8] It is a self-conscious, ecumenical renovation of religious tradition, as is his *Daily Practice of the Hindus* of 1904, conceived as a manual of ritual observance for Hindus everywhere. Vasu's translations of *haṭha* yoga texts should be understood as part of his broader project to reinterpret and define the traditions of Hinduism to suit the requirements of the day.

The "Sacred Books of the Hindus" series itself may be seen to represent an Indian alternative to Max Müller's famous fifty-volume "Sacred Books of the East" (1879–1910). Not only is the series title virtually the same (with the crucial substitution of "Hindu" for "East"), but the volumes themselves, as objects, closely resemble those of Müller and present a very similar choice of "sacred" texts within Hinduism. Both series, moreover, were produced in English rather the vernacular languages of India. As high-quality, Indian-produced scholastic documents setting out the "canon" of Hinduism, by Hindus and for Hindus, these books are an important instance of the Indian intellectual and religious self-assertion that arose in response to the European doctrine of the "fulfillment" of Hinduism by Christianity. Like its European namesake, Basu's Sacred Books series is a landmark in the creation of a modern canonical vision of Hinduism based on a particular selection of "sacred" texts.

Vasu's translations of *haṭha* yoga texts were one of the very few accessible sources for English speakers wishing to find out more on the topic. The only other widely available, printed English translations of *haṭha* texts at this time were Ayangar's *Haṭha Yoga Pradīpikā* (Theosophical Society 1893); Ayangar and Iyer's *Occult Physiology. Notes on Hata Yoga* (Theosophical Society 1893); B. N. Bannerjee's *Practical Yoga Philosophy or Siva-Sanhita in English* (People's Press, Calcutta 1894); and Pancham Sinh's *Haṭha Yoga Pradīpikā* (Sacred Books Series, 1915). As some of the very earliest and most widely distributed English translations of *haṭha* yoga texts, therefore, Vasu's editions not only defined to a large extent the *choice* of texts that would henceforth be included within the *haṭha* "canon" but were also instrumental in mediating *haṭha* yoga's status both within modern anglophone yoga as a whole and within the new, "free-thinking" modern Hinduism identified by Basu. For many decades, indeed, these works continued to be the source texts for anyone interested in discovering more about *haṭha* yoga, and they are still republished and read today. For example, Vasant Rele (1927) relied on these translations for his well-known scientific exposition of the *kuṇḍalinī* phenomenon (see next chapter), and Theos Bernard uses them as the textual basis for his landmark 1946 account of a *haṭha* yoga *sādhana* (course of practice). The same translations are reprinted today in cheap paperback editions (e.g., Vasu 1996a, 1996b, 2005).

Vasu and the *Haṭha* Yogin

So how does Vasu reconcile the widespread condemnation of the *haṭha* yogin within scholarship and his decision to translate some of the primary texts of that tradition? In his "Introduction to Yoga Philosophy" which prefaces the 1915 combined volume of the ŚS and the GhS (entitled *The Yoga Śāstra*) Vasu repeatedly condemns "those hideous specimens of humanity who parade through our streets bedaubed with dirt and ash—frightening the children, and extorting money from timid and good-natured folk" (2). In India, he confirms, this grotesque beggar-figure is what "many understand by the word Yogi" in spite of the apparent fact that "all true Yogis renounce any fraternity with these" (2). What Vasu is attempting with his vignettes of sinister holy men (and indeed in his introduction as a whole) is a reclamation of the very signifiers "Yogi" and "Yoga" from what they *do* mean in popular parlance and practice to what they *should* mean.

By dint of their "bigotry and ignorance" the *haṭha* yogis appear in Vasu's vision as the natural enemy of the *true Yogi* and have moreover "proved a great stumbling-block to the progress of this science [of Yoga]" (Vasu 1915: 2). This semantic and ideological maneuver on Vasu's part epitomizes Narayan's observation that "if the self-torturing holy man was denigrated in his embodiedness, the yogī was a disembodied textual ideal" (1993: 490). What is being attempted here in Vasu's Sacred Books translation is a redefinition of the yogin, in which the grassroots practitioner of *haṭha* methods has no part. The modern yogin must be scientific where the *haṭha* yogin is not.

Vasu offers stern warnings against the inherent perils of engaging in these practices: those impetuous ones who venture alone into the kind of "occult books" that the author here translates "are always exposed to the danger of *degenerating into haṭha Yoga*" (1915: 42, my emphasis). In this, Vasu is largely in agreement with the pronouncements of Müller on the "degeneration" caused by *haṭha* yogins as well as with the hard-line Theosophical rejection of *haṭha* practices (see below). He even goes so far as to entirely omit the description of certain traditional *haṭha* yoga techniques from his translation, such as *vajrolīmudrā*, in which the practitioner sucks vaginal and seminal fluids back into the penis during the act of sexual intercourse (ŚS IV; *HYP* III.82–89; IV.14). He dismisses *vajrolī* as "an obscene practice indulged in by low class Tantrists" (1915: 51). It is worth noting that the practice of *vajrolī* has continued to be censored in modern editions of *haṭha* yoga texts. Vishnudevananda cuts it from his translation of HYP, considering that, like the related practices of *sahajolī* and *amarolī*, it falls outside the bounds of wholesome practice, or "sattvic sadhana" (1999: 138); Rieker, a student of B. K. S. Iyengar, deems the same three practices to be "obscure and repugnant" and omits them entirely (1989: 127).[9]

Vasu's introduction seems to flatly condemn the very practices of which his translation is a document. If these practices, and those who undertake them, are morally suspect, why bother representing them for an English-speaking audience at all? Why not simply omit them, as Müller had done? What is surprising is that Vasu's original 1895 translation of his *Gheraṇḍa Saṃhitā* opens with a dedication by the "humble sevaka" Vasu to the well-known guru Haridas, "whose

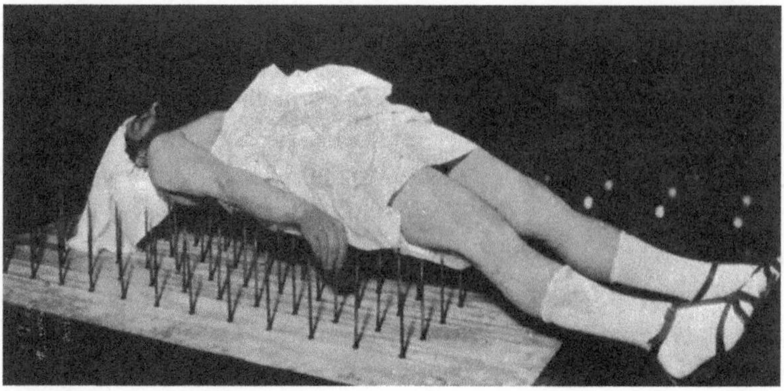

Yogin on a Bed of Nails, from Eliade 1963

practical illustrations and teachings convinced the translator of the reality, utility, and the immense advantages of Hatha Yoga." In this earlier edition, therefore, Vasu presents himself as a "humble servant" (i.e., student and devotee) of a renowned *haṭha* yogin—an insider rather than a mere impartial or critical commentator on *haṭha* yoga. There are none of the doom-filled warnings of the 1915 edition but rather a marked emphasis on the benefits of the practices, as well as a long account of the miraculous, forty day "burial" of his guru under "scientific" supervision at the court of Maharaja Ranjeet Singh, taken verbatim from J. M. Honigberger's famous travelogue *Thirty-five Years in the East* of 1852 (Honigberger 1852: 129).

It is worth noting that this incident crops up as a standard illustration of *haṭha* yogic feats during the early twentieth century. Carrington (1909: 41), for example, retells the story of Haridas but assumes that "doubtless the details are familiar to most of my readers," pointing to the story's widespread currency. Remarkably, Mircea Eliade is still using the burial story as a negative example of yogic imposture as late as 1963 in his *Patañjali et le Yoga*. Here, Haridas is presented as an infamous charlatan and "man of loose morals" whose "mastery of Yoga does not in the least imply spiritual superiority" (1963: 3, trans. mine). An accompanying photograph of a sock- and sandal-wearing yogin on a bed of nails functions by association to confirm Haridas as a mere purveyor of cheap fakir tricks. As Narayan (1993) points out, the yogi's bed of nails quickly became, in official and popular ethnography, the stock symbol of India's moral and spiritual backwardness, and the intention behind Eliade's odd juxtaposition of this image and the story of Haridas's burial is clear.

Vasu's apparent change of policy with regard to the practices of *haṭha* yoga between the 1895 and the 1915 editions may reflect the formalization of the new

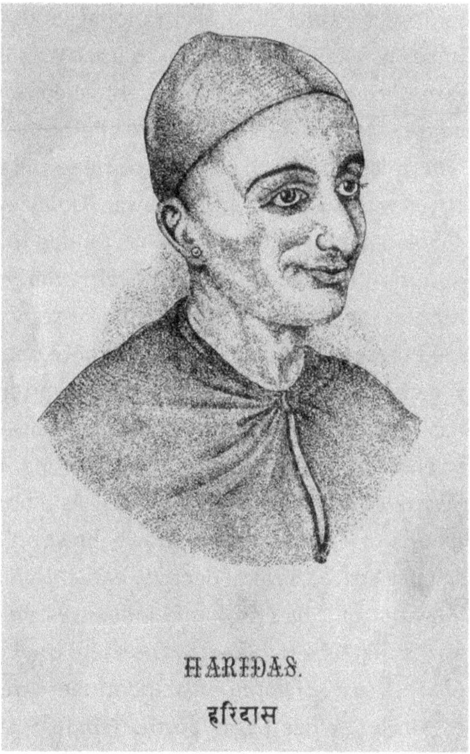

Haridas (as pictured in Vasu 1895)

creed of Hinduism during this twenty year period. The Sacred Books series, if it was to be taken seriously by scholars or modern Hindus, could not permit the acknowledgment of a morally suspect *haṭha* yoga guru as a source of inspiration to the author. The earlier volume was published in the year immediately prior to Vivekananda's *Raja Yoga*, a book that was to usher in a new, public age for yoga and in which (as we shall see) there was no room for the *haṭha* yogin. By 1915, it was probably clear to Vasu and his fraternal editor that if *haṭha* texts themselves were available for appropriation and modernization, *haṭha* yogis themselves remained embarrassing, impure guests at the modern Hindu table. *Haṭha* yoga had to be appropriated from the yogin, and one of the ways this occurred was through appeals to modern science and medicine.

Basu, Dayananda, Paul: The Roots of Medical *Haṭha* Yoga

Vasu's intention in the 1915 volume is not simply to decry *haṭha* yogins but to fashion an ideal of what a *real* practitioner of yoga should be—an ideal thoroughly informed by the scientific, rational, and "classical" values of the day. Yoga, implores Vasu, must be looked upon as a legitimate science and should not be disdained by the (Western) scientific community (4).[10] S. C. Vasu's brother and editor, Major Basu, was in fact one of the early, leading lights of the scientific enterprise of yoga that would come to full flower in India during the 1920s and 1930s with Sri Yogendra and Swami Kuvalayananda. We should note that recent scholarship on modern yoga has tended to overlook these early ventures and to assume that "scientific," medical *haṭha* yoga began with the experiments of Kuvalayananda and Yogendra. For instance, Joseph Alter (2004a) has considered these later developments in more detail than any other scholar of modern yoga but has not looked into their important precedents. Similarly, De Michelis has recently asserted that "the 'medicalisation' of yoga, and its dialogue with science, started in the 1920s in India, primarily with the work of Sri Yogendra . . . and Swami Kuvalayananda" (2007: 12). As a brief review of the early scientific orientations of Vasu and Basu shows, however, the dawn of *haṭha* yoga as medical science arrived several decades earlier than has been supposed. The model that grew out of it had profound influences on the shape of the transnational yoga forms that would follow. Let us therefore briefly review some of these early rapprochements of *haṭha* yoga and modern medical science.

In his "Prize Essay on the Hindu System of Medicine," published in the *Guy's Hospital Gazette* (London) in 1889 and cited in Vasu's 1915 foreword to the ŚS, Major Basu asserts—in what is one of the very first public and international claims of tantric yoga's scientific, medical status—that "better anatomy is given in the Tantras than in the medical works of the Hindus" (Vasu 1915: i). According to him, the *Śiva Saṃhitā* gives "a description of the several ganglia and plexuses of the nervous system" (i) and is proof that the Hindus were acquainted with the spinal cord, brain, and central nervous system. In this essay, and in a paper on the "Anatomy of the Tantras" published a year earlier in the *Theosophist* (March 1888), Basu commenced a mapping of tantric body symbolism onto Western anatomy that would keep the later pioneers of "scientific" *haṭha* yogic phenomena occupied for many decades to come. Kuvalayananda himself, indeed, identified Basu's *Theosophist* article as "the oldest attempt in the direction of scientifically interpreting the Yogic anatomy" (1935: 3). It is here, perhaps, that for the first time a "scientific" attempt is made to "identify the *Nâdîs, Chakras* and *Padmas*" of *haṭha* yoga with the conduits of the spine and the plexuses of the anatomical body—an identification that is still pervasive in popular transnational *haṭha* yoga today. Captain Basu's enquiry is based on the eminently empirical, rationalistic question, "Are [the *padmas* and *chakras*] real, or do they only exist in the imagination of the Tântrists?" (Vasu 1915: ii). It is clear that for the "lotuses" and "wheels" of the *haṭha* system to be taken seriously by his readers, they must be shown to have issued from proto-scientific observation rather than mere fancy ("imagination" here unmistakably connoting "nonrational"). On this basis, Basu professes, "we nevertheless believe that the Tântrists obtained their knowledge about them by dissection" (ii).

Contrary to Basu's assertion, we should note, there is no evidence whatever that "Tântrists," or any other religious group in India, ever engaged in the dissection of corpses. In fact, the first dissection by a Hindu was probably undertaken in 1836 by Madhusūdana Gupta in Calcutta (Wujastyk 2002: 74). As Bharati writes, "Ancient Indians never opened up dead bodies to study organs empirically.... The horror of defilement and ritual pollution was so strong in India that anatomical and physiological experimentation seemed until recently out of the question" (1976: 165). As far back as 1670, indeed, Bernier had noted the same horror among Indians with regard to anatomical dissection (1968 [1670]: 339). Basu's claim should therefore be understood as a projection of the scientific present onto the screen of tradition and as an expression of the modern need to view the *haṭha* yogic body as anatomical and "real." It is this need that forms the impetus and rationale for the *haṭha* experimentation of the twentieth century.

This point can be illustrated further by a (possibly apocryphal) anecdote from the life of Hindu firebrand and founder of the Ārya Samāj, Dayananda Saraswati (1824–1883). On a tour of India in 1855, Dayananda pulls a corpse from the river and dissects it to ascertain the truth of the tantric *cakras* he has been reading about. When his search fails, he scornfully tosses his yogic texts (including the *Haṭha Yoga Pradīpikā*) into the water (Yadav 2003 [1976]: 46). His experiment leads him to "the conclusion that with the exception of the *Vedas, Patanjali* and *Sankhya* all other works on the science of yoga are false" (Yadav 2003 [1976]: 41). While Basu's optimism and Dayananada's pessimism regarding the truth-value of *haṭha* yogic texts are clearly at odds, they nonetheless have in common that they enthrone rational empiricism as monarch in the kingdom of yoga.

Both the failed search of 1855 and the confident credo of 1888 are modern projects that stand in a contradictory relationship with a traditional conception of the tantric body as a constructed, "entextualised" entity, in which "imagination becomes a kind of action... and the forms that the body takes in ritual are a kind of knowing" (Flood 2006: 6). From the tantric perspective, the *cakras* are simply not observable physical phenomena but inscribed ritual processes: a notion that has largely escaped the attention of popular writers on *haṭha* yoga from Basu onward. As Bharati argues, the yogic subtle body "is an object our imagination has to create" (1976: 164).[11] This is not to say that *cakras* are not "real" in a very particular way: the point is that one would be hard-pressed to find them with a dissection scalpel or a camera. They are not, in other words, available for empirical or medical testing in the way that, say, ganglia are. As Wujastyk notes, the kind of thinking that prompts Dayananda to undertake his dissection, and which also lies behind Basu's project to find *cakras* in plexuses, is based on the notion that the world is one and that the traditional and modern explanations of it are both true and can be made to coincide (2002: 75). Such thinking informs research on the yogic body through the twentieth century, from Kuvalayananda's physiological experiments "between science and philosophy" in the 1920s and 1930s (Alter 2004a) up to and beyond Hiroshi Motoyama's cakra-detecting machines of the 1970s and 1980s (Motoyama 1981).[12]

Another vitally important early moment in the reconciliation of tradition and science is *A Treatise on the Yoga Philosophy* by Dr. N. C. Paul (also known as Navīna Candra Pāla), originally published in 1850 but saved from obscurity by the Theosophical Society reprint of 1888. Perhaps even more than Basu's work, this study might be credited as the first attempt to marry *haṭha* yoga practice and theory with modern medical science. Paul considers *haṭha* yogic suspension of the breath and the circulation of blood in Western medical terms, once again (like Vasu) evoking the interment of the guru Haridas as the paradigm of yogic physiological control (Paul 1888 [1850]: 49–50). As Blavatsky notes, the book's appearance in 1850 "produced a sensation amongst the representatives of medicine in India, and a lively polemic between the Anglo-Indian and native journalists" (Neff and Blavatsky 1937: 94–95). Copies were even burned on the grounds that the text was "offensive to the science of physiology and pathology" (95). However, its republication by the Theosophical Society, in the same year as Basu's seminal article in the Society's journal, relaunched it as a key text in the early formulation of *haṭha* yoga as science, and it was used as an authoritative source on *haṭha* yoga by some European scholars. For example, Hermann Walter's 1893 dissertation on the *Haṭhayogapradīpikā* at the University of Munich is, like Paul's work, greatly concerned with the "extent to which the chakras correspond to an anatomical reality" (1893: xv, my trans.). He notes the enormous therapeutic potential that an investigation into these matters might yield. Paul's book, he declares, is "the only work that goes into more detail on the topic [of *haṭha* yoga and anatomy]" (1893: i) and he seems to derive his notion of the potential medical applications offered by *haṭha* yoga principally from Paul's book.

Significantly, Paul did not glean his information about yoga directly from Indian yogins themselves but from textual sources and from one Captain Seymour, who had deserted the British army and escaped several mental institutions in England to "[become] a Yogi" (Neff and Blavatsky 1937: 95). It may indeed seem ironic that this earliest study of *haṭha* yoga as medical science is based on the account of a "gone-native" English informant as recorded by an anglicized Indian, but it is nonetheless typical of the way modern, anglophone interpretations of yoga are filtered through apparently disparate cultural lenses, and of the lack of direct ethnographic contact and engagement with lineages of practicing yogins. Apart from Paul's mediated experience of yogins through Seymour, information about *haṭha* yoga practice in this period tends to remain exclusively textual.

The scientific imperative given expression by S. C. Vasu, Major Basu, and N. C. Paul and (in his own way) by Dayananda represents a new departure for yoga and tantra along scientific, rational lines and sets the agenda for the scientific study of yogic phenomena throughout the twentieth century. Indeed, Vasant Rele's renowned physiological search for the *kuṇḍalinī* in the 1920s is itself based on Vasu's translations of *haṭha* yogic texts. These translations, shot through as they are with medical and scientific material (such as excerpts from the *British Medical Journal* on the benefits of respiratory exercises (Vasu 1915: 46–48), represent a landmark in the popular promulgation of *haṭha* yoga as medical science.[13] Geoffrey Samuel notes with regard to Tibetan medicine's encounter with the West that only those elements that can be readily assimilated into a materialist epistemology are retained, while those that do not "fit" are forgotten or rejected (Samuel 2006). It is clear that similar forces are at work in anglophone *haṭha* yoga as it negotiates its way into the Western scientific paradigm. That today some fourteen million Americans are recommended yoga by their therapist or doctor (Yoga Journal 2008) is in many respects a late consequence of yoga's assimilation into medical science that began in the mid-nineteenth century.

3

◇◇◇◇◇◇◇

Popular Portrayals of the Yogin

> From the time it was discovered, more than four thousand years ago Yoga was perfectly delineated, formulated and preached in India...the more ancient the writer, the more rational he is.
>
> (Vivekananda 2001 [1896]: 134)

The Topos of the Performing Yogi

The swell of disenfranchised *nāgas* during the nineteenth century ushered in a heyday for yogic showmanship and provided a wealth of material for newspapers and popular ethnographers. The emergence of the yogi as panhandling entertainer was a response to the uncompromising British clampdown on ascetic trade soldiers from the nineteenth century onward. To survive, large numbers were forced into mendicancy and yogic showmanship, thereby fulfilling post hoc well-established expectations about what a yogi ought to be:

> the intensifying market competition for ever-greater feats of austerity ensured that *nagas* would live up to the image of the mysterious *yogi* that had settled in comfortable urban, middle-class imaginations—Indian as well as British—as a wild throwback to a pre-modern form of religious asceticism. (Pinch 2006: 237)

The socioeconomic predicament that *nāgas* found themselves in during the nineteenth century made them the most visible representatives of this kind of asceticism and rich source material for Western journalists and travel writers. The ascetic had always tended to be presented in the West as the embodiment of both the sacred, mystical, and ecstatic dimensions of experience—*and* of those dimensions that were "backward, uncivilised, or dangerous" (Urban 2003:

277); and the representations of ascetic contortion at this time were a function of this well-established discourse. Ascetic busking had long been the province of the *haṭha* yogi, who was predominantly perceived, in Will's felicitous phrase, as "the carnival 'swami' or 'fakir'" (1996: 384). Such figures appear as early as Peter Mundy's eyewitness accounts of 1628–1634, in the form of "Bazighurres," or "bāzīgars," who "use dauncinge, tumblinge, etts. Feats" (Mundy 1914: 254). The acrobatic and balancing tricks of these men—such as swinging into a hand-stand position from a seated lotus pose (254)—are increasingly associated with yogins in the early modern period and continue to be features of modern trans-national *āsana* practice today. As mass-circulation print media brought images of yogic austerities to a wider audience, the *haṭha* yogin's reputation as the eccentric extreme of the Indian religious spectrum was increasingly cemented.

"The Most Stoopendous Marvel of the Age": Yogi Bava Lachman Dass

The case of Yogi Bava Lachman Dass is exemplary here.[1] When he arrived in London in 1897 to perform his forty-eight postures at a sideshow of London's Westminster Aquarium, his repertoire was already well inscribed within a bicentennial British imaginary of mendicant Indian fakirism fused with Western contortionist vaudeville. Dass's "picturesque" performance was reported by journalist Framley Steelcroft in Britain's preeminent illustrated journal of contemporary life, *The Strand*. It may well be the first ever photo-documented *haṭha yogāsana* demonstration on European soil and is quite possibly the first public demonstration by an Indian in Britain of *postural manipulation conceived as* yoga. The article reveals much about prevailing attitudes of the time toward religious mendicancy in India. Steelcroft presents Dass's *āsanas* as mere contortions for cash, as exhibits from the "repulsive" gallery of Indian religion (1897: 176). Dass, he notes, blithely broke Brahminical prohibitions on crossing oceans for the sake of "vulgar £. s. d. [pounds, shillings and pence]"; passing Londoners are heard to speculate that instead of meditating, Dass spends his evenings counting his takings (176). With heavy irony, Steelcroft expresses respectful awe of the yogin's sanctity while at the same time painting for his readers an Indian Tartuffe, an emissary of the disreputable phonies and holy swindlers who, we are given to understand, abound in India. Dass is presented primarily as a circus performer whose livelihood is earned through a display of renunciation in return for material gain: a ruse that fools Indians, perhaps, but not the savvy Cockney (178).

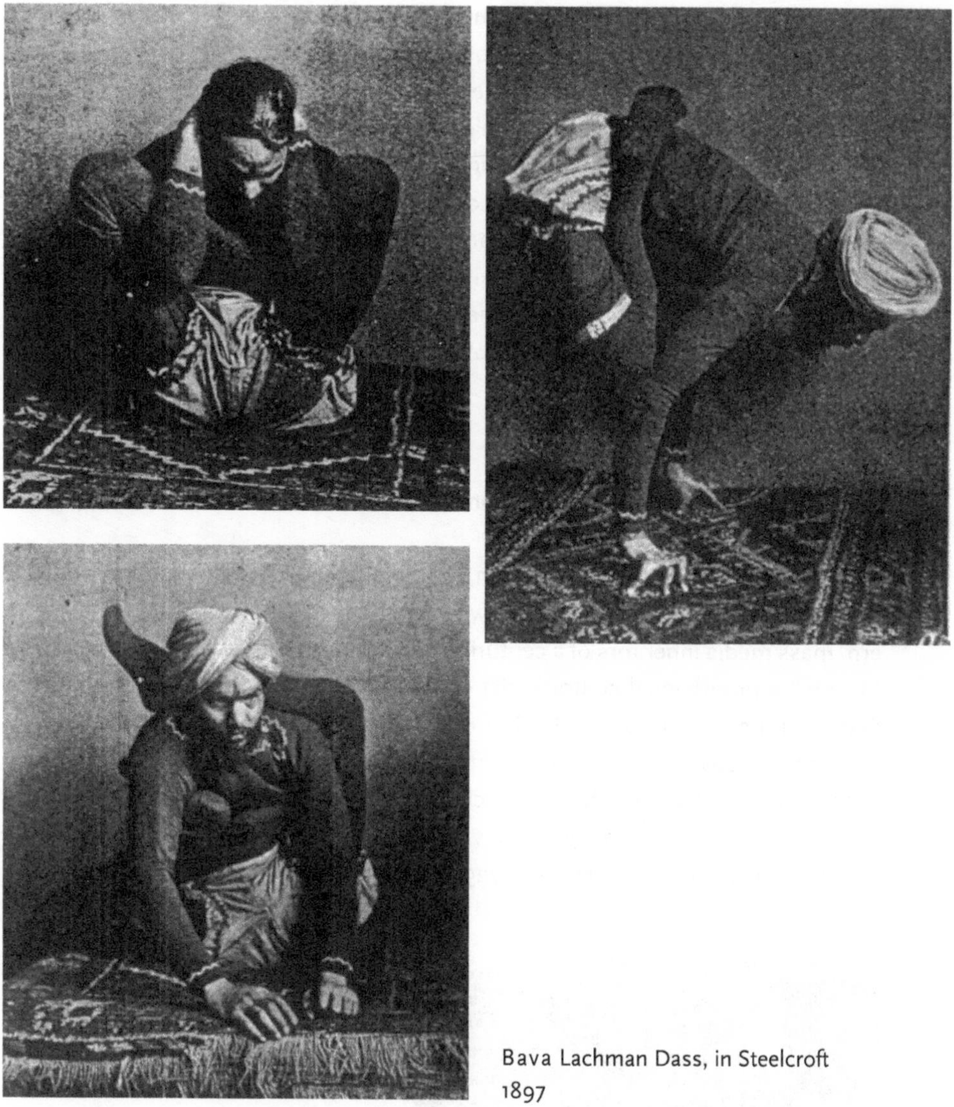

Bava Lachman Dass, in Steelcroft 1897

Strand readers of the time would have been very familiar with the topos of postural contortion as entertainment: it was not necessary to go to India to encounter such things. Steelcroft himself was something of a chronicler of freakish bodies, having one year earlier reported on the Western contortionists Walter Wentworth and "Ames, the boneless wonder," alongside Cliquot the sword-swallower, the iron-skinned Sri Lankan performer Rannin, and a variety of other human marvels (Steelcroft 1896). In the same year as the article on Dass, *Strand* journalist William G. Fitzgerald wrote pieces on the female contortionists Knotella and Leonora, and the "premier contortionist of the world" Marinelli the Man Snake (Fitzgerald 1897a, Fitzgerald 1897b). Other popular illustrated British weeklies of the time, like *Pearson's Magazine*, also commonly pictured contorted bodies, such as "The King of Contortionists" Pablo Diaz (Carnac 1897). Similar images were featured in the American popular press, as in Thomas Dwight's article "The Anatomy of the Contortionist," which appeared in *Scribner's Magazine* in 1898. Evidently, the British and American reading public were well primed to understand Dass's display as a form of contortionism, albeit enhanced with the magical glow of the East.

The Posture Master and European Contortionism

We should note also that the freakish, contorted characters who feature in the periodicals of the 1890s are not a new phenomenon. They are in fact the modern, mass media inheritors of a centuries-old European tradition of the "Posture Master," a professional contortionist commonly found at fairs and saturnalia, and entertaining in royal courts. There is a whole history to be written on this topic and no space to enter into the matter at any length here, but suffice it to say that famous Posture Masters, such as Englishmen Joseph Clarke (d. 1697) and the employees of Master Fawkes (or "Faux," who had his own theater in James's Street in London between 1729 and 1731), had been entertaining British

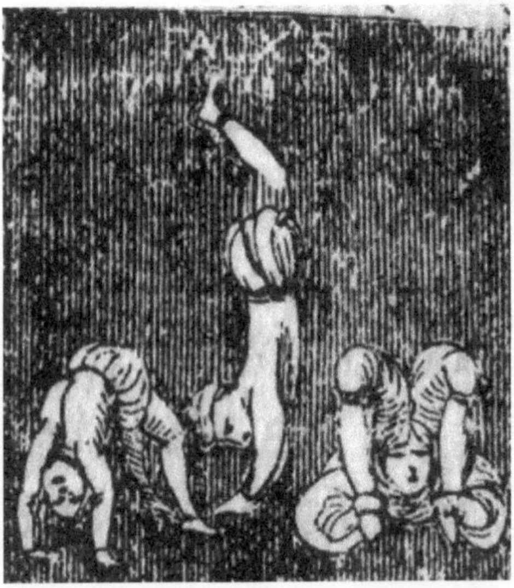

Detail from "Faux the Conjuror's Booth, Bartholomew Fair," in Chambers (ed.) 1862–1864, 2: 265

and European audiences with outlandish contortions for hundreds of years prior to the arrival of Yogi Dass.[2]

While the new mass photographic media of the nineteenth century made images of extreme postural manipulations available to a far wider audience, the topos of contortion-as-entertainment is far older and more deeply ingrained in the British and European consciousness than the encounter with posture-practicing yogins and fakirs. With this in mind, it is easy to see how the *āsanas* of *haṭha* yoga would readily have been interpreted by readers as the Indian equivalent of Western sideshow contortionist routines. The increasing numbers and high profile of yogin-entertainers in India from the mid-1800s onward also contributed to such interpretations.

There is a clear, circumscribed vocabulary of postural forms both within the posture-master tradition and among later performers such as those depicted in *The Strand*. Many of the most common positions are a perfect match with the advanced postures of popular postural yoga today, coincidences that may be at least partially due to the structure and limitations of the human body itself. As Elkins remarks, "despite whatever meanings are elided by the fantasy of bonelessness, it won't be possible to evade the basic possibilities of the normal body" (Elkins 1999: 105). While the apparent similarities between modern yoga postures and contortionist turns are to some degree a function of these basic possibilities, they remain nonetheless suggestive. The most frequently occurring postures are, to use Iyengar's 1966 nomenclature, *gaṇḍabheruṇḍāsana, naṭarājāsana, hanumānāsana, ṭiṭṭibhāsana, samakoṇāsana*, and *pādāṅguṣṭha dhanurāsana*. For instance, the postures in Faux's advertisement in the figure above correspond (left to right) to *ūrdhvadhanurāsana, adhomukhavṛkṣāsana*, and *gaṇḍabheruṇḍāsana* in Iyengar's nomenclature (1966). As further visual evidence of this formal proximity, I include here a photo-montage of standard Western contortionist poses from the late nineteenth century alongside some advanced *āsana* performed by B. K. S. Iyengar himself.

I point out these similarities not to suggest any *causal* link between the postural forms of the Western sideshow contortionist and the *āsanas* of modern postural yoga but to further emphasize the strong associations that extreme postural forms, such as those demonstrated by Dass, would have naturally had in the European (and American) psyche. If Western ethnographic journalism, as one modern postural yoga writer asserts, helped to make *āsanas* "the laughing stock of the world by spot-lighting their cheapness and vulgarity" (Sondhi 1962: 38), this was facilitated by their ready association with European traditions of contortionism. Articles like Steelcroft's sustained and reinforced the image of the "postural yogin" as India's addition to the menagerie of European sideshows. These associations with "vulgar" popular entertainment contributed to

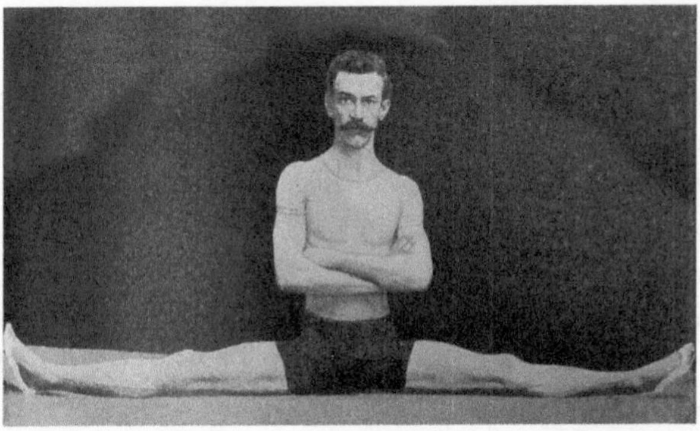

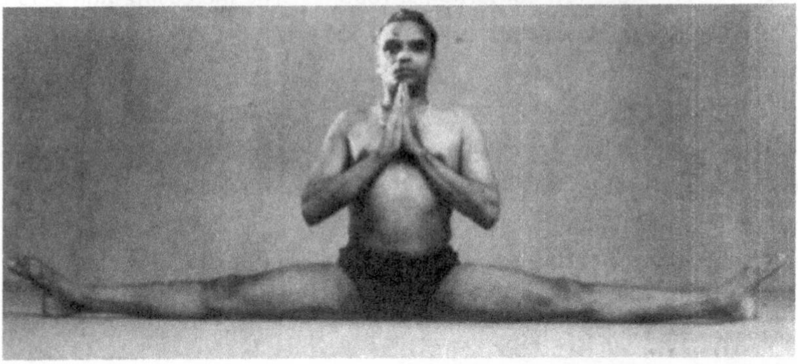

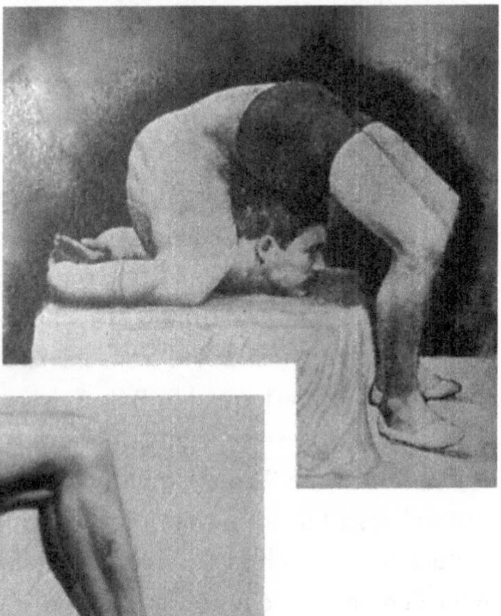

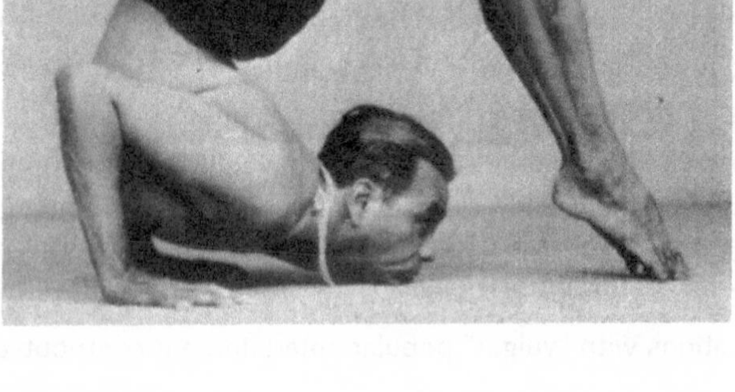

Montage from Thomas Dwight's "Anatomy of a Contortionist," *Scribner's Magazine*, April 1889, and B. K. S. Iyengar's *Light on Yoga* (with permission of HarperCollins Publishers Ltd, ©1966 and George Allen & Unwin and [Publishers] Limited)

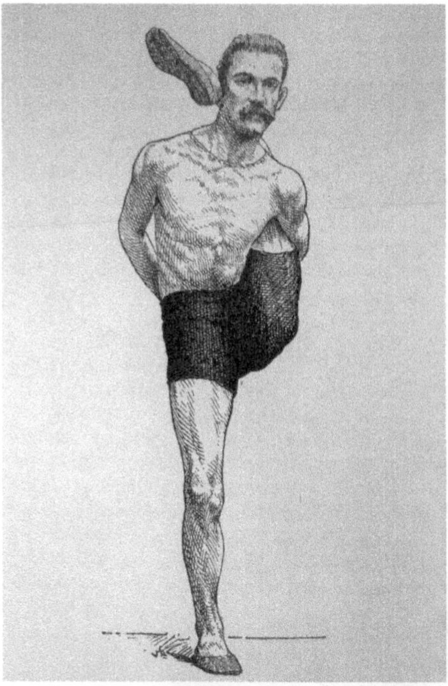

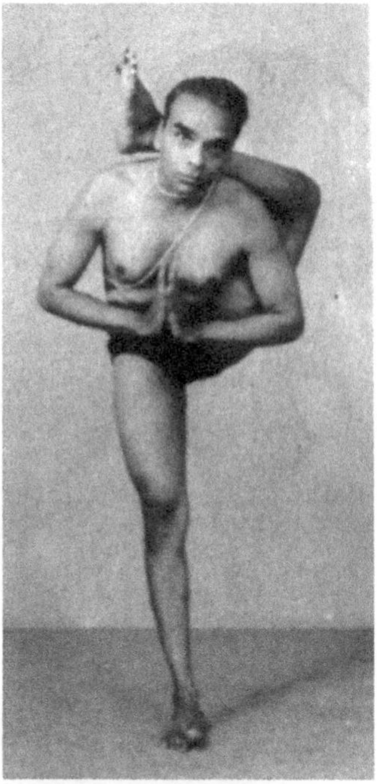

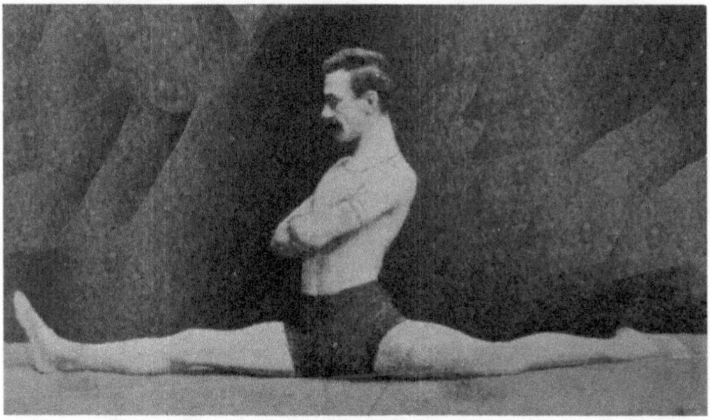

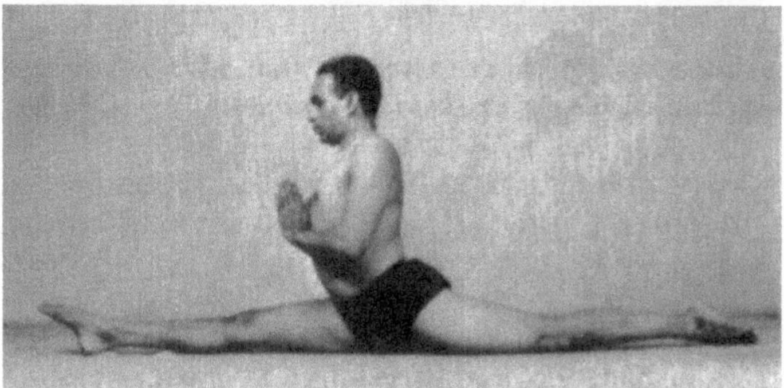

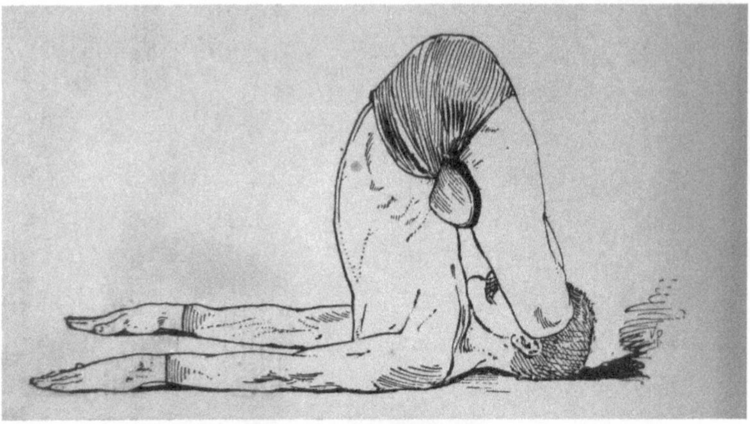

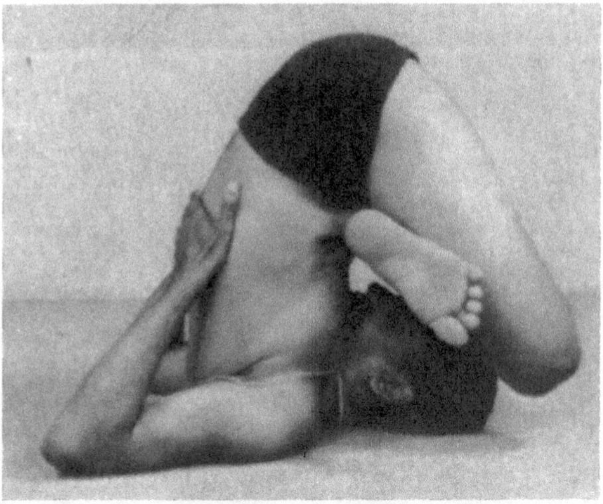

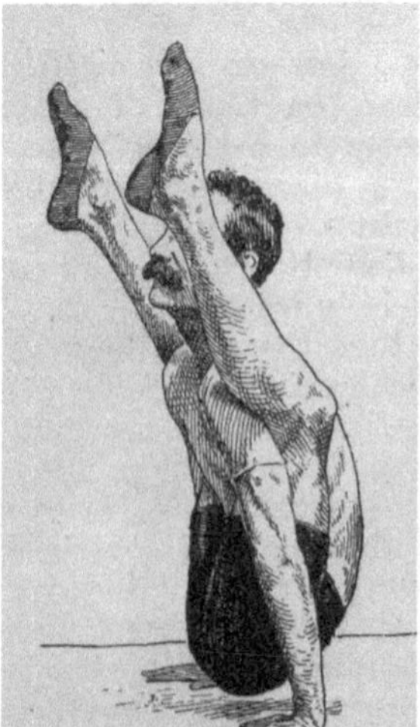

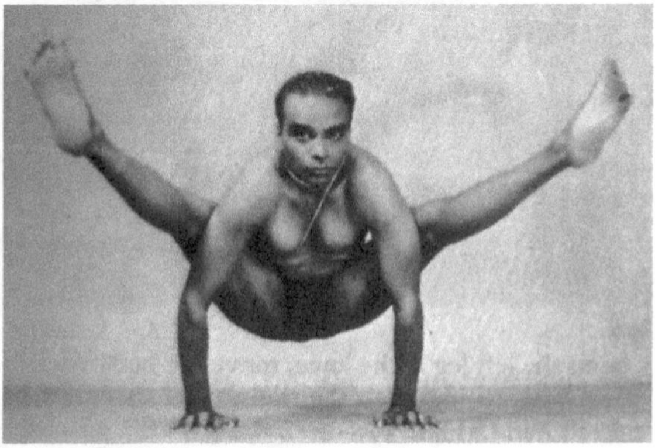

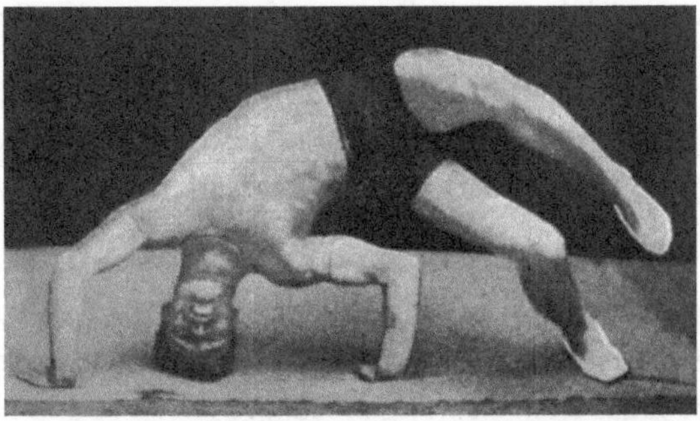
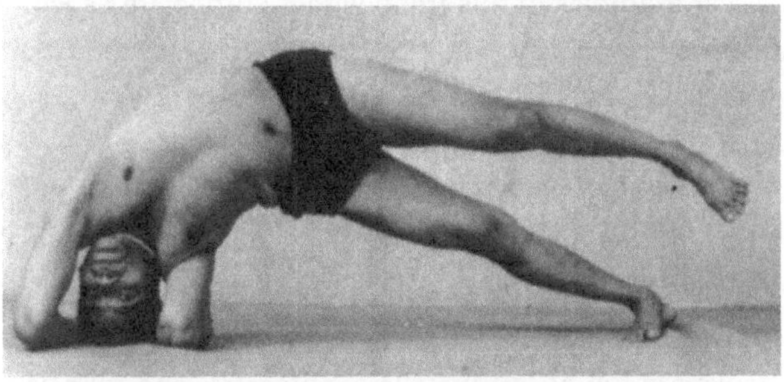
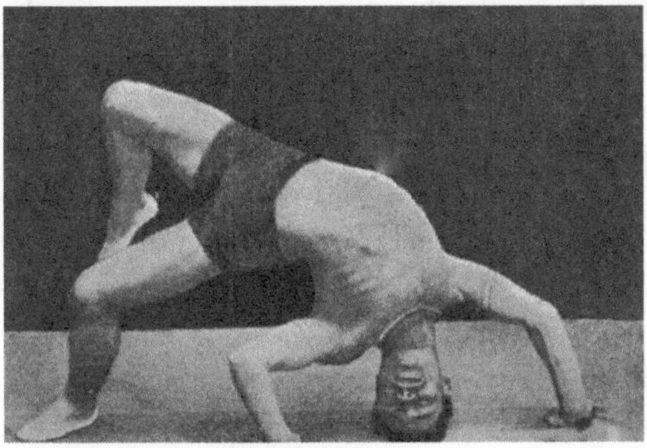
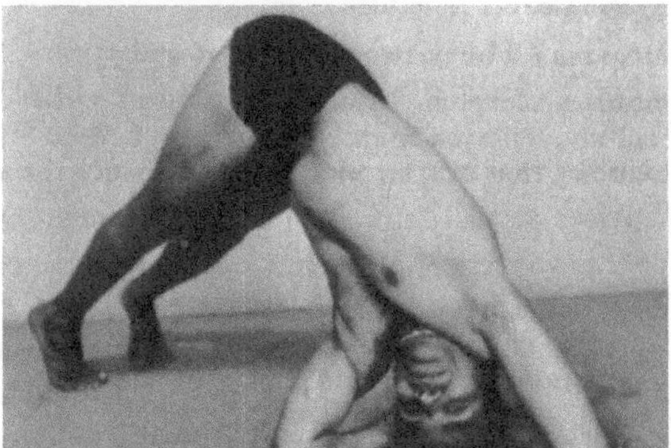

keeping *āsanas* beyond the pale of the export forms of yoga that began to develop from 1893 onward.

The Yogi-Fakir as Magician

The fakir-yogi was the object of an intense fascination for European occultists, who naturally emphasized the wondrous magical powers that such figures could acquire through yoga, often claiming personal experience and mastery of these techniques. Clear examples of this trend within Europe are *Le Fakirisme Hindou* by Paul Sédir (also known as Yves Le Loup), published by the Librarie Générale des Sciences Occultes in Paris in 1906; O. Hashnu Hara's *Practical Yoga, with a chapter devoted to Persian Magic*, also of 1906; Fairfax Asturel et al.'s *Wunder Indischer Fakire* (Berlin 1912); Ernest Bosc's *Yoghisme et Fakirisme Hindous* (in the series Librairie Internationale de la Pensée Nouvelle, Paris 1913); and Max Wilke's *Hatha-Yoga. Die indische Fakir-Lehre zur Entwicklung magischer Gewalten im Menschen* (Dresden 1926).

These books are full of fortunetellers, sorcerers, and miracle workers and are clearly designed to enthrall and entertain in a way that the scholarly treatments of the yogi-fakir considered in the previous chapter are not. They appeal to an esoteric audience thirsty for stories about the yogic magicians of the mystical East and are rarely reliable when it comes to information regarding the techniques and belief frameworks of yogins. Even works that set out to debunk the authenticity of yogic feats, such as Hereward-Carrington's *Hindu Magic: An Exposé of the Tricks of the Yogis and Fakirs of India* of 1909, nevertheless contribute to the continued identification of yoga with sideshow entertainment and with the various systems of para-religious illusionism in India. It is in keeping with this kind of juxtaposition, indeed, that the 1913 American reprint of Carrington's book is bound together with two of his other exposés, *Handcuff Tricks* and *Sideshow and Animal Tricks*.

The more or less fantastical works of Louis Jacolliot, such as his book on "occult science" in India of 1884 (and in particular chapter XI titled "The Yoguys"), should also be mentioned here. As David Smith has shown, Jacolliot's books were often used as source material for information on India and Hindu texts, in spite of their scholarly inadequacy (Smith 2004), and purvey a version of India (including yogins) imbued with occult magic.

The role of the British black magician Aleister Crowley, famously referred to in Hemingway's *A Moveable Feast* as the most evil man in the world, is also noteworthy. J. Gordon Melton credits Crowley with assisting "in the introduction of yoga by authoring a textbook on the eight-step yoga path, *Book 4* in 1913" and

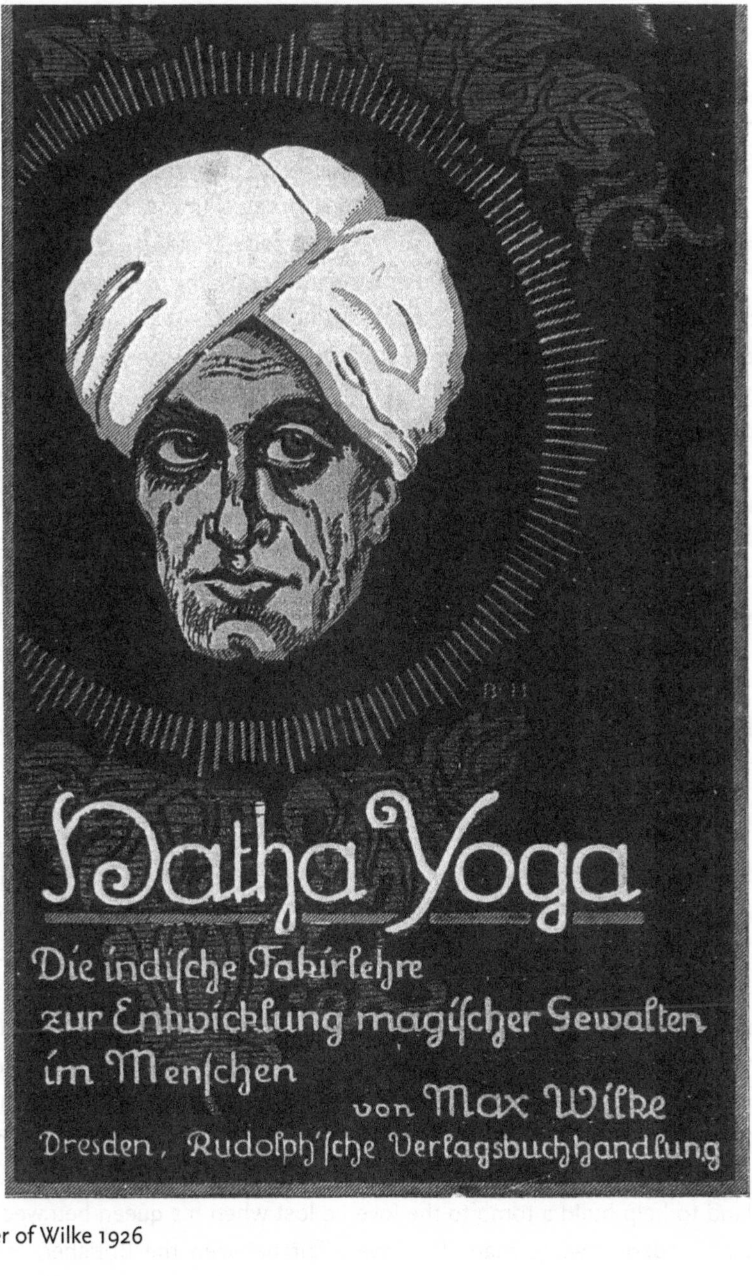

Cover of Wilke 1926

by integrating yoga into his occult training (Melton 1990: 503). Crowley's *Eight Lectures on Yoga*, published under the modest pseudonym Mahatma Guru Sri Paramahansa Shivaji in 1939, is further evidence of a deep-seated fascination with yoga as a component of the occult. There is little doubt that Crowley, as well as other occult authors who were trying their hand at yoga, greatly contributed to a generalized identification of yogins with magicians. According to Hugh Urban, Crowley actually did have a fairly good grasp of Patañjali and knew some postures of *haṭha* yoga (2006: 123). However, his enduring legacy was the merging of Tantric yoga with Western esoteric sexual practices, based on "secondary, superficial and distorted sources that are deeply colored by the Orientalist biases of the nineteenth century" (111). Tantra thereafter became "largely confused in the popular imagination with Crowleyian-style sex magick" (111).

In this light, anti-India polemicist William Archer's judgment of the practices of the yogin as "very patently a branch of magic" (1918: 79) are quite understandable. As Bharati points out, *haṭha* yoga is, during the late nineteenth century, negatively polarized insofar as it is seen to lead toward *siddhis* (supernormal powers) and "to support occult rather than salvational ambitions" (1976: 163). Indeed, in the modern Hindu context, *āsana* practice, when performed by and for itself, "is supposed to generate occult powers" and tends to be avoided for that reason (163). Given this situation, it is hardly surprising that the modern forms of postural practice that we will consider from chapter 5 onward make little or no reference to the attainment of such powers.[3]

We might also briefly note that the yogi-fakir is an important presence in early filmic representations of India. Indeed, the first ever American film about India was a 1902 Edison documentary entitled "Hindu Fakir" (Narayan 1993: 487), and there is a body of early twentieth-century films concerned uniquely with the figure of the yogi-fakir.[4] The 1921 production, *The Indian Tomb*, produced and directed by Joe May, with a scenario by Fritz Lang and Thea von Harbou, is a particularly interesting instance of (fictitious) yogins on film. It begins with the revival of an interred yogin, Ramigani (played by Bernhard Goetzke), who magically transports himself to Europe with orders from the Maharaja to return with the architect Herbert Rowland. The Maharaja wants Rowland to help build a tomb to the love he lost when his queen betrayed him for a philandering white man. The love affair between the Britisher, Harold Berger, and the Maharaja's "queen" (actually a temple dancer named Seetha) had been the subject of Lang's *The Tiger of Eschnapur*, of which *The Indian Tomb* is the sequel. A key moment in the plot of *The Indian Tomb* is when Herbert's fiancée, and then Herbert himself, precipitately enter a cavernous room of the Maharaja's palace occupied by a group of yogi-fakirs in stock ascetic poses: some are hanging upside down, some are lying on beds of nails, others are bent

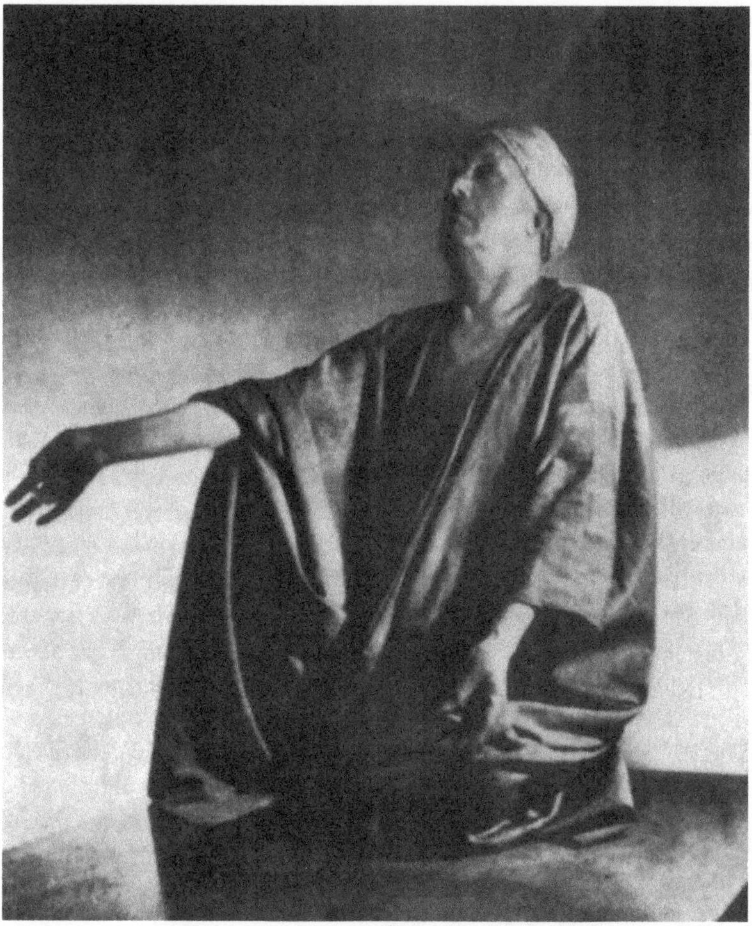

Aleister Crowley as Paramahansa Shivaji (© Ordo Templi Orientis 2009)

backward over rocks or standing with arms raised. Herbert narrowly avoids standing on the head of a yogin buried up to his neck, who utters the curse, "Leprosy shall eat away your white skin." Practitioners of yogic austerities, we are given to understand, are powerful, dangerous, and irascible beings, capable of supernatural feats and horrific maledictions against Europeans.

The European fakir-yogi genre continues well into the twentieth century, with works like Victor Dane's *Naked Ascetic* (1933) and Edmond Demaître's *Fakirs et Yogis des Indes* (1936). Dane's book is replete with mysterious yogins and magicians, such as the poison-eating, bullet-proof *haṭha* guru Nara Singh (32). Dane himself claims to be a master of "the systems of Hatha and Raja Yoga" (17) who writes from his own experience. Indeed, his mesmeric powers were well known in England, and he had been featured in national newspapers such as the *Sunday Graphic* and the *Daily Mirror* under the label "The Only White Yogi."[5] Like other esotericists of the early twentieth century, Dane's mystique derives from the fantastical figure of the yogi-fakir. We should also note, however, that Dane was an ardent physical culturist. He authored a book entitled *Modern Fitness* (1934) and was the editor of the magazine *The Sporting Arena*. His vision of yoga, while firmly rooted in Asian-inspired esoterica, was also deeply influenced by modern physical culture, and his yoga writings exhibit a marked concern for the hygienic perfection of the body (see epigraph to chapter 5).

Demaître's semi-scholarly ethnography of 1936 is a later example of the continued European fascination with the Indian ascetic. Unlike Dane, however, Demaître styles himself as an outsider, a sympathetic though hardheaded observer of the Indian religious fringes, and his book lies at the moderately less lurid end of the spectrum of the yogi/fakir genre. Although he prefaces his book with a "Letter to a Yogi" condemning the "macabre rites," "excesses," "horrors," and "perversions" of the said yogin's religion (14–16), he is nonetheless clearly fascinated by such displays and dedicates many words to describing them (translations mine). The one "yogi" in the study to meet with his approval is, significantly, a Vivekananda-quoting *bhakta* who leads a quiet life of devotional

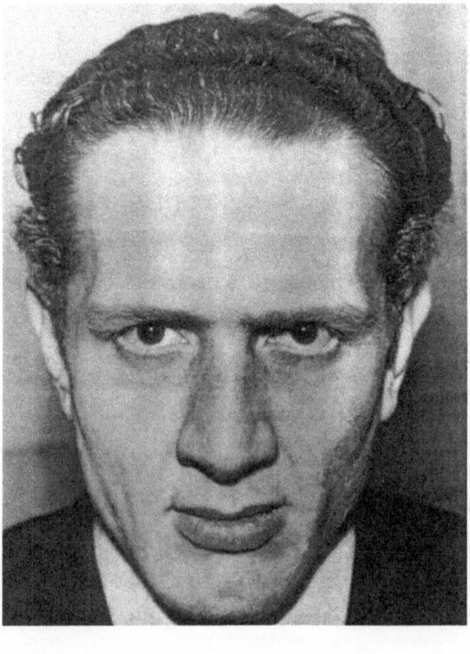

"The Only White Yogi," Victor Dane, in Dane 1933

prayer and study near the Golden Temple in Benares and declares to the (apparently concurring) ethnographer that Jesus himself must have been "a Bhakti-Yogi" (35). This yogin is in stark, positive contrast to the picturesque śaiva ascetics who pepper the pages of much of the rest of the book and who remain squarely within the realm of voiceless ethnographic objects.

One particularly revealing episode deserves our attention. Demaître's observation of an "ourdamoukhi" (i.e., an inverted ascetic) at Assi Ghat in Benares is interrupted by an angry "young Hindu, dressed like a European and visibly belonging to the *badralogh* class" (i.e., the gentlemanly, educated class: lit. "good people" or "proper folk," 40). The young man demands to know why the author is photographing "these clowns" (47). The young man, assuming that the author is there to make "anti-Hindu propaganda" aggressively affirms that individuals like these "fanatics" "exercise no influence whatsoever on the mentality of today's Hindus," or at least not on those who are, like him, "modern and educated" (48). This momentary constellation—of the young *bhadralok* Hindu vociferously protesting that sensationalized ascetic practices have nothing to do with the real Indian religion; the European observer also sharply critical of "fakirism" but eager to document it for his readers at home; and the *sadhu* himself who displays his ascetic practices for monetary gain in a public forum frequented by tourists—is particularly revealing of several dynamics that work around and against the yogi (or more generally the fakir). While the young man's outburst is given short, gallic shrift by the sagacious Demaître, it is clear that they share a common mistrust of the ascetic before them—although for the latter, one suspects that this attitude is a component part of the fun. And while Demaître's book as a whole is not at all of the same order as the damning textual and photographic productions of anti-fakir (and often simply anti-Indian) propagandists like Kathleen Mayo (1927 and 1928), it is easy to see how it might contribute to the continued association of yoga with flamboyant ascetic displays.

Demaître's altercation with the young man at Assi Ghat is illustrative of the critical distance that modern Hindus had taken from the Śaiva ascetics and yogins who exerted such a lurid fascination on the European mind. If Hindus were to be taken seriously and their religion given due respect, it was vital that they dissociate themselves from the contortions and austerities of figures such as these. As John Campbell Oman remarks in his colorful study of *The Mystics, Ascetics and Saints of India* (1903), the yogi "has been accepted in the West as the type or representative of the religious ascetics of India" (168) and the struggle to decouple yoga from the "irresponsible indolence and mendicancy" and "devious wanderings" that Oman himself describes

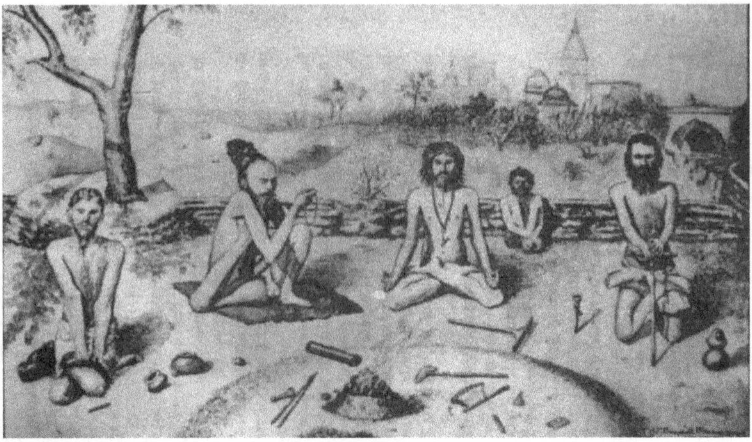

"Sadhus in Various Prescribed Postures," from Oman 1903

(36)—and from the penances of the yogi-fakir with which his book is richly illustrated—underpins the structure of modern anglophone yoga from Vivekananda onward. We should also briefly note here Oman's puzzling remark that "there are âsans and *âsans* known to the Indian people, and they are not all connected with *sadhuism* nor with religious practices; many of them quite the reverse. A book descriptive of these latter exists, but it is, I believe, on the Index *librorum prohibitorum* of the Indian police" (51 n.2). One might speculate that this banned book of *āsanas* describes sexual tantric practices that Oman (and the judiciary) deemed outside the domain of religion; or perhaps Oman is confusing yoga postures with the sexual positions of the *Kāmasūtra*. Whatever the case, the association of postural yoga with profanity and licentiousness is clear.

Anti-*Haṭha* Sentiment in Vivekananda

The foregoing survey of the yogin in scholarship and popular media should leave us in no doubt that the *haṭha* yogin, inextricably associated with the mendicant, performing fakir, was an unacceptable facet of modern Hinduism. This brings us to the way in which *haṭha* yoga was mediated in the early years of the modern international yoga movement. It was Swami Vivekananda and those who followed him who represented the public face of the yoga renaissance (De Michelis 2004). Perhaps more than any other single work, his *Raja Yoga* of 1896 was influential in giving shape to the cluster of methods and belief frameworks that make up, in De Michelis's 2004 typology, "Modern Yoga." What is important for our purposes is that in *Raja Yoga* Vivekananda uncompromisingly rejects the "entirely" physical practices of *haṭha* yoga: "we have nothing to do with it here, because its practices are very difficult, and cannot be learned in a day, and, after all, do not lead to much spiritual growth" (1992 [1896]: 20). He concedes that while "one or two ordinary lessons of the Hatha-Yogis are very useful" (viz. *neti krīya*, or nasal douche, for headaches), the chief aim and result of *haṭha* yoga—"to make men live long" and endow them with perfect health—is an inferior goal for the seeker after *spiritual* attainment (20). Vivekanada makes an emphatic distinction between the *merely physical* exercises of *haṭha* yoga, and the *spiritual* ones of "raja yoga," a dichotomy that obtains in modern yoga up to the present day. As we shall see, this is in no way due to a dislike of physical culture per se on his part but to an antipathy toward *haṭha* yogins. Moreover, he declares that these practices, such as "placing the body in different postures," can be found in "Delsarte and other teachers" (1896: 20) and are thus mere secular exercise. As we shall see in chapter 7, the reciprocal influence of "harmonial" gymnastic systems (like the American Delsartism of Genevieve Stebbins to which Vivekananda is most likely referring) and modern *haṭha* yoga is enormous. But for now suffice it to note that an explicit rapprochement of postural yoga and "Western" esoteric exercise seems already to have been under way by the time Vivekananda penned *Raja Yoga*.

Vivekananda expresses similarly negative sentiments in a talk delivered at the Washington Hall, San Francisco, on March 16, 1900: "There are some sects called Hatha-Yogis.... They say the greatest good is to keep the body from dying.... Their whole process is clinging to the body. Twelve years training! And they begin with little children, otherwise it is impossible" (1992 [1900]: 225). Evoking a *haṭha* yogi reputed to have lived for five hundred years, he exclaims, "What of that? I would not want to live so long: 'sufficient unto the day is the evil thereof.' [Matthew 6.34]. One little body, with all its delusions and limitations, is enough" (225). Ironically, or perhaps prophetically, Vivekananda would die just two years later at the age of forty. This passage exemplifies an other-worldly rhetoric in Vivekananda's writing that is strangely at odds with the focus on the accumulation of personal power and control over nature that we find in *Raja Yoga*. "Knowledge is power," he notes. "We have to get this power" (2001 [1896]: 145). While emphasis on power in yoga is associated with the *haṭha* yogin, I would argue that it primarily derives in Vivekananda's writing from the "personal power" rhetoric of American New Thought (see in chapter 6).

During his intensive study of the *Yogasūtras* in 1895, in preparation for the lectures upon which *Raja Yoga* is based, Vivekananda requested of E. T. Sturdy in New York that he acquire on his behalf several works on yoga—"the originals of course"—including what have come to be considered among the fundamental texts of premodern *haṭha* yoga: *Haṭha Yoga Pradīpikā* and *Śiva Saṃhitā* (1992 [1895]: 361). Clearly Vivekananda thought the *haṭha* tradition important enough to take these texts into consideration in the concoction of his modern yoga doctrine, but he ultimately rejected the ends and means of *haṭha* practitioners as an impediment to and distraction from the real work of the mind and spirit. This desire and willingness to scrutinize the basic texts of medieval *haṭha* yoga alongside Patañjali's *Yogasūtras* during the crucial period of the conception and composition of "Modern Yoga's" foundational document does not, in other words, entail a concomitant valorization of the goals and methods of *haṭha* yogins. On the contrary, in his writings before and after *Raja Yoga*, the *haṭha* practitioner is consistently qualified by Vivekananda as essentially deluded with regard to the true meaning of yoga.

Among the allusions to *haṭha* yoga in Vivekananda's life and works is an anecdote recounted by the Swami to his Indian disciples shortly before his death, during the 1902 anniversary celebration of his guru Ramakrishna. It describes what seems to have been not only a decisive moment in his future attitude toward *haṭha* yoga but also in the prevailing tenor of his missionary career. A disciple asks him whether he has ever had a vision of Ramakrishna after Ramakrishna's death. In reply, Vivekananda relates that shortly after his master's death he had formed a close relationship with the Vaiṣṇava saint Pavhari Baba of Ghazipur, noting that "I liked him very much, and he also came to love me deeply" (1992 [1902]: 242). In *The Life of Swami Vivekananda by His Eastern and Western Disciples* (1979), this encounter is dated to the third week of January 1890. Max Müller, in his study of the life and sayings of Ramakrishna, notes that the guru's name "is explained as a contraction of Pavanahari, 'he who lives on air'" and writes that Pavhari's self-immolation in his house in Ghazipur in, or shortly before, 1898 had "created a painful sensation all over India" (1974 [1898]: 10–11).

After two months of "severe ascetic practices" under Pavhari's guidance (Disciples 1979: 230), Vivekananda, suffering from agonizing lumbago and deteriorating health, resolved to undertake a training in the *haṭha vidyā* with this guru to complement what he had received from Ramakrishna:

> I thought that I did not learn any art for making this weak body strong, even though I lived with Shri Ramakrishna for many years. I had heard that Pavhari Baba knew the science of Hatha-Yoga. So I thought I would learn the practices of Hatha-Yoga from him, and through them strengthen the body. (Disciples 1979: 230)

However, on the eve of his initiation, Ramakrishna appears to him in a vision, "looking steadfastly at me, as if very much grieved" and remains in this attitude for "perhaps two or three hours" (243). Vivekananda returns his gaze in shamed silence and subsequently postpones the initiation. After a day or two, however, the idea of undergoing a *haṭha* apprenticeship with Pavhari Baba rises once again in his mind and is again quickly followed by the silent vision of a reproachful Ramakrishna. When this happens several times in succession, Vivekananda finally and decisively gives up the desire for initiation, "thinking that as every time I resolved on it, I was getting a vision, then no good but harm would come from it" (230).

The anecdote is interesting from several points of view. The only vision granted to Vivekananda of his deceased master functions to definitively forestall his acquisition of an "embodied" *haṭha* transmission via a living guru. While Ramakrishna's disapprobation is interpreted by Vivekananda principally as a jealous assertion of an exclusive (and posthumous) guru-chela relationship, it effectively serves as a dramatic lesson for him against following the path of *haṭha* yoga. It is also significant that the spectral saint does not make an appearance during the months-long, intimate relationship with Pavhari Baba prior to Vivekananda's sudden interest in *haṭha* yoga, indicating that the silent admonition (at least in Vivekananda's mind) is aimed specifically at his involvement in *haṭha* yoga. In a letter to Akhandananda written in Ghazipur shortly after the apparitions, there is a notable change in Vivekananda's attitude toward *haṭha* yoga:.

> Our Bengal is the land of Bhakti and Jnana. Yoga is scarcely mentioned there. What little there is, is but the queer breathing exercises of the Hatha-Yoga—which is nothing but a kind of gymnastics. Therefore I am staying with this wonderful Raja-Yogi [i.e. Pavhari Baba]. (Disciples 1979: 236)

What is remarkable is the rapidity with which Vivekananda's fancy for *haṭha* yoga as a system of curative or strengthening physical culture turns to a wholesale rejection of its "queer breathing exercises" and "gymnastics." Also notable is the apparent paradox that although Bengal is "the land of Bhakti and Jnana," the only "yoga" that appears to be actually practiced there is the bizarre, rudimentary *haṭha*! Vivekananda's idealized image of spiritual Bengal, then, contradicts the actual, lamentable situation he sees there with his own eyes. From this time onward Vivekananda would consistently reject or ignore *haṭha* yoga as the most inferior aspect of yoga. This is not to say that *haṭha* methodology and theory do not have a part to play: *haṭha*'s symbolic spirito-physiology, though not named as such, is recast in *Raja Yoga* itself as an empirical epistemology accessible to scientific and proprioceptive scrutiny (De Michelis 2004: 166). However, these *haṭha* elements are included only insofar as they can be subsumed and assimilated into Vivekananda's wider project.

Also initially puzzling here is that Pavhari Baba's stature in Vivekananda's mind remains undiminished (although not unaltered) after this volte-face on *haṭha* yoga: at the end of these troubled months the guru is a "wonderful Raja-Yogi," in spite of being simultaneously an acknowledged adept of *haṭha* yoga. Bharati (1976) argues that prior to modern times there was always a considerable *haṭha* component in practical yoga, but that "since the turn of the century...we find a clear polarization into *dhyāna* or meditation oriented and *haṭha-* or *āsana-* and body-oriented practitioners" (163). This encounter between Pavhari Baba and Vivekananda in the last decade of the nineteenth century represents the historical cusp of this change. Pavhari himself is able to combine *haṭha* and non-*haṭha* practice within himself with no apparent contradiction whereas Vivekananda shies away from those methods that do not fit within his conception of "raja yoga." The perplexing ambiguity of the "therefore" in Vivekananda's statement ("Therefore I am staying with this wonderful Raja-Yogi") may, I suggest, point to a similar kind of selective forgetting (or hagiographic censorship?) that Urban (2003) and Kripal (1995) have convincingly pinpointed in Vivekananda's management of the memory of Ramakrishna—in particular the latter's obvious proximity to tantric practices. In a single stroke here, *haṭha* yoga is cast out while Pavhari Baba is appropriated (or expropriated?) as an exemplar of "raja yoga"—the implication being that he shares his student's contempt for *haṭha* yoga, in spite of his noted, apparently contradictory, mastery of that discipline. Increasingly in the years to come Vivekananda would forge a vision of yoga in which this polarization between "raja" and *haṭha* practice would become permanently reified and in which his respective gurus would be rewritten to fit this modern orientation.

An 1894 interview with *The Memphis Commercial* will serve as a final example of Vivekananda's attitude toward *haṭha* yoga. Vivekananda is speaking to the reporter about the astounding longevity of *haṭha* practitioners when a local woman asks him if he is himself able to perform the kinds of feats she associates with the figure of the yogi, such as the rope trick and being buried alive (1992 [1894] 184).[6] Vivekananda is incensed: "'What have those things to do with religion?' he asked. 'Do they make a man purer? The Satan of your Bible is powerful, but differs from God in not being pure'" (184). Vivekananda's outburst is illustrative for a number of reasons. First, the performing fakir-yogi—so familiar in North America and Europe through popular ethnography and nineteenth-century orientalist scholarship—is seen not only as impure but as embodying the very principle of evil.[7] This is a particularly literal instance of the "demonization" that was directed toward the *haṭha* yogi in the modern formulation of yoga and of the urgent necessity for Vivekananda and those who emulated him to reverse the widespread associations of yoga with magic and religious mendicancy. Second, putting to one side the obvious self-contradiction (Satan having *everything* to do with religion in a Christian context), the response is significant in revealing an underlying assumption as to what counts as religion and what does not—an assumption that shaped many modern versions of yoga and assured that the *haṭha* yogi remain on its margins. As we have seen, this is the second time Matthew's Gospel is used by Vivekananda against *haṭha* yoga. In the previous instance, Vivekananda invokes the section of the Sermon on the Mount in which Jesus urges his listeners to set their mind on God's kingdom and not worry for the morrow (6.33–34) in order to turn his audience away from *haṭha* longevity practices (including, it seems, *āsana*).[8]

Vivekananda and Müller

In 1899, Max Müller published a small book celebrating the life and sayings of Ramakrishna. If Ramakrishna himself is presented as an exemplar of Indian saintliness, Müller reserves characteristic scorn for certain types of Indian ascetic, and the

> tortures which some of them, who hardly deserve to be called Samnyasins, for they are not much better than jugglers or Hathayogins, inflict on themselves, the ascetic methods by which they try to subdue and annihilate their passions, and bring themselves to a state of extreme nervous exaltation accompanied by trances or fainting fits of long duration. (Müller 1974 [1898]: vii)

What is striking is that these reprehensible ascetics are nevertheless not quite so bad as the "Hathayogins" who, we must assume, are quite simply the lowest of the low. As we have already seen, Müller was not opposed to yoga as such but specifically to those kinds that departed from the intellectual schema he so admired in the Vedānta and Sāṃkhya systems. Indeed, in a moment of enthusiasm later in the book he even declares that "within certain limits Yoga seems to be an excellent discipline, and, in one sense, we ought all to be Yogins" (6). While we need not labor the point that the *haṭha* yogin lies far outside these limits, the suggestion that his readers should themselves become yogins is nevertheless remarkable. Müller's respectful treatment of his subject, based as it is on Vivekananda's version of Ramakrishna's life, is blind to the unorthodox, tantric elements that were so central to the latter's religious life and were excised from Vivekananda's public presentation of his guru (Kripal 1995). But it is still striking that Müller is actually prepared to promote a particular aspect of yoga doctrine as a universally valid way of being.

Vivekananda wrote a review of Müller's book in which he praises the professor as a "well-wisher of India" who "has a strong faith in Indian philosophy and Indian religion" (in Müller 1974 [1898]: 139). Müller has, he avers, helped to dispel,

> the wrong ideas of the civilized West about India as a country full of naked, infanticidal, ignorant, cowardly race of men who were cannibals, and little removed from beasts, who forcibly burnt their widows and were steeped in all sorts of sin and darkness. (141)

As the world's most authoritative arbiter of taste in matters of Indian religion, Müller is in certain regards a vital ally for Vivekananda in gaining acceptance for yoga. His insistence on the philosophical sophistication of Indian thought and his uncompromising rejection of exemplars of "sin and darkness" like *haṭha* yogins, contributed (as Vivekananda acknowledges here) to changing prevailing opinion about Indians and their religion and may have helped to make Vivekananda's job easier.

This does not indicate, however, that Müller in any way sanctioned Vivekananda's practical modern yoga project. We have already seen Müller's disdain for practical (i.e., nonintellectual) yoga, and he frankly deplored the 1893 Parliament of World Religions in Chicago (at which Vivekananda made his sensational American debut) as being based on the kind of "respectful tolerance" that "engendered a false, even gushing, enthusiasm for a religious unity not subject to any certain documentary standards of signification" (Girardot 2002: 234 n.42). Indeed, we might recognize an implicit criticism of Vivekananda's new yoga synthesis in Müller's lamentation that yoga has, in modern times, descended into "its purely practical and most degenerate form" (1899: xx). Müller even, it seems, wrote directly to Vivekananda with criticisms concerning this latter's over-enthusiastic (if edifying) renderings of Ramakrishna's life (Müller 1974 [1898]: 22). There can be little doubt that, for Müller, Vivekananda's doctrine and example would not concur with his conception of an acceptable, proper kind of yoga. Nevertheless, the professor and the Swami are in complete agreement that the *haṭha* yogin has nothing whatever to do with what a yogin "ought to be."

Fakir's Avenue: Blavatsky and *Haṭha* Yoga

> In Jubblepore we saw much great wonders. Strolling along the bank of the river, we reached the so-called Fakirs' Avenue, and the Takur invited

> us to visit the courtyard of the pagoda.... We left this "holy of holies" of the secular mysteries, with our minds more perplexed than before.
>
> (Mme. Blavatsky relating her first visit to India in 1852–1853, Neff and Blavatsky 1937: 92–94)

Theosophical constructions of yoga were profoundly influential in shaping contemporary ideas, and Blavatsky's claim in 1881—that "neither modern Europe nor America had so much as heard" of yoga "until the Theosophists began to speak and write"—while hyperbolic, is not made without reason (1982b: 104). Blavatsky disciple and "in-house" yoga author Rama Prasad, in a 1907 Theosophical edition of the *Yogasūtras*, even goes so far as to claim that whatever knowledge Hindus within the Society possess "is due to their contact with and the influence of Western brothers" (1907: 11). Expressions of disdain and distrust for *haṭha* yoga and *haṭha* yogis are frequent in Blavatsky's writings and often function as rhetorical foils for Theosophical renditions of true yoga. For Blavatsky the *haṭha* yogi is a common, ignorant sorcerer, the embodiment of "a *triply distilled* SELFISHNESS" (1982d: 160), who converses with the devil and in whom ascetic practices are "une maladie héréditaire" (1982e: 51). Members of the "Esoteric Section" of the Theosophical Society (i.e., those initiates actually practicing the "secret doctrine") are strongly urged to avoid "attempting any of these Hatha Yoga practices" lest they succumb to the inevitable demise that had already befallen several foolhardy disciples of her acquaintance (1982f: 604 and 615).[9] Baleful propaganda such as this from the doyenne of late nineteenth-century Asian esoterica substantially contributed to shaping the attitudes that show up in contemporaneous translations of *haṭha* texts and which create the notional ambiguities we find in sometime *haṭha* commentators like Vasu.

Anti-Haṭha Tendencies in Early Popular Yoga Primers

For at least three decades following the publication of *Raja Yoga*, popular yoga literature both in India and the West would often continue to cast suspicion upon, or simply ignore, *haṭha* yoga. As Krishnan Lal Sondhi writes in the journal of Sri Yogendra's pioneering Yoga Institute:

> The tendency in recent times in India has been to shun Hatha Yoga as something undesirable and even dangerous. Even great minds like Swami Vivekananda, Sri Aurobindo, Swami Dayanand Saraswati, Raman Maharshi talk only of Raja Yoga and Bhakti Yoga and Jnana Yoga etc.—that is about those Yogas only which concern the higher

> mental processes and disciplines and they have regarded Hatha Yoga as something either dangerous or superfluous. (Sondhi 1962: 63)

Because of its association with mercenary yogi terror and the risible contortions of the mendicant fakir, the practices of *haṭha* yoga (the most visible of which was *āsana*) were excluded from the yoga revival initiated by Vivekananda. As the exemplary *public sannyasin* working to transmute "a space previously accessible only to initiates into something that would admit the general public" (Chowdhury-Sengupta 1996: 135), Vivekananda was beset by the anxiety to maintain a respectable face. The "menacing image of the sannyasi-fakir" (128) had no place in this reconstruction of "spiritual heroism," and in spite of his own proselytizing on behalf of physical culture in India—and his own one-time fascination for a *haṭha* guru—Vivekananda's yoga was stripped of the dangerous associations of *haṭha* sannyasins and wild tantric sects like the Kāpālikas, who would nevertheless remain a skeleton in the cupboard of modern yoga for many years to come.[10] Although Vivekananda did everything he could to dissociate himself from these figures, there were still those (like Kathleen Mayo) who persisted in seeing him, and the English-speaking gurus who visited Europe and North America in his wake, as disguised fakir-yogis who cynically duped their naïve female audience before returning to India and reassuming their natural state.

If in succeeding decades certain *haṭha* practices reentered the arena of international yoga as exercise science and movement therapy, the disreputable legacy of the *haṭha* yogi was simultaneously excised thanks to the kind of puritanism expressed, and thereby consolidated, by Vivekananda himself. As Green also concurs, the programmatic sanitization of the *haṭha* method and spirit "ignored the living practice of large numbers of Yogi practitioners to create a sober and restrained Yoga" (Green 2008: 312) that sought "classical" authenticity in what was presented as authoritative textual precedent. This required a rewriting of the yoga tradition to assimilate, in radically modified form, "*haṭha*" modes of practice.

Western yoga tracts in the wake of Vivekananda's *Raja Yoga* also generally echo the sentiments that the Swami expresses with regard to *haṭha* yoga. As we would expect, the physical postures of yoga (associated overwhelmingly with *haṭha* practitioners) tend to be reviled, ignored, or significantly downplayed. For instance, O. Hashnu Hara's *Practical Yoga with a Chapter Devoted to Persian Magic* of 1906 calls the "postures and contortions" of *haṭha* yoga "disgusting and repellant [*sic*]" (vi), "impossible and ridiculous" (6), and "repulsive" (10) in what is clearly a conditioned response to the sensationalized postural austerities of the yogi-fakir. R. Dimsdale Stocker's *Yoga Methods* of the same year simply

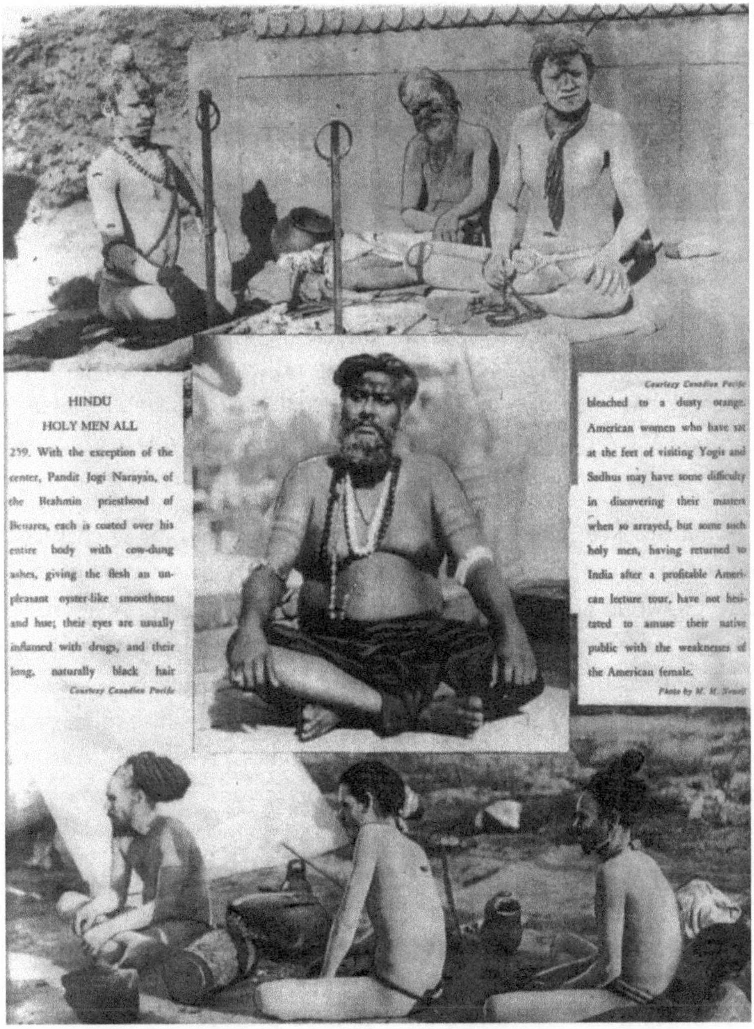

HINDU
HOLY MEN ALL

259. With the exception of the center, Pandit Jogi Narayan, of the Brahmin priesthood of Benares, each is coated over his entire body with cow-dung ashes, giving the flesh an unpleasant oyster-like smoothness and hue; their eyes are usually inflamed with drugs, and their long, naturally black hair

Courtesy Canadian Pacific

Courtesy Canadian Pacific

bleached to a dusty orange. American women who have sat at the feet of visiting Yogis and Sadhus may have some difficulty in discovering their masters when so arrayed, but some such holy men, having returned to India after a profitable American lecture tour, have not hesitated to amuse their native public with the weaknesses of the American female.

Photo by M. M. Newell

Yogis who amuse their "native public" with stories of "the weaknesses of the American female," in Mayo 1928

omits any mention of them: "attention to diet, regularity in meals and sleep, relaxation, cleanliness, and the art of respiration may be said to constitute the sum total of Hatha Yoga or physical regeneration" (1906: 29). Hara and Stocker's books belong to a genre of cheap, do-it-yourself yoga primers comprising variable measures of fact and fantasy about yoga, which began to appear on the esoteric book market from the beginning of the twentieth century. Until the pioneering publications of Yogendra and Kuvalayananda in the 1920s, one was very unlikely to encounter much mention of, or instruction in, the postures of yoga. Authors, like Hara, who do mention *āsanas* tend to dismiss them out of hand and to echo the negative attitudes of Vivekananda and Blavatsky toward practices of *haṭha* yoga such as *āsana*.

Popular author and Chicago-based guru Swami Bhakta Vishita summarizes the situation as follows:

> The prejudice existing in the Western mind against Asana, or Postures, which, as we have said, arises by reason of the fanatical excesses of the lower class devotees in India who carry to abnormal extremes the methods of Hatha Yoga, or rather of certain phases thereof, has tended to cause most of the Hindu Yogis who travel in Europe and America to say very little concerning this phase of Practical Yoga. (1918: 48)

Haṭha practice (and in particular *āsana*) was taboo for English-speaking, transnational gurus from Vivekananda onward, as they were at pains to present yoga to the world as the flower of Indian culture and Hindu religion. Western and Indian imitators of these successful gurus tended to echo these judgments about *haṭha* yoga. The latter was expunged from their teaching, or selectively reformulated, as it is with Bhakta Vishita, as a simple health tool or as a methodological precursor to the real work of the mind. Perhaps as a result of this tendency during the early stage of the history of transnational modern yoga, there was little interest in the postural practices that would later come to dominate its popular form, either in India or the West. Even as late as the 1930s—in many respects the heyday of the *āsana* revival—postural yoga "was ridiculed so much that only a few select people were practising it" (Iyengar 2000: 60). The pioneers of modern *haṭha* yoga had to contend with a deep-seated, inherited attitude of scorn and fear toward these physical practices.

4

India and the International Physical Culture Movement

> You were meant to have a fine looking strong and super healthy body. God cannot be pleased with the ugly, unhealthy, weak and flabby bodies. It is a sacrilege not to possess a fine, shapely, healthy body. It is a crime against oneself and against our country to be weak and ailing. Our own future and that of your Nation depend upon good health and enough strength.
>
> (Mujumdar, *Encyclopedia of Indian Physical Culture*, 1950: ii)

To a large extent, popular postural yoga came into being in the first half of the twentieth century as a hybridized product of colonial India's dialogical encounter with the worldwide physical culture movement. The forms of physical practice that predominate in popular international yoga today were developed in a climate of intense experimentation and research around a suitable regimen for Indian bodies and minds. "Yoga," foregrounded in certain quarters as the epitome of Hindu physical culture, became one of the names of this new national physical culture. The launching of the popular physical culture self-instruction genre and the staging of the first modern Olympics coincide chronologically with the appearance of Vivekananda's *Raja Yoga* (1896), which ushered in a new phase of yoga's long history (De Michelis 2004). Moreover, the first ever modern bodybuilding display took place on August 1, 1893 (Dutton 1995: 9), *the very day* that Vivekananda himself arrived on Western soil. Transnational anglophone yoga was born at the peak of an unprecedented enthusiasm for physical culture, and the meaning of yoga itself would not remain unaltered by the encounter.

As a vital contextual prelude to our examination of modern postural yoga, I now offer an overview of physical culture in India from the late nineteenth century to the 1930s. An unprecedented enthusiasm for athletic and gymnastic disciplines swept Britain and Europe during the nineteenth century. These disciplines—and the values that underpinned them—found their way to British India, where they at once reinforced stereotypes of Indian effeminacy and at the same time offered methods to rebut that image. Several key types of Western gymnastics and body culture radically impacted Indian physical consciousness during this period (Ling, Sandow, YMCA), leading to the creation or revival of "indigenous" exercise forms distinct (though often borrowing) from these imported systems. The swell of Indian physical culture was to some extent nationalistically motivated, and highly organized campaigns of militant physical resistance to colonial rule were commonly run out of local gymnasia and physical culture clubs. Often, nativized exercise such as this was also referred to as "yoga."

The Dawn of Nationalist Physical Culture in Britain and Europe

> But as one looks back now from the vantage of the turn of the century, one can appreciate how speedily and successfully somatic nationalism became an unquestioned feature of a shared global grammar of modernity manifested through many local varieties.
>
> (Uberoi 2006)

> We should strive to develop our youthful Indians physically as well as mentally, morally and religiously. We should endeavour to introduce something of our public-school manliness of tone into Indian seminaries.
>
> (Monier Williams 1879: 329)

The nineteenth century saw an eruption of European interest in the cultivation of the body as a means of regenerating the moral and physical mettle of the nation. J. F. C. Gutsmuth's *Gymnastik für Jugend* of 1793 was to become the basic text of this physical revivalism in Germany, followed by the work of his influential younger contemporary F. L. "Turnvater" Jahn. Their gymnastic exercises "were not only meant to form healthy and beautiful bodies that would express a proper morality, but were designed in fact to create new Germans" (Mosse 1996: 42). During the century to come, nationalistic "man-making" gymnastics building on Germany's example burgeoned throughout Europe, with the most enduringly influential forms issuing from France, Prussia, and Scandinavia. During the 1830s and 1840s Britain also began to assimilate a variety of continental gymnastics and to place a similar emphasis on the cultivation of national brawn through exercise. Donald Walker's *British Manly Exercises* of 1834 is one of the earliest examples of this trend. Walker's book includes a treatment of the new sports of rowing, sailing, riding, and driving "as well as the usual subjects of walking, balancing, wrestling, running, scating [*sic*], boxing, leaping, climbing, training, vaulting [and] swimming" (Walker 1834, frontispiece). The enthusiasm for strength-building exercise and sport grew exponentially from this time onward, and by about 1860, a "New Athleticism" with a "society-wide organisation of games and sports" was becoming well established in Britain (Budd 1997: 17). This zeal for physical fitness was *economically* as well as patriotically motivated: to survive and earn a livelihood in the new industrial world one could not afford a weak constitution.

It was not until the end of the century, however, that these various fitness and exercise regimens were "beginning to be known by the catchphrase 'physical culture'" (Budd 1997: 43). The appearance of a new pan-European genre of health and fitness magazine, starting with Edmond Desbonnet's *L'Athlète* in 1896, consolidated physical culture's populist status and extolled the benefits of bodily cultivation through gymnastics and weight resistance exercises. The same year saw the first large-scale gymnastics competition at the first modern Olympics in Athens.

The beginning of the twentieth century saw an "efflorescence of periodicals" (Dutton 1995: 125), which provoked an unparalleled concern for the health of the body among British middle-class men and "a surge of support for building and disciplining the body" among the working classes (125). The doctrine of *mens sana in corpore sano* ("a sound mind in a sound body") underpinned a wide range of physical innovations in British society, in particular the 1830s reformation of English public schools to include more games and sports and the ongoing modification of military training in the British army and navy under the influence of continental gymnastics (notably the Ling system). Physical culture in the nineteenth century bound together a cluster of ideological items, including manliness, morality, patriotism, fair play, and faith, and it was "a means for moulding the perfect Englishman" (Collingham 2001: 124).

Nurtured largely within the English public schools and Oxbridge, these values came to be together known as *Muscular Christianity*. The term was first used in a review of Charles Kingsley's 1857 novel *Two Years Ago* and was reprised shortly afterward by Kingsley's friend Thomas Hughes in his *Tom Brown at Oxford* (1860) to denote the subjection of the body for the advancement of just, godly causes. Proponents of Muscular Christianity took the *mens sana* principle and turned it into an article of faith, "a battle cry against all sinfulness, and against those who stood in the way of England's greatness" (Mosse 1996: 49). This new ethos of athleticism was not confined to the public school system, however, but spread far and wide into the populace through organizations such as the Salvation Army and, most significantly for this study, the YMCA. The body, with its cultivated capacity for moral engagement in the world, housed a *somatic imperative* for all who belonged to nation, religion, and empire and was negatively defined in contrast to those races and lands that did not share this common ideology of purpose.

In the late nineteenth century (and throughout the twentieth), individuals, like states, became "transfixed with the idea of improving their own bodies and were often equally obsessed with the vision of improving the collective national or racial body" (Ross 2005: 5). This eugenic compulsion often grew from a perceived imbalance of "body-mind-soul" that had occurred from an over-development of the intellect at the expense of the spiritual and physical aspects of man. Like modern yoga today, early physical culture was often based on a pronounced anti-intellectualism, and a (re-)valorization of the neglected parts of the triadic human model. It was not conceived as a merely mechanical pursuit of strength but as a project to restore wholeness to individual and collective life. By the dawn of the twentieth century,.

> the body had become a source of amazement and pride, a symbol of human strength, ability and endurance. Culminating with the invention of the Modern Olympics in the 1890s, the growth of sport culture in the nineteenth century made the body the main attraction in the great age of athletic competition and exhibitions, a position it continues to hold. (Ross 2005: 7)

This foregrounding of the body in modern times as the locus of individual and nationalist nostalgia for wholeness is an essential indicator of the conditions underlying the *haṭha* yoga renaissance. New forms of *haṭha* yoga came into being during this period in response to these same longings and aspirations, and promised a similar dream of self-fulfillment (or rather "self-realization") to many forms of Western nationalist physical culture.

Scandinavian Gymnastics

Perhaps more than any other single system of physical culture, the Swedish gymnastics built on the pioneering work of Ling (1766–1839) has oriented the development of modern physical culture in the West and postural yoga in its modern, export forms. Ling's method, following in the "medical gymnastics" tradition developed by C. J. Tissot and others, was primarily therapeutic, aiming at the conquest of disease through movement, and for this reason it was commonly known as "movement cure" (Dixon and McIntosh 1957: 88). Ling's successor, L. G. Branting, "brought medical gymnastics to a high level of efficiency and worked out a terminology for gymnastics which persisted well into the twentieth century" (Dixon and McIntosh 1957: 94; cf. Branting 1882). Ling-based training was concerned with the development of the "whole person" in a way that prefigures the "mind, body, and spirit" emphasis of yoga-associated practices in the New Age and in the YMCA. One early English apostle of the system considered that "the oneness of the human organism, and the harmony between mind and body, and between the various parts of the same body, constitute the great principle of Ling's gymnastics" (Roth 1856: 5).[1]

These and similar free-standing holistic exercise systems grew in popularity and spread rapidly. In the early years of the twentieth century, Swedish exercises based on Ling's method, as well as more aerobic forms of Danish gymnastics, displaced the apparatus-based system of Oxford's Archibald Maclaren as the official physical training program of the British army and navy (Leonard 1947: 212) and became the basis for physical education in schools and colleges in Britain. As G. V. Sibley, director of physical education at Loughborough College, notes in 1939, "Physical education in England has been built up, in the main, on Swedish gymnastics, except that they have been greatly modified to suit English conditions" (in Leonard 1947: 421). The Swedish pedagogical regimen also attained prominence in late nineteenth-century America (Leonard 1947: 329; Ruyter 1999: 94), influencing the development of YMCA physical education programs and the "harmonial gymnastic" work of Genevieve Stebbins (which we will consider separately later), both of which had a significant effect on the shaping of postural modern yoga.

Via an anglicized schooling system and military service, Ling and its offshoots became extremely widespread in Indian education establishments where, as in Britain, they eventually prevailed over the previously dominant Maclaren system because they did not require costly apparatus and purpose-built gymnasia. Maclaren gymnastics had been promoted as part of the "muscular Christian" reforms of George Campbell, lieutenant-governor of Bengal in 1871–1874; but in spite of its great popularity it eventually proved economically unviable in India (Rosselli 1980: 137). Indeed, one of the major selling points of the "free movements" of Ling—as for the new *haṭha* yoga—had always been that "the expense of the apparatus and machines is saved" (Roth 1852: 5). Maclaren's system lost out to Ling gymnastics, which Maclaren himself had once scornfully rated as a "system of bodily exercise in its main characteristic suitable to invalids only" (1869: 77).[2]

Physical education drillmasters in Indian schools were largely low-ranking ex-military men, "ordinarily chosen from among 'vastads' or super-annuated army gymnasts who knew a little of modified Swedish gymnastics" and who had a reputation for brutality and ignorance (Govindarajulu 1949: 21). The Indian physical culture luminary, Professor K. Ramamurthy, writing in 1923, paints a similar picture of "the ill-paid and meagrely clad (mostly in the relics of bygone military glory) Drill teacher or Gymnastic instructor, often a pensioned, half-famished and weather-beaten sepoy [i.e., an Indian soldier serving under British command]" (ix). Indian YMCA physical culture director H. C. Buck (1936: 13) and physical culture historian Van Dalen (Van Dalen and Bennett 1953: 620) give further evidence that the Indian gymnastic instructor was in the main a reviled and pitiable figure. It was nevertheless *his* forms of mass-drill Western gymnastics that prevailed as the default form of physical culture for Indian youth well into the twentieth century. Unsurprisingly, such forms would influence the pedagogical structure of modernized *haṭha* yoga, as we shall see in chapter 9 with regard to Kuvalayananda and Krishnamacharya.

Ling and Yoga

From its earliest stages, modern *āsana* was perceived as *a health and hygiene regime for body and mind based on posture and "free" movement* (free as it is performed with the body only, without the constraints of equipment, and also as it doesn't require any expenditure on apparatus). This situation owes much to the establishment of Ling as the paradigm of postural exercise in India. As far back as the middle of the nineteenth century, indeed, therapeutic gymnastics were being compared with what were perceived as "oriental" methods of movement cure. George Taylor in *An Exposition of the Swedish Movement Cure* of 1860 compares Chinese "Cong Fou"—in which the patient assumes certain postures and breathes in particular ways according to the disease to be treated—with Ling (33), and he also credits the "many bodily exercises" of India with therapeutic effects similar to those achieved by the movement cure method (39). Although he admits these systems may appear superstitious to the European, he insists that they are not only effective in the treatment of disease but are susceptible to scientific examination like Ling itself: "All that was required was a larger amount of the science of physiology with which to direct and extend the application, to render this resource legitimate and complete" (40). It is clear to see that well before the "medicalization" of *haṭha* yoga as therapeutic gymnastics by Kuvalayananda and Yogendra (see chapter 6), the assumption that *āsana* was an Asian version of the Swedish movement cure was already gaining currency. Taylor's book was published by Fowler and Wells (New York) who, throughout the first decades of the twentieth century, produced many paperback editions on yoga, "alternative" health, and New Thought. At this time, then, Ling gymnastics filled a niche in the book market that would later be filled by yoga.

Other examples of *āsana* presented as curative gymnastics are not hard to find: S. C. Vasu, in his 1895 translation of the *Gheraṇḍa Saṃhitā*, for instance, asserts that the various *āsanas* in the book "are gymnastic exercises, good for general health, and peace of mind" (xxv), in what is a fairly standard assimilation of *haṭha* postures into a post-Lingian model of physical and mental therapeutics. Similarly, an early American dilettante of Asian esoterica, William Flagg, describes the *haṭha* yoga procedures of *nauli* (abdominal "churning") and *uḍḍiyāna bandha* (diaphragmatic vacuum) as Swedish gymnastics (1898: 169–76). Gymnastics in the Lingian and post-Lingian paradigm provided a convenient and intelligible explanation of the function and form of *āsana*, which to some extent circumvented the need to engage with the complexities of *haṭha* yoga theory. Instead, *yogāsanas* were reconfigured as ancient forms of movement cure, with individual postures prescribed for specific diseases.

An unattributed article of 1927 in the Maharastrian physical culture magazine *Vyāyam*, entitled "Athletic and Gymnastic Exercise," asserts, for example, that.

> formerly gymnastics (such as Asans i.e. particular postures of the bodily limbs etc.) formed a part of medicine, for the purpose of counteracting the sad and injurious effects of luxury and indolence...particular movements of the limbs of the body are antidotes against particular diseases which are declared incurable by means of any medicine. (n.a. 1927: 146)

This widespread understanding that *āsanas* were essentially medical and curative in function had the effect of relegating the esoteric specifics of *haṭha* yoga to a subsidiary position. While my primary concern here is with physical culture, we should also note in this regard the close historical links that postural yoga has with modern Nature Cure. The integration of *āsana* into Nature Cure, especially during the 1930s and 1940s was, as Joseph Alter has shown, an important factor in yoga's secularization and demystification, and was crucial in terms of the production of a theory of why and how *āsana* were of physiological benefit (Alter 2000 and 2004a).

Norman Sjoman argues, "the therapeutic cause-effect relation [of *āsana*] is a later superimposition on what was originally a spiritual discipline only" (1996: 48).[3] While we might well take issue with Sjoman's notion of "spiritual only" here, it is true that in the twentieth century individual yoga postures came to be explicitly associated with the cure of particular conditions. The rigorous and elaborate development of this relationship in the 1920s by the pioneering modern *haṭha* yogins Shri Yogendra and Swami Kuvalayananda only consolidated an earlier, generalized acceptance of yoga as an Indian system of therapeutic movement cure. An early student of Kuvalayananda recalls how, prior to meeting his teacher, yoga had been for him "medical and chamber gymnastics pure and simple" (Muzumdar 1949: v), indicating that this was one standard paradigm during the 1920s for the physical practices of yoga. Twelve years earlier,

Muzumdar had in fact argued that the very source of Swedish gymnastics is ultimately yoga itself. The similarities between yoga and Ling, he claims, can be explained in terms of a westward knowledge transmission from India to Europe which is thousands of years old. "Swedish exercises are not original," we learn, but derive from ancient therapeutic techniques of Indian yoga (1937a: 816).

When Mircea Eliade protests that *haṭha* yoga "is neither athletic nor hygienic perfection" and that it "cannot and must not be confused with gymnastics" (Eliade 1969: 228), he is responding to what had, even by the 1930s, become a standard equation of the physiological exercises of *haṭha* yoga and gymnastics.[4] The appeal of postural yoga lay to a great extent precisely in this reputation as an accessible Indian alternative to the Western systems that dominated physical education in India from the last third of the nineteenth century. The very authors who were synthesizing modern gymnastic technique and theory with *haṭha* yoga nevertheless tended to present Western gymnastics as impoverished with regard to the "spiritual" and the "holistic" (Yogendra 1988 [1928]; Sundaram 1989 [1928]). But while these allegations may have been true for the gymnastic drills that were the standard in Indian schools at the turn of the century, they are not (as we will continue to see) an accurate depiction of much modern physical culture, which presented itself as an inherently spiritual pursuit.

This kind of negative comparison endures in practical yoga primers well into the twentieth century. In the most influential do-it-yourself yoga book of all time, Iyengar's *Light on Yoga*, we read for example that "Āsanas are not merely gymnastic exercises; they are postures" (1966: 10). Iyengar then goes on to present *āsana* as essentially a health and fitness regime comparable to gymnastics but without the need for costly equipment (10). In essence, Iyengar's message is the same as those of his predecessors from the 1930s. Even when they are at pains to demonstrate that yoga is not gymnastics, modern English-medium authors rarely draw a *qualitative* distinction between gymnastic exercise and *āsana*. The pervasive message is that *āsana* is an indigenous, democratic form of Indian gymnastics, requiring no apparatus and essentially comparable in function and goal to Western physical culture—but with more and better to offer.

Sandow and Bodybuilding

The term *bodybuilding* was first coined in 1881 by YMCA physical culturalist Robert J. Roberts (see Brink 1916). However, it was the great Eugene Sandow (1867–1925), who must be credited with initiating a worldwide revolution in bodybuilding through the many demonstrations and lecture tours that he undertook at the beginning of the twentieth century as well as through his popular periodical, *Sandow's Magazine of Physical Culture*, first published in 1898. His advice on health and fitness helped to make "physical culture" a household phrase. Sandow left an indelible mark not only on the European and American exercise regimes but also in India, where he had a wide and enthusiastic following within the nascent physical culture movement (Segel 1998: 206). By the time of his trip to the Far East in 1905, Sandow was already a cultural hero in India, and his successful tour of the subcontinent served to further disseminate his system (Budd 1997: 85). Many of the popular physical culture authors of the next decades (e.g., Ramamurthy 1923; Ghose 1925; Gupta 1925) recall this tour as a defining moment in their own, or their countrymen's, physical culture history. Bodybuilding, under the influence of Sandow and others—such as the American physical culturalist Bernarr Macfadden—enjoyed an unparalleled vogue in India from the turn of the century. In combination with home-grown health and fitness regimes, it was instrumental in shaping the "indigenous" exercise revival from which modern postural yoga would issue. We might recall here Joseph Alter's "heretical," though undeveloped, statement that it was Sandow, rather than Vivekananda or Aurobindo, who exerted the greatest influence on popular modern yoga (Alter 2004a: 28). In the hands of many, yoga was conceived as a form of bodybuilding, and vice versa, although it is worth remembering that during the early years of the century the latter term had a much greater semantic breadth than it does today, connoting a whole range of health and fitness activities that included, but were not confined to, the genre of weight-resistance body sculpting.

Sandow's trip to India "indicated the politically subversive potential of physical culture as well as its inherent malleability" (Budd 1997: 85) in that his methods were transformed into tools for independence. In the hands of nationalist leaders such as Sarala Debi (see below) physical culture such as that popularized by Sandow "was not considered inherently or uniquely Western, but as separated from its user, and capable of serving any master" (85). It could be used, in other words, both as a symbolic rebuttal of colonial degeneracy narratives and—at times—as an underpinning for violent, forcible resistance. Sandow's rhetoric was shot through with notions of exercise as religious practice, which made it all the more compatible with Indian nationalistic fusions of religion and bodybuilding, such as the heady blends of patriotic Hinduism and physical culture in the Bengali *samitis* considered in chapter 5. For Sandow, "the moral strictures of religion and mortification of the flesh were to be replaced by the physical regimen of exercise and the body's liberation" (Budd 1997: 67), and techniques of physical self-improvement became "quasi-religious substitutes" (128). The resacralization of the body through ritualized techniques of physical culture was of course also an extremely important element in the creation of a

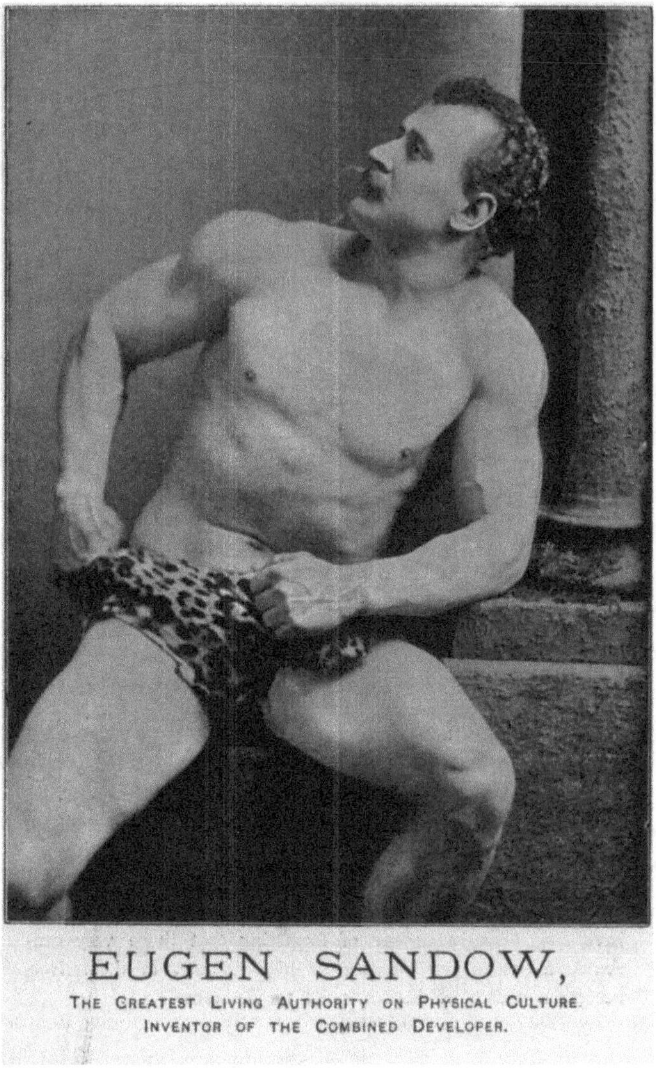
EUGEN SANDOW,
THE GREATEST LIVING AUTHORITY ON PHYSICAL CULTURE.
INVENTOR OF THE COMBINED DEVELOPER.

Eugene Sandow (courtesy of Roger Fillary)

postural modern yoga. We will consider several key examples of modern bodybuilding yogins in the next chapter, but for the moment we may simply note that "spiritual" discourses of physical culture such as Sandow's found a natural place within the Indian movement. The new, or revived, *yogāsana* systems—with their supposed millennia-long pedigree in the orthodox *darśanas* of Hinduism and their apparent parallels with holistic European gymnastics and bodybuilding—inevitably lent themselves to expression by way of these same discourses.

Young Men's Christian Association

> There is no single "system" or "brand" of Physical Training, Culture or Education that can adequately or satisfactorily meet India's need. What then is India to do? Clearly she should and must be eclectic and fall back on a group of essentially fundamental principles and on them build her own programme.
>
> ("India's Physical Education, What Shall It Be?" Gray 1930: 8)

No organization had a greater influence on the international diffusion of physical culture than the YMCA. Indeed, it was in the creation of a hybridized but distinctly Indian culture of sport and exercise that the YMCA offered its most significant contribution "to the making of modern India" (David 1992: 17). Its physical culture programs were explicitly intended to function as a somatic tool of moral reform, whose core values were those of the Christian West, and in particular Christian America. The emphasis was on "wholesome living" and on the power of "physical education [as] a socializing agency" ("Curriculum of Studies," n.a. 1931: 29–30). Physical culture, as conceived by the Indian YMCA, was education *through* the body, not *of* the body (Gray 1931: 15) and was intended to contribute to the even development of the three-fold nature of man—mind, body, and spirit—as symbolized by the famous inverted red triangle logo devised by the influential YMCA thinker Luther Halsey Gulick (1865–1918), head of the YMCA training school in Springfield, Massachusetts.[5] As such, it was of a piece with the holistic preoccupations of much of early European gymnastics. It was meant, furthermore, in no uncertain terms "to inculcate in young people the ideals, value structures and behavioural patterns implicit in the Christian way of life" (Johnson 1979: 13).

If, prior to the 1920s, "physical education was a term unknown to this country [i.e., India] and its educational system" (Govindarajalu 1949: 21), by 1930 the national physical director of the organization, J. H. Gray, could confidently declare that with regard to physical education, "India is perhaps the '*hotspot*' of all the nations in the world" (Gray 1930: 5). In Gray's assessment of the relative popularity of physical training systems in India at the time, Ling ranks first, followed by the "primary gymnastics" of Niels Bukh (1880–1950) which, as I shall argue later with regard to T. Krishnamacharya and Swami Kuvalayananda, exercised considerable influence on the modern "power yoga" movement. Significantly, even at this relatively late date, neither "yoga" nor "*āsana*" appears in Gray's catalogue of physical culture, indicating that the semantic and practical merger of "exercise" and "yoga" was yet to become pervasive, as it would in the next two decades.

The "Physical awakening of India" (Johnson 1979: 14) initiated by Gray was greatly furthered by H. C. Buck, who set up the first school for Indian physical directors in 1919 and trained the first Indian national athletics team for the Paris Olympics of 1924.[6] He also helped launch a popular sports and exercise quarterly, *Vyāyam*, in the summer of 1929 and served as its editor for the next twenty-three years. (Buck's journal should not be confused with the Maharastrian journal *Vyāyam, the Bodybuilder*, discussed below, edited by Katdare.) Broad-ranging and adaptable in his choice of fitness regimes, Buck "devised programmes and courses which combined both Indian and Western physical exercise so that the YMCA college offered the best of the East and the West" (Johnson 1979: 177). In the hands of the YMCA, physical culture was eventually elevated to a position of social and moral respectability, a status that it had not previously enjoyed in India.

Buck and his organization were "constantly searching for attractive indigenous activities which are suitable for physical education" (Buck 1930: 2), and the eclectic and wide-ranging syllabi they devised largely became the face of Indian physical education in the early to mid-twentieth century. Buck made postural yoga "an integral part of the YMCA physical education programme" (Johnson 1979: 177), promoting *āsana* as a component of the overarching ethos of Christian piety and service at the heart of the "Y" ideology. N. Vasudeva Bhat, who wrote his Ph.D. thesis on Buck and is now an officer at the YMCA College of Physical Education in Bangalore, learned his *āsanas* in the early 1960s from one Shri Kallesha, who received them directly from Buck in Madras during the 1930s. However, it was, according to Bhat, Buck's successor, P. M. Joseph, who finally made *āsana* a part of the Y's national syllabus (interview, N. Vasudeva Bhat, September 9, 2005).

While there is evidence to suggest that Buck had misgivings about the ultimate value of *āsanas* (he sometimes complained, for instance, that they are too "subjective" and therefore inferior to group games and sports; cf. Buck 1939: 77),[7] there is little doubt that his efforts to meld indigenous Indian exercises with YMCA philosophical principles (alongside the efforts of other physical fitness directors like A. G. Noehren) did much to create an environment favorable to the emergence of athletic postural yoga conceived as a system for the holistic development of the individual. That is to say, the enormous and pervasive influence of YMCA physical education in India altered not only the cultural status of exercise but brought its ontological function into line with "Y" policy. Partially as a result of this, international postural yoga became (and remains) perceived as a system for the holistic development of the "mind, body, and spirit" of the individual—a feature it has in common with a whole gamut of gymnastic systems (including Ling) that developed within and outside India in the first half of the twentieth century.

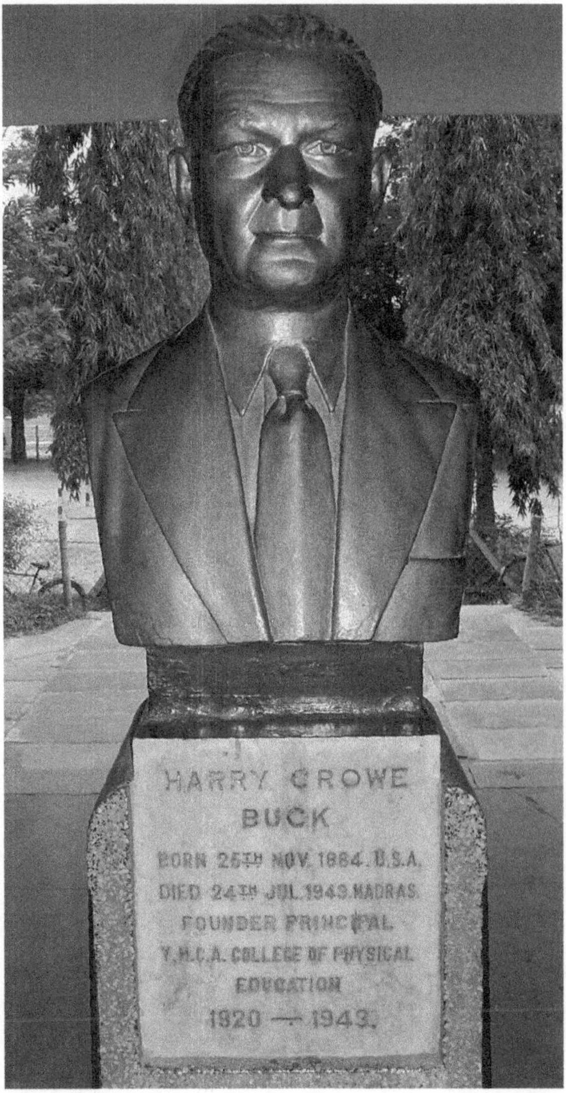
HARRY CROWE
BUCK
FOUNDER PRINCIPAL
Y.M.C.A. COLLEGE OF PHYSICAL
EDUCATION
1920 — 1943.

Bust of H. C. Buck at the YMCA College of Physical Education in Chennai (photo by author)

It is worth reiterating, furthermore, that J. H. Gray's explicitly eclectic vision for physical education in India is mirrored in the spirit of radical experimentalism embraced by the pioneers of modern postural yoga. Their endeavor was self-conscious and possibly conceived as a Hindu rival to the YMCA itself. Indeed, Bhat claims that the world-renowned spokesman of modern *haṭha* yoga, Swami Kuvalayananda, developed his system of rigorous posture work at least partially to refute Buck's assertion of the inadequacy of *āsana* as a complete physical culture program. Whatever the case, the creation of modern postural yoga was an admixture of rejection and assimilation with regard to foreign modes of exercise. At the time—as Gray declares of physical education in general—*there simply was no "system" or "brand" of physicalized yoga that could satisfactorily meet India's need*. This had to be created out of what was available, including a large number of exercises that had not hitherto been considered part of yoga (most significantly, nature cure, therapeutic gymnastics, callisthenics, and bodybuilding). When India built "her own programme" of physical culture, one of the names she gave it was "yoga."

5

Modern Indian Physical Culture: Degeneracy and Experimentation

> In the new yoga there is no room for the physically unfit, for the lazy, the neurotic, the weedy. Both men and women who wish to practise and be of use to humanity, if such is their wish, must have strong and healthy bodies. Without this perfection of body we cannot have a pure functioning of all our actions.
>
> (Dane 1933: 279–80)

From the middle of the nineteenth century, there was a growing awareness of the possibilities for a national physical culture that would raise Indian individuals and society from the degeneracy into which they were perceived to be sunk. For example, from the 1850s until at least the 1930s the nationalistic Bengali Hindu elite, "strove to overcome its supposed degeneracy through the pursuit of physical culture" (Rosselli 1980: 121). The "supreme aim" of Maharashtrian physical culture movement, as expressed in the mission statement of the popular journal *Vyāyam, the Body Builder* was to "[uplift] India from the mire of physical decadence" (Katdare 1927a: 25). Sentiments such as these are found throughout Indian physical culture publications of the period.

This sense of physical and racial degradation was in large part the result of a stereotype promulgated by the colonial powers and internalized by Indians themselves, often via the anglicized education system. One function of this myth of Indian effeminacy was to justify in the minds of the colonizers continued British subjugation. Baden-Powell, the founder of the international scout movement, considered the task of colonial education in India as "that great work of developing the bodies, the character and the souls of an otherwise feeble people" (Sen 2004: 94). His view is typical of the British conviction of the physical, moral, and spiritual inferiority of Indians, as judged against the idealized masculine body and perfect conduct of the English gentleman. The "degeneracy narrative" in the nineteenth and early twentieth centuries served as "an explanation of otherness, securing the identity of, variously, the scientist, (white) man, bourgeoisie against superstition, fiction, darkness, femininity, the masses, effete aristocracy" (Pick 1989: 230), and here it is applied by a renowned advocate of colonial man-making as an account of the otherness of the very humanity he seeks to reform.

One of the outcomes of the colonial man-making project was that programs of formal physical exercise reinforced such stereotypes but also helped to undermine them, insofar as they transformed and strengthened Indian bodies—thus the mandatory rhetorical exhortations that preface so many popular Indian exercise manuals of the time. The pervasive discourse of Indian effeminacy "generated an obsessive search on the part of Indian males for properly masculine bodies, and this search led them to the gymnasium, the wrestling *akhara*, the playing field and the military recruitment office" (Sen 2004: 70). It became vitally important to reverse the debility myth by representing Indian bodies not only as strong in themselves but also as capable of vanquishing the champions of Europe: physical fitness and strength thus became a potent expression of cultural politics.

Physical culture manuals are replete with figures such as the wrestler Ahmad Bux who beat the regnant champions of France and Switzerland but whose challenge to the American world champion Frank Gotch was refused due, it is implied, to the latter's cowardice (Ghose 1925: 19). Similarly, both Gholam Rusom Hind and the famous K. Ramamurthy (who claimed to be able to deadlift three times more than Sandow; see below) challenged Sandow to a trial of strength during his 1905 visit to India, but the great pioneer of world physical culture balked on both occasions (Ghose 1925: 18; Ramamurthy 1923: ii). We should also mention here the world champion wrestler Gama the Great (c. 1882–1960) who, like Ramamurthy, became a heroic symbol of the Indian freedom struggle (see Alter 2000, chapter 5). Such anecdotes of the "Indian Hercules"[1] function to counter the stereotype of the flimsy Indian and create a myth of bodily power. They also suggest the grip that Grecian ideals of strength and beauty had on the imagination of Indian youth in the wake of the first modern Olympics in Athens in 1896. We shall see that these ideals are also transmitted into the new forms of *haṭha* yoga that emerge around this time.

The woeful sense of deterioration in physical, moral, and spiritual vigor is, however, by no means exclusive to the Indian situation but is also a dominant theme in Western exercise culture generally at the beginning of the century. It contributes extensively to the perceived need for bodybuilding regimes in Europe and America. Part of Sandow's success, indeed, "resulted from the increased currency of degeneracy rhetoric at the century's end" (Budd 1997: 37), and magazines and books devoted to building better bodies constantly hark back to a preindustrial state of virile physical perfection. As Bernarr Macfadden, America's most popular physical culture author, puts it, "our ancestors were strong, virile and conquering because they lived close to Nature and so absorbed her inexhaustible vitality. *But we are losing our inherited vitality, slowly perhaps, but none the less surely*" (Macfadden 1904b: 15).[2]

The motif of degeneracy in the modern urban age sold. Sandow's enormous success in India, and that of bodybuilding and gymnastic culture in general, is no doubt partly due to the painful chord that such themes struck among the country's youth and to their embrace of a peculiarly modernist (nationalist) physicality. The dire diagnostics of the Western bodybuilding mandarins appeared to be addressed directly to Indians: not only were their bodies weak, but "physical effeteness seemed often a mere index of spiritual downfall" (Rosselli 1980: 125). The twin myths of physical degeneration and prelapsarian vigor were used as goads by Hindu nationalist leaders and physical culture revivalists alike.

The struggle to define an Indian form of body discipline was rendered ambivalent by the adoption of certain core ideological values of a Western, and ultimately imperialist, discourse on manliness and the body. The *akhāṛa* and the Hindu *melā* worked alongside (and sometimes squarely within) the current of colonial education reform and "indigenous" physical culture movements maintained a permeability to Western influence, based on a deep appreciation of the cultural and political potential of the nationalistic gymnastic movements of Europe. Indeed, even in the schools and gurukuls of the Ārya Samāj, that most ardently "swadeshi" of the Indian Samajs and "perhaps the greatest indigenous educational agency" (Rai 1967: 145), the students would arise before dawn and immediately perform "dumbbell exercises and calisthenics" (145), a regime clearly borrowed from the methods of physical culture in vogue in Europe at the time and widely disseminated throughout India.[3] It was through experiments such as these that physical culture became "a central part of the educational programme" in India (Watt 1997: 367). Physically fit, healthy citizens of good character dedicating themselves to the betterment of Mother India thereby became "important symbols of a strong and vibrant nation in an age when Hindus felt that they lacked 'manliness,' were 'weak,' 'lacking in courage,' were a 'lethargic race'" (367).

Physical Culture as Eugenics

This degeneration anxiety is also closely linked to the histories of Social Darwinism and the eugenics movement. By the turn of the nineteenth century, Social Darwinism and the eugenic fervor had taken a powerful grip on the Western psyche and had quickly spread beyond the boundaries of Europe. In India, Social Darwinist discourses underpinned the rhetoric of the nascent nationalist movement, and Indian eugenics societies sprang up from the 1920s onward in response to the collective sense of the physical, moral, and spiritual degeneration of the nation. In Europe, as in India, modern physical culture was at the heart of the eugenics movement.

The nationalistic gymnastics of Europe, such as J. P. Müller's phenomenally popular "System,"[4] were built on narratives such as the degeneration of the "stock" and the Lamarckian mythos of inherited acquired characteristics. Lamarckism was one of the most important ingredients in the stew of social Darwinism and eugenics, and it made popular the belief that the individual could manipulate his or her own evolutionary processes. Lamarck (1744–1829) held that particular changes wrought in the human constitution during one's lifetime (such as a blacksmith's acquisition of muscular arms through constant wielding of a hammer) are passed on in the same form to one's children (who will also, ergo, have muscular arms). Although largely discredited after the discoveries of Darwin, Lamarck's theory continued to hold sway well into the twentieth century and influenced many expressions of the international physical culture movement, of which modern postural yoga is so clearly a part. Müller's System exemplifies this Lamarckian/eugenicist bent, and it is not surprising that "Müllerites" were regulars at British eugenics meetings from at least 1913 (Kevles 1995: 58).

To take but one example from his work, Müller encourages citizens to practice physical culture in order that they "may have children who are improved editions of their parents," thereby rendering the "noblest service to the State, namely, that of contributing to raising the level of the race as a whole" (1905: 44). Such notions, known as the "law of exercise," were standard fare in the physical culture prose of the late nineteenth and early twentieth centuries—and were often the principal motivation to take up physical exercise in the first place. Indeed it is well known that Lamarckianism "dramatically influenced the push for women's physical training" (Todd 1998: 24). Modern physical culture was Larmarckianism in action, and in colonial India the two were rarely long apart. And since, as we shall see, the history of modern physical culture cannot be separated from the history of modern yoga, it is hardly surprising that many modern transnational, anglophone yoga teachers were very receptive to core eugenic beliefs. As I have demonstrated at length elsewhere (Singleton 2007p), and as we shall see in ensuing chapters (especially in the section on Yogendra in chapter 6), yoga came to be seen in some quarters as a kind of transgenerational fast track to genetic and spiritual perfection.

Nationalist Physical Culture

Bankimcandra Chatterji's novel *Ānandamaṭh*, published in the early 1880s amid a growing nationalist fervor in India, did much to popularize the ideal of the patriotic Hindu *sannyasin* fighting against the foreign oppressor and to promote the ideal of a national physical culture. As Julius Lipner points out in the introduction to his recent translation of the novel, the characters are "all upper-class Hindus, relatively few in number, literate, disciplined, and imbued with a specific patriotic purpose," and therefore quite distinct from the yogins, ascetics, and "starving and desperate villagers" who swelled their ranks during the novel's central episode, the so-called sannyasi Rebellion (in Chatterjee and Lipner 2005: 29–30). Furthermore, whereas the wandering *sannyasins* tended to be Śaiva, the initiated "*sāntans*" of Bankim's novel "belonged to a kind of Vaiṣṇava order" (29 n. 51). Bankim's *santān* represented a partial, consciously constructed asceticism for the modern, literate *bhadralok* or "gentle folk" who formed the vanguard of Indian nationalist consciousness in late nineteenth- and early twentieth-century Bengal. Bankim's novel has often been interpreted as the assertion of a new religio-nationalist heroic identity for (Hindu) Indians, and therefore as a key factor in the creation of a belligerent modern nationalist consciousness. I refer the reader to Lipner's introduction (especially pp. 59–84) for an extensive history of the tactical political uses *Ānandamaṭh* has been put to and an account of what would become the national song of independent India, "Bande Mātaram," both in proto-nationalism and subsequent Hindu-Muslim antagonism.

The religious and political imagery of *Ānandamaṭh* inspired many young nationalists to enter violent struggle against British rule in the name of a timeless and unchanging Hindu religious protocol: the *sanātana dharma*.[5] This religious code transcends intra-Hindu sectarian divisions such that the *santāns*, although nominally identified as Vaiṣṇavas, "are not Vaiṣṇava in any narrow sense" (Lipner in Chatterjee and Lipner 2005: 73) and instead combine Vaiṣṇava, Śaiva, and Śakta elements to constitute their nationalist-ascetic religious identity.

Wakankar notes that

> It was Bankim Chandra who defined for physical education both its precise location in the larger movement for what is called, in textbook histories, "socio-religious reform" in Bengal, as well as the exact nature of the regime it described. At the core of the program lay the notion of *anushilam*, and its locus was the (bourgeois, Hindu) male body. (Wakankar 1995: 48)

One key figure in this physical culture revival was Sarala Debi Ghosal (1872–1946), a niece of Rabindranath Tagore who, as well as being an ardent supporter of women's rights and one-time Brahmo (Southard 1993; Kumar 1993), gained prominence from 1905 as an extremist leader and campaigner for a militant nationalist physical culture. Debi was galvanized by the example of Bankim's heroine Shanti[6] to organize a physical culture campaign and exhorted young men to undertake martial training for their own defense "and for the defence of their women against molestation by British soldiers" (Kumar 1993: 39). She organized parades of "physical prowess," opened an academy of martial arts at her father's house in Calcutta in 1902 (under one Professor Murtaza), and was an influential presence behind the establishment of similar centers across Bengal. Sarkar notes similarly that "gymnastic displays formed an important part of the Birastami and Pratapaditya festivals organised by this remarkable young lady" (1973: 470). In all her activities, then, Sarala Debi's main aim was to bring forth a "nationalist warrior hero" based on figures from Indian history and myth (Kumar 1993: 39).

Debi was in touch with Vivekananda on the topic of nationalist physical culture after his triumphal return from America. The Swami was himself an ardent supporter of the Indian physical culture campaign, and he even reportedly held the view that one can get closer to God through football than through the *Bhagavad Gīta* (Nikhilananda 1953: 167). Certainly, Vivekananda was outspoken in his belief in the necessity of physical culture for Indian youth and at times insisted on its sequential priority over mental and spiritual development, such as in the following dialogue recorded in 1897:.

> *Swamiji:* How will you struggle with the mind unless the physique be strong? Do you deserve to be called men any longer—the highest evolution in the world?... First build up your physique. Then only you can get control over the mind.... "This Self is not to be attained by the weak" (*Katha Upanishad*, 1. ii. 23). (Vivekananda 1992 [1897]: 155)

It is difficult to see how Vivekananda extracts his translation from this Upaniṣad,[7] but his message is clear: the development of bodily strength is of the utmost importance for the spiritual evolution of the modern Hindu. It is the urgency of this task, indeed, that seems to be sufficient motive for his innovative reading of traditional Hindu scripture. The exchange that follows this statement, indeed, suggests that Vivekananda is well aware of the departure he is making from orthodox interpretation:

> *Disciple:* But, sir, the commentator (Shankara) has interpreted the word "weak" to mean "devoid of Brahmacharya or continence."
>
> *Swamiji:* Let him. I say "the physically weak are unfit for the realisation of the Self." (1992 [1897]: 155–156)

This cavalier approach to interpretation suggests that the exigencies of the age prevail to some degree over any rigid fidelity to commentatorial tradition. Vivekananda requires scriptural endorsement for his promotion of physical culture and seems determined to find it in this verse. His creative use of the teachings of Ramakrishna during this same exchange of 1898 suggests a similar determination. Summarizing the matter for his disciple, Vivekananda declares, "The gist of the thing is that unless one has a good physique one can never aspire to Self-realisation. Shri Ramakrishna used to say, 'one fails to attain realisation if there be but a slight defect of the body'" (156). Ramakrishna may well have spoken of certain physical disability as an impediment to spiritual progress, but it is probable that the notion of a muscular body as being in itself the vehicle of realization belongs to Vivekananda. While, as we have seen, Vivekananda scorned the practices of *haṭha* yoga and does not seem to have made the link between *āsana* and physical culture, the same equation of bodily strength and spiritual merit that we see here was to become central to the merger between the physical culture movement and *haṭha* yoga itself.

Vivekananda, along with associates like Sarala Debi and Sister Nivedita,[8] was instrumental in pushing forward the physical culture agenda among the nationalist youth of the country, and it is clear to see that a close relationship obtained from the beginning between the ideological milieu in which modern yoga had its genesis and the militant nationalist physical culture movement. We might also note in this regard that the men trained at Debi's gymnasium often collaborated with Aurobindo Ghosh (Sarkar 1973: 470), the vociferous pamphleteer, radical extremist, and future modern yoga guru, who was himself inspired to translate Bankim's novel in 1909. This is one more example of the atmosphere of nationalist physical culture from which modern yoga would emerge.

Modern, physical culture *akhāṛas* ("clubs," "gymnasia") of the kind organized by Debi often functioned as centers of a political struggle that *self-consciously emulated* the militancy of the institutionalized violent yogin. This is not to say that all physical culture clubs across India were nuclei of patriotic terror nor that they were generally patronized by the majority of Indians. However, just as the "Indian independence movement involved not only Gandhian strategies of non-violent protest and civil disobedience but also acts and threats of violence by revolutionary groups" (McKean 1996: 73), so too the physiological nationalism of the modern politicized *akhāṛa* included both moderate and extremist elements. Indeed, according to Gharote and Gharote (1999), such *akhāṛas* quickly acquired a reputation as "centres of goondaism" and hence were opposed and avoided by the educated classes (6). However, since Gharote and Gharote are themselves writing from the perspective of middle-class modern yoga, this assertion should perhaps be taken with a grain of salt.

Another, possibly key, instance of the intersection of militant political struggle and exercise is the advocacy for physical culture of extremist social reformer and "Father of the Indian Unrest" B. G. Tilak (1856–1920). Tilak was himself an avid physical culturist and even lent a helping hand to the pioneer of yogic physical culture, Professor K. Ramamurthy, at an early stage in his career (Ketkar 1927: 230, and below). He also appears to have had a direct influence on the Rajah of Aundh, the founder of the modern *sūryanamaskār* system (Sen 1974: 307).

The partial emulation of the violent yogin was based on an extensive and pragmatic re-visioning of the recent past to fit current needs and future aspirations. The growth of the new clandestine, fighting "yogin" was encouraged by the 1908 publication of Savarkar's *Indian War of Independence 1857*, ostensibly a history of the same rebellion that was given literary treatment by Bankim in *Ānandamaṭh* but in fact a manual of violent resistance to British rule, including "instructions on how religious personages—pandits, sadhus, sannyasis, swamis, fakirs, and maulvis—can be used by revolutionaries as publicists of the cause"

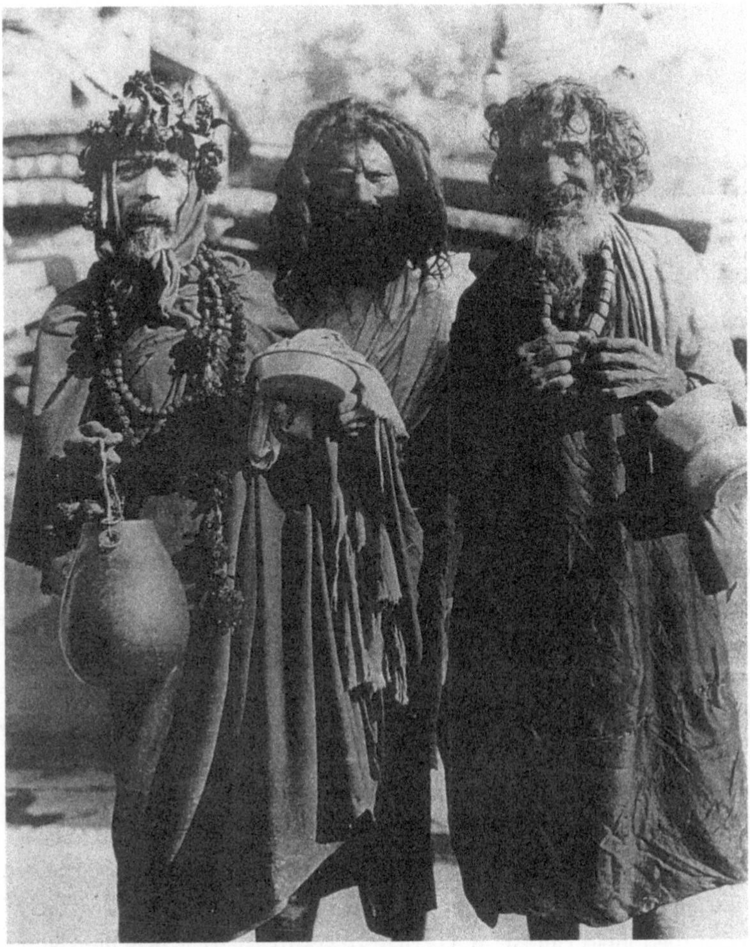

"Secret Agents of the Terrorists," in Mayo 1928

(McKean 1996: 77). These "secret agents of the Terrorists"—as they are branded by the controversial opponent of Indian self-rule, Kathleen Mayo—were demonized by the colonial media as murderers and brigands (see Mayo 1927, 1928).

The practice of *yoga*, in certain milieux, became an alibi for training in violent, militant resistance. Militant *akhāṛas* posing as centers of "Yogic instruction" were often in trouble with the British authorities (Green 2008: 310) in much the same way their forebears (imagined and actual) had incurred the wrath of Company and Raj (see chapter 2). It was in this way that "yoga" could come to signify insurrection. A striking example of the tripartite constellation of yoga, physical culture, and violence in the lead up to Independence is afforded by the modern yoga author "Tiruka" (also known as Sri Raghavendra Rao) who, while masquerading as an itinerant guru, traveled around India in the early 1930s assimilating an array of exercise and combat techniques that he then disseminated to future freedom fighters as "yoga."

One of his main teachers during this period was the famous wrestler, gymnast, and militant revolutionary Rajaratna Manick Rao who, writes Tiruka, "believed that India could free herself from foreign domination only by revolution and never by the Gandhian non-violent method. Therefore, he preached, that it was essential to build an army of strong bodied soldiers to wrest our freedom and to keep it" (Tiruka 1977: v). Rao was one of the key figures in the reformation of the *akhāṛa* along physical culture lines, restyling many of them as *vyāyam mandirs*,

Tiruka (Sri Raghavendra Swami), in Tiruka 1971

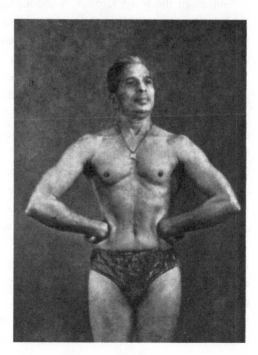

or "exercise associations," for the promotion of indigenous exercise in the service of social welfare (Gharote and Gharote 1998: 19), and Tiruka's blend of exercise conceived as yoga was in large part a product of Rao's innovations. Tiruka also studied with the renowned Swami Kuvalayananda, pioneer of yogic physical culture and founder of the Kaivalyadhama institute for scientific research into yoga (see chapter 6), and himself a student of the same Manick Rao.

Also included among Tiruka's teachers are Swami Sivananda of Rishikesh, one of the most important "transnational" modern yoga gurus (Strauss 2005); the Rajah of Aundh, whose "*sūryanamaskār*" sequence forms the basis of several of the most important postural yoga systems of today (cf. chapters 6 and 9 below); and Paramahaṃsa Yogananda, renowned author of *Autobiography of a Yogi* (Tiruka 1977: v). His account is a fascinating if brief insight into the clandestine yogic physical culture milieu of the pre-Independence era and the close relationship that obtained between nationalist struggle on the one hand and the early formulations of modern (postural) yoga on the other.

After his training, Tiruka toured Karnataka State for seven years disguised as a yoga guru, narrowly avoiding arrest and using the methods he had garnered to prepare people for liberation of a distinctly worldly kind: "Outwardly, it was the teaching of yogasana, suryanamaskara, pranayama and dhyana; at the core it was much more: preparation in physical fitness and personal combat methods.... Thus yoga training and physical culture became household words" (1983: x).

Although the most famous "freedom-fighting yogi" remains Aurobindo, Tiruka's story is exemplary of the way in which violent nationalist physical culture came to be associated with yoga and *thousands* of "freedom fighters... were formed side by side of [*sic*] yoga propaganda" (Tiruka 1983: x). If we are to give credence to his historical assessment of the process, yoga *as physical culture* would have entered the sociocultural vocabulary of India partly as a specific signifier of violent, physical resistance to British rule. To "do yoga" or to be a yogi in this sense meant to train oneself as a guerilla, using whichever martial and body-strengthening techniques were to hand, and it is thus that the yoga tradition itself, as Rosselli puts it, "could be used to underwrite both violence and non-violence" (1980: 147). Furthermore, the long list of Indian and Western methods acquired under Manick Rao indicates at once the proliferation of exercise activities within this milieu and the ease with which they could be combined under the heading of "yoga."[9] It is clear that the "canon" of modern *āsana* that we know today was still very much in a state of flux. In other words, it was the martial exercise revival of the early "physiological nationalists" (Mcdonald 1999), whether extremist or moderate, that initially created the conditions for the popular understanding of yoga as physical culture and for the eventual ascendancy of *āsana* as its principal branch. We might also note in passing that this secret

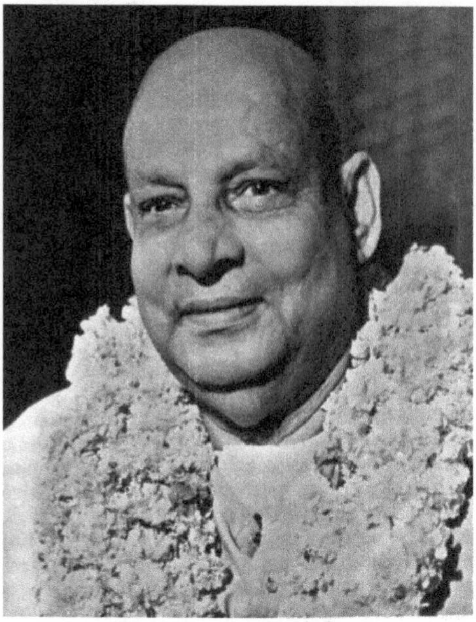

Swami Sivananda of Rishikesh (with permission of the Divine Life Society, Rishikesh)

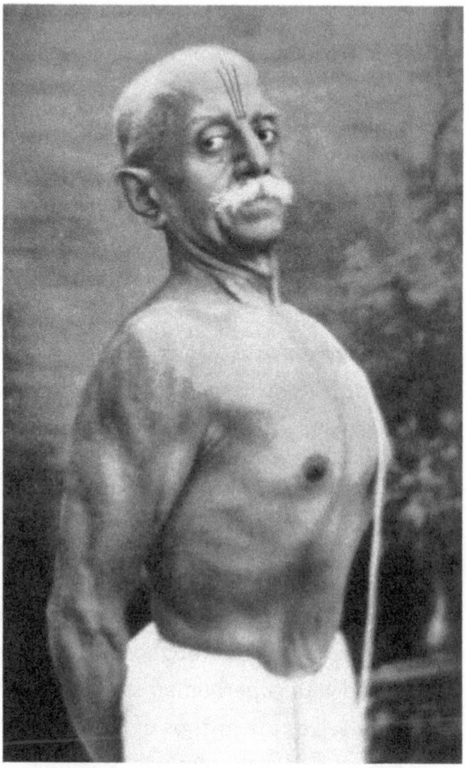

Pratinidhi, Raja of Aundh (courtesy of Elizabeth De Michelis)

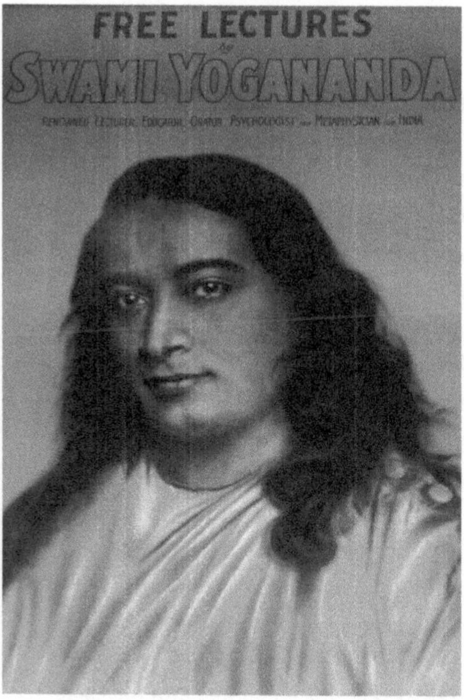

Swami Yogananda, early U.S. lecture poster

honing of martial skill under the guise of *yogāsana* bears comparison with the development of nineteenth-century Brazilian capoeira as an indigeous combat technique disguised as dance (see Chvaicer 2002).

This reconstruction of the spirit and practice of the violent *saṃnyāsin* led to a continued association of *haṭha* yoga with the culture of martial exercise exemplified by the militant ascetic. But just as the yogi figure underwent an ideological and religious sea change in this process, so too did the the orientation of the physical practices themselves, largely as a result of a sustained dialogue with the worldwide physical culture movement.

Haṭha Yoga and Feats of Strength

The narrative of degeneration within the physical culture movement was plural, ambiguous, and subject to appropriation. A similar situation obtains within modern *haṭha* yoga. If *haṭha* yogins were exemplars of degeneracy for scholars like S. C. Vasu, it is not unusual to find their craft invoked in physical culture discourse as the propulsive force and very basis of strength-building regimes. This contradictory role of *haṭha* practice—as prime suspect in the crime of racial degeneracy *and* the agent of rehabilitation—reflects a tension at the heart of modern *haṭha* itself, insofar as the *yogi* can function as both reviled other and the ideal of embodied power in the world.

It was common (especially in Bengal) to find modern Indian physical culturalists demonstrating "exceptional physical feats" that they claimed to have learned through the practice of *haṭha* yoga (Rosselli 1980: 137). White (1996) has pointed out that throughout history the practices of yoga have always been associated with superhuman strength. But these latter-day Indian yogis combined in themselves the mythos of the medieval *siddha* with the modern day strong man. Vasant G. Rele's seminal "scientific" *haṭha* yoga tract *The Mysterious Kundalini* (1927), for example, evokes the youths of the day who "perform the daring feat of allowing a loaded cart to pass over their chests without suffering any injury" thanks to their knowledge of yoga (Rele 1927: 8). He dedicates most of his introduction to the formidable Deshbandhu who, in front of an audience of Bombay medics in 1926, split a hair with an arrow from twenty feet and broke iron chains "by a mere tug of his body" thanks to his knowledge of "Yogic Science and Prānāyāma" (xxi).[10] The superiority of yogic physical training over Western methods, he avers, is that it increases powers of physical endurance, as is "amply proved by the exploits of the Indian army in the recent war" (xxii).

In this regard, we must also consider the prodigious showman and physical culture icon, Professor K. Ramamurthy, who dazzled audiences in India and

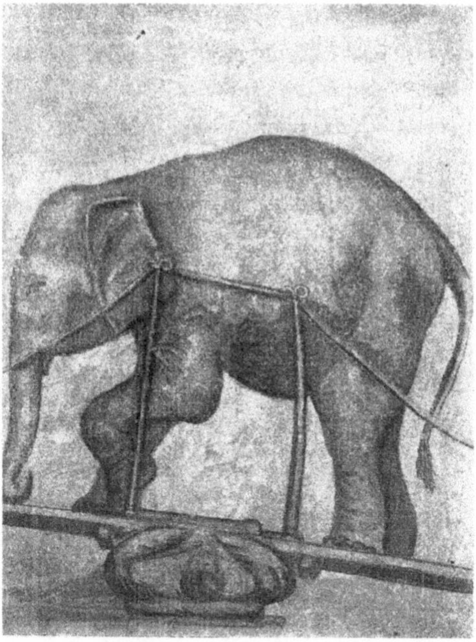

"Professor Ramamurti supporting an elephant on his chest," in Nadkarni 1927

Europe with his "phenomenal strength and endurance," acquired "through Pranayama and Asanas" (Muzumdar 1949: 10). During his 1911 performances in London, for example, the professor broke large iron chains with his neck and allowed carts loaded with sixty people each to pass over his body, as well as a three-ton elephant and a motor car (Nadkarni 1927: 107).

His flamboyant example would inspire many others to take up yogic strength training, including the well-known "muscular Āsana" guru S. S. Goswami (Goswami 1959: 15). *Āsana* and *prāṇāyāma* underpinned Ramamurthy's widely eclectic array of international exercise techniques refashioned along "cultural lines" (Ramamurthy 1923: 37). Having (he claimed) personally practiced all the available systems of world physical culture, Ramamurthy concluded that the "Indian System of Physical Culture" was the most effective in bringing about "permanent health and muscular development" (i). In spite of his vehement rejection of "Western ideas," however, it is more than clear that this "Indian System" is itself thoroughly imbued with the characteristic ideals of British physical culture, such as sportsmanship, "chivalry and gallantry," and the "manliness" of exercise (x). Indeed, his depictions of "ancient ashram education," with its physical and martial emphases, evokes vividly the militarily inclined, muscular, Christian, public schools of nineteenth-century England.

Ramamurthy's trip to England in 1911 was, according to one of his younger contemporaries, intended "to prove the supreme worth of the Indian method of exercise and at the same time to learn the English method so that the happy blending of both may bring about much improvement in [the] Physical Department in general" (Nadkarni 1927: 106). This receptivity to foreign (especially British) influences, combined with an aggressive assertion of the superiority of the Indian methods, is a common trope across physical culture and modern *haṭha* yoga. Ramamurthy navigates this apparent conflict by radically widening the definition of the "Indian System" to include "*all the various systems of Physical Culture practiced outside India*" including dumbells, chest expanders, hockey, cricket, tennis, billiards, and boxing. For, he insists, such systems "have their origins in India" (Ramamurthy 1923: 3, my emphasis). This kind of reappropriation of what is rightfully Indian is also a hallmark of the new *haṭha* yoga. In this respect, Ramamurthy is an important predecessor of the *haṭha* pioneers we consider in chapter 6, in particular the "bodybuilding yogis," K. V. Iyer, Yogācarya Sundaram, and Ramesh Balsekar.

Ramamurthy's drive to stamp the Indian cultural seal on apparently European systems is one aspect of a wider, ongoing effort among exercise educationalists to define the elements of a national Indian physical culture. To take one example, in the Presidential Address to the Maharashtra Physical Culture Conference of 1927, Sardar Abasaheb Mujumdar urges his listeners to turn toward physical practices from within the cradle of Hinduism, which he presents as "a happy combination of religion and physical culture" (Mujumdar 1927: 188). Hindu physical culture is, according to him, a complete and integrated system of health and fitness that has the capacity to overcome the damage wrought by a reliance on foreign systems of exercise. While Mujumdar's speech is a clear example of the condemnation of "the exclusive practice of Western activities as a symptom of denationalisation" (Gharote and Gharote 1999: 107), calls for self-sufficiency such as his almost always exist alongside a recognition that it was necessary to blend Indian and Western systems of physical culture to develop the richest possible program for India. And indeed, a survey of the popular Mahrashtrian magazine *Vyāyam, the Bodybuilder* shows clearly that in practice nationalist aspirations *were* compatible with adapted Western techniques. These synthetic techniques of nationalist strength training, indeed, are even referred to as "Yogi-ism" (Katdare 1927b: 89).

Other Early Syntheses

The first decades of the twentieth century, then, were a period of intense and eclectic experimentation within nationalist physical culture, with manifold techniques and systems being borrowed, adapted, and naturalized to suit Indian needs. Modern *āsana* practice emerged from this crucible as the imagined essence of Hindu physical training. The physical education author P. K. Ghose notes that in the first decade of the century, there was a multitude of experiments seeking to combine foreign and indigenous methods of practice. One Professor Mohun C. R. D. Naidu, indeed, "had invented a method of physical culture, a combination of Western and Eastern, based on the principles of Yoga philosophy and which, on experiment for years, was found to be eminently suitable to our young men" (Ghose 1925: 25). The system never flourished, however, due to the pervasive fear among young Indian men of government repression of physical culture clubs, following the violent agitation surrounding Viceroy Lord Curzon's partition of Bengal in 1905 (25). "Our young men," notes Ghose, "were so much demoralised by the repressions of the Government following the partition of Bengal that they began to dread any form of physical exercise as a red rag before a bull" (25), the clumsy simile perhaps suggesting the element of rage that went along with this dread.

However, *as an alloy of local and foreign gymnastics, rationalized as a counterpart of "yoga philosophy"* (itself interpreted through a modern Hindu lens), Naidu's system is a clear precursor of the later postural forms that helped to make popular transnational yoga what it is today. It is also a concrete example of the political function of body disciplines within the British regime and what happens when this function is challenged. Naidu's was, according to Ghose (25), one among many similar experimental syntheses of yoga and physical culture at the time, such as those of Captain C. P. K. Gupta (see figure below and Gupta 1925); the previously mentioned wrestler-hero Gama the Great; and M. V. Krishna Rao of Bangalore who, as we shall see in chapter 9, was the full-time organizer of "indigenous physical culture" in the state of Mysore during the years immediately prior to Krishnamacharya's vastly influential experiments in melding physical culture and *āsana*. It is not hard to see that the early gurus of modern postural yoga were themselves participants in a developmental arc that had begun with early experiments like these. Although Ghose doesn't mention him in this particular list, we should also include Ramamurthy's syntheses as a vital moment in the rapprochement of physical culture and yoga.

Curzon himself, like other prominent Victorian colonialists, was an ardent supporter of physical culture and

> firmly believed in sports as a means of developing character, morality and a sense of discipline combined with fair play that provided training for war, for life and for the building of civilised society. These ideas were implemented through pedagogical games played in schools and

in religious settings; they sought to change Indian physical culture and to bring it under colonial control and discipline. (Dimeo 2004: 40)

Sport and exercise were explicitly conceived as a writing of the values of Empire on the Indian body—and when experiments in physical culture exceeded, or subverted, this project, they were emphatically repressed. The attempt on Curzon's life by extremists in 1912 (cf. Hay 1988: 129) might therefore be understood as a violent, symbolic assertion of an Indian's right to use *his* body in the way he sees fit rather than as dictated by an outside authority.

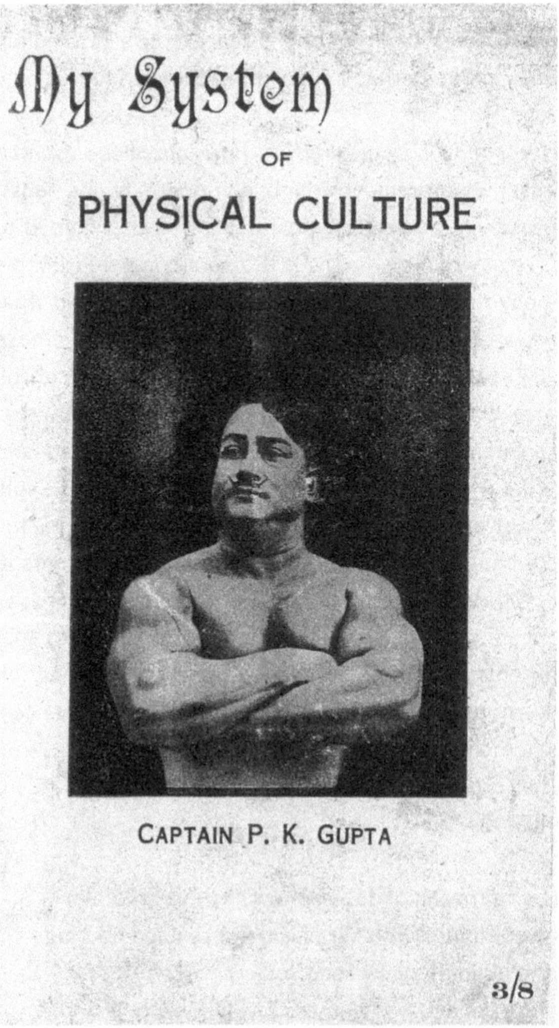

Captain C. P. K. Gupta (as pictured in Gupta 1925)

The revival of physical culture clubs around 1905 was also met, notes Ghose, with a massive propaganda campaign in the Anglo-Indian press intended to "kill these honest efforts" and "to give a political colouring to the movement as a whole" (1925: 4). Popular enthusiasm for physical culture quickly waned in response to the "wholesale crusade... directed against these organisations" (4). These glimpses of smear campaigns and the forceful repression of physical culture in Bengal in the early twentieth century also help to explain why the new forms of *haṭha* yoga did not really come into their own prior to the mid-1920s. Another crucial factor is probably the immense resistance to physical exercise among many sections of Indian society. As Kuvalayananda disciples and scholars Gharote and Gharote note, members of educated society considered that "taking physical exercise was the concern of illiterate people" (1999: 7); D. S. R. Rao, in his study of "health, strength and longevity in Modern India" asserts that "a pandit or a philosopher in the orient would consider it derogatory to be in any way associated with sportsmen and athletes" (1913: 10); and Kathleen Mayo diagnoses the Kashmiri Brahmin's distaste for physical culture "lest he grow muscular arms and legs like a coolie" (1928, plate 277).

Experiments such as those mentioned by Ghose were the forerunners of the *āsana* revival of the 1920s and 1930s and created the conditions for later innovators like Krishnamacharya, Kuvalayananda, and Yogendra to seamlessly incorporate elements of physical culture into their systems of "yoga." By the time they came to formulate their methods, the process was already well under way, largely thanks to the mushrooming of local "health associations," clubs, and *akhāṛa* across the country teaching "Indian methods of health culture" (Ghose 1925: 4). What had until then been dispersed, heterogeneous arenas of physical culture and group exercise—subsisting sometimes for centuries in an unconnected way as fora of traditional physical disciplines like wrestling, stave (*lathi*), *kabaddi*, and indigenous martial arts—were increasingly organized and assimilated into the nationalist elite's agenda to create "a culture of physical education" (Wakankar 1995: 47). This recasting of body discipline as physical culture involved a high degree of experimentation and innovation. The systems of gymnastic posture work that today pass for timeless modalities of "yoga" were yet to be brought into existence, and developed in an atmosphere of radical experimentalism that encouraged new combinations of Eastern and Western physical culture methods, albeit naturalized as ancient Hindu knowledge.

6

Yoga as Physical Culture I: Strength and Vigor

> May God who is omniscient shower health and strength on all! May *He* create in the hearts of the sons and Daughters of India a burning desire for Physical Regeneration.
>
> (Sundaram, *Yogic Physical Culture* (1989 [1931]: 130)

> From the beginning of this century, *Āsana* or yoga postural exercise became popular as Yoga. These posture-exercises were avidly absorbed, in the early stages, by the physical culturalists and seekers of health, as some curious addendum. Because of their inherent physiological and, to some extent, psychological merit, the study of *Āsanas* gained popularity in India and elsewhere.
>
> (Publisher's note, Yogendra 1989 [1928]: 5)

> Here begin those bodily exercises which do not profit.
>
> (*Hindu Philosophy Popularly Explained, the Orthodox Systems*, Bose 1884b: 117)

This chapter presents for the first time a survey of early textual and photographic expressions of *haṭha* yoga conceived as physical culture. While some of my examples date from the turn of the century, most are from the succeeding decades and derive mainly from popular do-it-yourself manuals and magazines. It was not until the 1920s that gymnastics and physical culture really began to establish themselves as a contemporary expression of the *haṭha* tradition and to significantly influence the semantic and practical plurality of modern yoga itself—the genre of popular, self-help yoga books reflects this shifting tendency. A glance at the yoga marketplace of today shows just how complete the operation has become, with "yoga" now virtually synonymous in common parlance in the West with posture practice. The foundations of these postural forms, however, were laid during the first four decades of the twentieth century. In the main, my chronological ceiling in this chapter is the end of the 1930s, by which time *āsana* had definitively taken its place within the yoga renaissance as a whole (with a period of particularly intense production between 1925 and 1930). My purpose, however, is to map the emergence of a popular, physically oriented modern yoga in the early to mid-twentieth century through the publications used to promote these forms—a project that reveals much about the genesis of today's postural yoga. Note that I consider the implications of the heavy visual element in modern postural yoga in more detail in chapter 8.

This chapter and the next are two parts of a whole and are structured as follows: In this chapter, I present a brief examination of Kuvalayananda and Yogendra's use of physical culture as *āsana* and the latter's receptivity to physical culture influences that were abroad at the time. I then consider several examples of *āsana* reformulated as bodybuilding and gymnastics, most notably international body-beautiful sensation, K. V. Iyer and best-selling yoga author and Iyer's collaborator, Yogacarya Sundaram. Finally in this first part, I briefly consider a number of "export" *haṭha* yogis operating in America during the 1920s, the most famous of whom is undoubtedly Paramahaṃsa Yoganandada, author of *Autobiography of a Yogi*. These (mainly Indian) men purveyed a combination of New Thought (a popular reformulation of American Transcendentalism and Christian Science), naturopathy, adapted Swedish gymnastics, and "muscle control" techniques in a range of teachings specially adapted for their Western audience. Among them is the author of perhaps the earliest photographic manual of modern *haṭha* yoga, the prolific California-based guru, Yogi Rishi Singh Gherwal. The aim is to explore how the contextual frameworks of modern bodybuilding and New Thought pervaded yogic physical culture.

The second part (chapter 7) considers several variations of women's exercise regimes, beginning with what I will call the "harmonial gymnastics" tradition exemplified by the Americans Genevieve Stebbins, Annie Payson Call, and to a lesser extent the Dublin-born Molly Bagot-Stack. I also consider in this category the esoteric yoga gymnast Cajzoran Ali. My argument is that these women, and others like them, promoted modes of "spiritual stretching" and deep breathing that endure today (and among a similar demographic) as "yoga." Finally, in support of this thesis, I look at the presentation of yoga within Britain's most popular physical culture periodical of the time, *Health and Strength*, and compare today's forms with other techniques commonly presented within the magazine's covers. The conclusion from this general survey is that even in Western physical culture magazines, "yoga" simply did not, until very late in the day, principally signify anything like the *āsana*-heavy systems of today, whether in their "stretch and relax" mode or more aerobic forms. And, conversely, those techniques that we now recognize as "yoga" were then (i.e., by the 1930s) already a well-established part of Western physical culture—particularly that intended for women—and were not yet associated in any way with yoga.

Contexts of Physical Culture as Yoga

Kuvalayananda

> During the 43-year sad history of Yoga from 1928 to 1971 when Yoga was confused with *physical* education by the yoga gymnasts, including the official yogin at the Government level, it became imperative to call a halt to these quixotic official adventures in the field of Yoga.
>
> (*Facts about Yoga*, Śrī Yogendra 1971: 169)

Born in Dabhoi in Gujarat, Swami Kuvalayananda (also known as Jagannath G. Gune, 1883–1966) became one of the most important figures in the modern "renaissance" of yoga as therapeutics and physical culture. His first training, from 1907, was in combat techniques and gymnastics under the nationalist physical culture reformist, Rājaratna Manik Rao of Baroda. He also studied yoga for two years with the Vaiṣṇava sage Paramahaṃsa Shri Madhvadasji (1789–1921) and with this latter's blessing established the teaching and research institute Kaivalyadhama, in Lonavla (near Mumbai) in 1921. Using the paraphernalia of modern science, he and his group of researchers set about measuring the physiological effects of *āsana*, *prāṇāyāma*, *kriyā*, and *bandha*, and they used their findings to develop therapeutic approaches to disease.

The profound early influence of Manik Rao manifested itself in an ongoing concern for Indian physical culture. As early as 1914, Kuvalayananda had introduced various types of indigenous and foreign physical exercises and resolved "to evolve a system of *physical culture based on Yoga* and to take steps to popularise that system" (Gharote and Gharote 1999: 14; 37; my emphasis). Between 1927 and 1937, Kuvalayananda worked on physical education committees for the Bombay government, devising mass "yogic" exercise schemes that were subsequently employed in schools across the United Provinces (marking the beginning of the "quixotic official adventures" so disdained by Yogendra). His *Yaugik Saṅgh Vyāyam* of 1936 is a fascinating record of these curricula, the particularities of which I will examine in relation to T. Krishnamacharya's "Mysore style" in chapter 9. For the moment, however, suffice it to note that the Swāmi's influence on the general perception of yoga as physical culture, through publications and initiatives such as these, was enormous at both a national and and international level. Kaivalyadhama's literary output was prodigious. The Institute's journal, *Yoga Mīmāṃsā*, first published in 1924, was at once cutting-edge scientific review and practical illustrated instruction manual, and it was immediately taken up "as a practical guide by students all over India," by whom it was "looked upon as the most authoritative text-book on practical Yoga" (Kuvalayananda 1935: 8). The appearance of *Popular Yoga, Āsanas* in 1931, "intended only for those who have almost nothing but practical interest in Yoga" (Kuvalayananda 1972 [1931]: xiv), further consolidated the Swāmi's role as the champion of yogic physical culture. Kuvalayananda is constantly cited as an authority in later Indian *yogāsana* manuals. This short outline of Kuvalayananda's physical culture heritage will suffice for our present purposes, but those wishing to learn more should consult Joseph Alter's extensive studies of Kuvalayananda's role in creating a yoga of therapeutics, the account of which I will not reproduce here.[1] We will return to Kuvalayananda, and his likely influence on the T. Krishnamacharya's Mysore *āsana* tradition, in chapter 9.

Yogendra and the Domestication of Haṭha *Yoga*

> *Haṭha*yoga, or the physiological Yoga (*ghaṭastha yoga*) is in its entirety and essence the subliminal process of physical culture of which physical education is one aspect.
>
> (Yogendra 1989 [1928]: 38)

Shri Yogendra (also known as Manibhai Haribhai Desai, 1897–1989), like Kuvalayananda, entered the path of yoga after years of intensive immersion in modern physical culture. Also like Kuvalayananda, this reorientation was a direct result of an encounter with the guru Paramahaṃsa Mādhvadās-jī. As a youth, Yogendra's ruling passion was gymnastics, wrestling, and physical culture. He would skip school to train at the gymnasium he himself had established, gaining a reputation for extraordinary physical strength as well as the nickname "Mr. Muscle-man" (Rodrigues 1997: 20, 40). His biographer suggests that his fixation with "physical exercises, deep breathing and gymnastics" were "a forerunner of his involvement in Yoga" (Rodrigues 1997: 19) and indeed Yogendra's yoga teachings are saturated with the exercises and rhetoric of physical culture. His Yoga Institute at Santa Cruz (once a fairly rural setting, now a busy Mumbai suburb) was set up in 1918 for research into the health-giving aspects of yoga and, according to Yogendra himself, signaled the dawn of a proper understanding of "yoga physical education" (1989 [1928]: 39). In 1919, he traveled to the United States, where he established the Yoga Institute of America on Bear Mountain near New York. He stayed for four years, working with a number of avant-garde Western doctors and naturopaths, such as Benedict Lust and John Harvey Kellogg, and giving what may have been the first ever *āsana* demonstrations in America (beginning September 1921; Rodrigues 1997: 96). He was prevented from returning to the United States in 1924 by the newly implemented Asian Exclusion Act, a subsection of the wider Immigration Restriction Act, the intent of which was candidly racist and eugenic, as it aimed to preserve the dominance of Northern and Western European races in the United States. As President Calvin Coolidge said on signing the act, "America must remain American" (see Zolberg 2006). Thereafter, Yogendra turned his attention to the Indian institute. There is certainly some irony in Yogendra's exclusion from the United States on the grounds of "racial hygiene" when, as we shall see shortly, he was himself fascinated with the potential of *yoga* to effect permanent eugenic improvement in the individual and the race. One might speculate, indeed, that this fascination with racial evolution was itself in some measure a response to having been the victim of the draconian racial policies of the United States, which in so many ways prefigured those of 1930s European fascism.

Like Kuvalayananda, Yogendra was concerned with providing scientific corroboration for the health benefits of yoga and with creating simplified, accessible *Āsana* courses for the public. He and his institute published a large body of material on the practical benefits of yoga for fitness and health, such as *Yoga Āsanas Simplified* (1928) and *Yoga Personal Hygiene* (1931). As the self-styled "householder yogi," Yogendra perhaps did more than anyone (barring Kuvalayananda) to carve out the kind of public health and fitness regimen that today dominates the transnational yoga industry—often in explicit opposition to the secretive, mystical *haṭha* yogi. Three biographical episodes are illustrative here. Once almost kidnapped as a small child by "the dreaded *kanphatas*, known to practice obscure Yoga practices" (Rodrigues 1997: 12), Yogendra developed from an early age a pronounced "mistrust of the false prophets of Yoga" (12). In this, Yogendra shares a widespread, and apparently justified, suspicion of such yogins who, as Farquhar notes, "recruited their numbers by buying or stealing, during their raids, the healthiest children they could find" (Farquhar 1925: 446).

In a parallel incident later in life, three naked yogins arrived at Yogendra's door, offering to take him in and teach him the deeper secrets of yoga. The homely Yogendra refused, but the encounter steeled him in his will to "retrieve Yoga from the confies [*sic*] of self-mortifying cults and other jealous repositories of the Ultimate Truth" (Vijayadev 1962: 30), and gave him "the strength to revolt against age-old traditions, to bring about *reformation in the concept and practice of Yoga*" (30, my emphasis). The face of modern physical yoga would be benevolent, accessible, scientific, and safe, and its domesticated, democratic practice would be defined in contradistinction to the shameful, secret powers of the wandering *haṭha* yogis, powers that nevertheless remain as a signifier of yoga's magical potency within and beyond the scientific yogic project.[2]

Nile Green argues with regard to meditation that such modernized cultures of self-discipline "cannot be disentangled from colonial efforts towards taming the violence of the holy man" (2008: 298). Yogendra's work exemplifies this observation as it pertains to postural yoga. In this, Yogendra inherits elements of the late nineteenth-century Protestant discourses on *haṭha* yoga examined in chapter 2, as well as Max Müller's "Reformationist" vision of Indian religious history. Also evident in Yogendra's work is the influence of Vivekananda's distinctive anti-mysticism. "Anything that is secret and mysterious in these systems of Yoga," writes Vivekananda, "should be at once rejected," on the grounds that "mystery-mongering weakens the brain" (2001 [1896]: 134). As Alter points out—and as we saw in chapter 1—scholars of the period tended to foreground the magical and mystical within yoga (Alter 2004a: 7), and Vivekananda's emphasis on the rational and scientific is clearly intended to reverse the predilection for mystery which, he avers, has "well-nigh destroyed yoga" (2001 [1896]: 134). Yogendra's own democratizing mission—to give the "man-in-the-street" all the benefits hitherto denied him (Vijayadev 1962: 30)—is clearly in step with the Swami's injunction that yoga "ought to be preached in the public streets in broad daylight" (1991 [1896]: 134). But where Vivekananda had roundly dismissed *haṭha* yoga from his vision of what was useful and worthy, Yogendra salvages its curative aspects and refashions them as medicine and modern physical culture—at once "rational, utilitarian, and scientific" (1989 [1928]: 31).

In light of the growing enthusiasm for yoga as physical culture during these early years Yogendra took it on himself to publish "casual literature with more illustrations than exposition" to "fill the demand for information on *Āsana*" (1989 [1928]: 5, publisher's note). *Hatha Yoga Simplified* was one such publication and outlined "a very simple rational and scientific course of posture-exercises as an accessory to the study of classic Yoga" (5). These exercises, conceived as a preparation for more static postures, nonetheless "represent the essentials of yoga physical education," (62) which consists, in the main, of free-standing, dynamically performed exercises from Ling gymnastics and J. P. Müller's enormously influential "System" of callisthenics and personal hygiene (see Müller 1905 and chapter 5 of this volume). Although Yogendra himself dismisses Müller—along with Sandow, Delsarte, and MacFadden—as inferior fads (83), it is more than clear that the "posture-exercises" he chooses are inspired by and borrowed from these sources, with which he was clearly very familiar. It is worth noting, indeed, that Yogendra knew Macfadden personally from his years in New York (Rodrigues 1997: 105) and was almost certainly influenced by the health and fitness milieu that surrounded the American maestro.

Yogendra's repeated definitions through the book of "what yoga really is" tally to a large extent with the physical culture rhetoric of the time. To take a few examples: yoga is "a comprehensive practical system of self-culture...which through interchangeable harmonious development of one's body, mind and psychic potencies ultimately leads to physical well-being, mental harmony, moral elevation and habituation to spiritual consciousness" (1989 [1928]: 20). Yoga aims at the "interrelated harmonious development of one's body, mind and dormant psychic potencies" (25). A comparable "body-mind-spirit" model of "self-culture," with a strong moral subtext, underlies mainstream physical culture at this time. It underpins all YMCA sport and exercise, and in its more mystical guises is the rationale behind the Western tradition of "harmonial gymnastics" (see below).

Although Yogendra was in later decades at pains to stem yoga's identification with physical culture and gymnastics,[3] there seems little doubt that his own early publications fed the appetite for information about *āsana* among health and fitness faddists of the time. His dynamic course of "daily physical exercises for sedative and positive health" (69), as the epigraph to this chapter makes clear, filled a gap in the physical culture market and was taken up *as physical culture*. Yogendra's vision of *haṭha* yoga lent itself to incorporation within the fashionable, contemporary health and hygiene systems with which he had

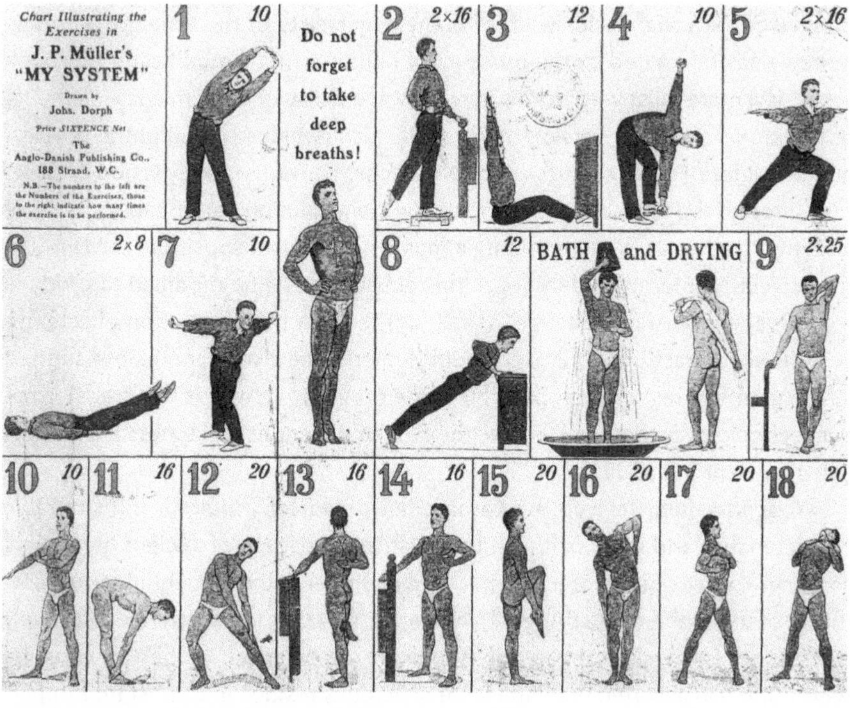

Fold-out exercise chart from Müller 1905

himself been once so enamored. For Yogendra, yoga exercises "have all the merits of medical and preventive gymnastics" (1989 [1928]: 162). His self-proclaimed "yoga renaissance" (see De Michelis 2004: xvii) should be understood as in large measure a holistic and scientific system of movement cure, conceived within the context of the modern "renaissance of gymnastics" (Dixon and McIntosh 1957: 92) but proclaimed as a uniquely indigenous Indian therapy—more ancient and effective than the European styles that had been imposed as the standard form of exercise in India during the nineteenth century.

Yogendra yogic teleology, like so much physical culture and modern yoga writing of this period, also manifests the influence of Social Darwinist and eugenic thought (see "Physical Culture as Eugenics" in chapter 5). The "technology of Yoga" functions for Yogendra as a fillip toward higher states of "physical, mental, moral and psychic" development which "the slow process of evolution" tarries in attaining (1978: 28).[4] Yogendra terms this process *śīghramokṣasyahetuḥ*, literally "the cause of swift liberation." That he equates *mokṣa* with the evolutionary project of "modern science" and eugenics shows the extent to which his vision of yoga diverges from "classical" yogic conceptions of liberation.

Similarly, Yogendra shares what is by then a fairly widespread belief that "the very concept of evolution originated and developed with (Sāṃkhya) Yoga" (1978: 27). While his committed populism would make it unlikely for him to partake of the racial exclusivism of many eugenicists of the time, Yogendra is nonetheless fascinated by the prospect of human genetic modification through yoga. As a materialist who from a very early age distrusted the magical elements of traditional yoga, his version of yoga eugenics remains rooted in the physical and biological. For Yogendra, as for Nietzsche, Darwin's stately vision of progress through the ages is not sufficient. Natural evolution, lamentably, does not alter the "germ plasm" determining a man's hereditary disposition, but through the project "contemplated by yoga" this substance *can* be modified to produce a "permanent germinal change" (1978: 29). Such a transformation effects not only the yoga practitioner himself "but by inheritance also becomes transmitted as the germinal instinct (propensity) of the progeny" (29). It is this transformative technology, he asserts, that is "the crux of the entire metaphysical perspective in ancient India" (29).

Yogendra here revives the Lamarckian dream of acquired, transmittable characteristics and imbues it with the mystical landscape of ancient India. This yogic neo-Lamarckism would seem to be a rejoinder to the influential *germ plasm* theory of the embryologist August Weismann (1834–1914) which had effectively discredited Lamarck's apparently simplistic cause-effect model of heredity. Weismann had asserted that "the force of heredity resided in a substance impermeable to environmental influence" (Kevles 1995: 19) and had proved his convictions through apparently incontrovertible experiment. As a result, the inviolability of the germ plasm became largely accepted as fact in the scientific community (see Maranto 1996: 99). The evolutionary biologist J. B. S. Haldane, for example, is evoking Weismann's experiments on multigenerational amputation of mice's tails when he notes, as evidence against Lamarck, that Jews "whose ancestors have been circumcised for thousands of years are born without any trace of this operation" (Haldane and Lunn 1935: 108). The term had also passed into the vocabulary of the eugenics movement and was in common use among the Indian eugenicists of the day (see, for example, N. D. Mehta's *Hindu Eugenics* of 1919: "The law of heredity or 'Nature' for practical Eugenics is to be sought in the germ-plasm of the parents" (19).

Yogendra reasons, then, that it is the practices of *haṭha* yoga alone that can overcome this impermeability of the germ plasm and lead to permanent and hereditary change in the individual and offspring. *Haṭha* yoga, in other words, is the unique force that can overcome Weismann's "barrier." The example of "recent experiments on certain receptive worms and their succeeding generations" (1978: 28), which apparently produced hereditary alterations comparable to the ones that he envisages through yoga, is further grist for his mill. Yogendra transmutes his fascination with the "science" of eugenics into one of the eternal truths of yoga, and his work represents a striking instance of *haṭha* practice married with modern biology.

Also very notable, and characteristic of many modern expressions of yoga, is his repeated conviction that yoga does not concern itself solely with the well-being or liberation of the individual but with "the germinal character within the whole society of mankind" (Yogendra 1978: 30). This is a perspective that is far more in keeping with the modern eugenic enterprise than with, say, the "classical" yoga of Patañjali. The empowerment afforded by this "germinal change" is furthermore identified with the human domination of "nature" (that is, *prakṛti*), which is in turn identified as the successful attainment of the four goals of Hindu life (*purṣārtha*)! Thus, Yogendra aligns his yoga project (and Hinduism itself) with the aspirations of modern science to control the natural world. And the means toward this end is self-directed eugenic mutation.

Yogendra's version of yoga as a system of curative gymnastics and fitness training makes his eugenic fantasy of societywide hereditary mutation through exercise more similar to Lamarckian aspirations of the kind espoused by J. P. Müller (whom Yogendra cites as an influence) than, for instance, to the alchemical yoga traditions studied by White (1996). One final example, taken from Yogendra's 1928 fusion of Western physical culture and yoga, *Yoga Āsanas Simplified*,[5] will have to suffice to indicate this orientation. Yoga insists, he writes, "that it is imperative in the interest of human evolution [*sic*]" that the seed be made strong, and that "this link [i.e., the reader] in the endless chain which connects the generations yet to come shall be made as healthy and strong as the environments, heredity and auto-inherited potentials (*saṃskāravāsana*) will permit" (1989 [1928]: 42). In Yogendra's hands, the gymnastic practices of yoga become a transgenerational insurance policy and the yogic enterprise an expanded and revised version of the Lamarckian eugenics promoted by the international physical culture movement.[6]

Iyer, Sundaram, Balsekar: Yoga Body Beautiful

> Who owns this system? Is the owner reaping its full benefit? And what is it? To the first the answer is India; the second, alas, No; And to the last, the reply echoes through centuries of neglect—YOGA-ASANA.
>
> (Sundaram 1989 [1928]: 3)

> A baffled mind steeped in Western Physical Culture turns to Hata-Yoga, India's heritage.
>
> (Iyer 1930: 43)

K. V. Iyer of Bangalore (1897–1980), possibly the most high-profile Indian advocate of physical culture in the first half of the twentieth century, set up his first gymnasium at Tippu Sultan's Palace (in the Fort area of the old city) in 1922, and after a series of further gymnasia finally moved to his famous *Vyāyamśālā* on J. C. Road in 1940.[7] During the 1930s, Iyer would often appear in international physical culture magazines such as *Health and Strength* and *The Superman*, striking classical Grecian poses. He also authored books on health and bodybuilding and was a regular contributor to the Maharastrian journal *Vyāyam*. He was a great admirer of Sandow, Macfadden, and the "muscle control" maestro Maxick (of whom more below) and later held an ongoing correspondence with Charles Atlas. Never one for modesty, Iyer declared himself to be possessed of "a body which Gods covet" and claimed for himself the title of "India's most perfectly developed man" (Iyer 1927: 163, 164; see also Goldberg forthcoming).

Although almost exclusively remembered as a bodybuilder, Iyer was an avid promoter of *haṭha* yogic exercise as part of a larger, highly aestheticized physical culture regime based on Western models. In his *Muscle Cult* of 1930 he declares that "Hata-Yoga, the ancient system of body-cult... had more to do in the making of me what I am to-day than all the bells, bars, steel-springs and strands I have used" (41–42).[8] Iyer epitomizes the manner in which *āsana* was "appended" (to use Yogendra's term) to physical culture as well

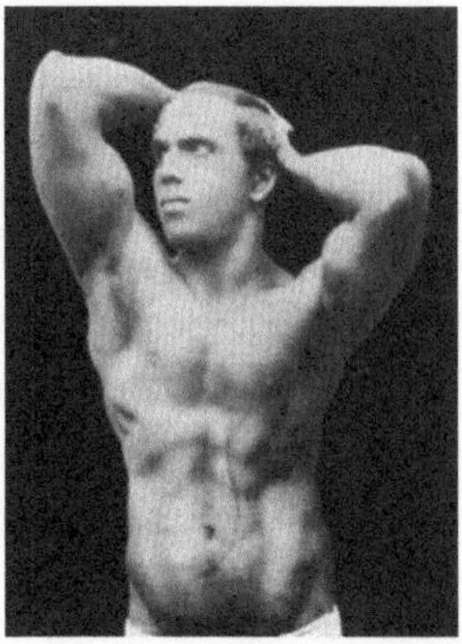

Iyer, in his *Muscle Cult* of 1930

as the shift identified by Alter from a *haṭha* yogic "perfection of the body" (conceived as the "conquest of the five material elements") to a modern cosmetic or fitness model (Alter 2005: 126).

His system was a self-conscious marriage of bodybuilding and yoga, and uses as a foundation the innovations of early synthesizers like Ramamurthy. The "conscientious incorporation of what I might term this INDIAN SPECIALITY as an organic part of My System" (Iyer 1930: 42) aimed to complement the external bodily emphasis of the Western physical culture techniques he also offered and eventually to bring forth the "ideally developed man," who would have "both the symmetry and strength of a Sandow" and the immunity to disease afforded by *haṭha* yoga (42). Importantly, and following from our discussion in chapter 4, Iyer (like many modern Indian physical culturists) considered Ling gymnastics wholly ineffectual and called for a boycott of "the Swedish drill" in Indian universities and educational institutions: "Years and years of these drill," he complains, "have not improved the physique of our Nation even a wee-bit" (Iyer 1927: 245–46). The new yogic synthesis was envisaged as an Indian hybrid alternative to the predominant but ineffectual Ling system and aimed at a national revolution in physical culture.

As this quotation suggests, and as one might expect given his affiliations with the international physical culture scene, Iyer's work also bears traces of the eugenic bent that characterizes so much writing of this period (see chapter 5 above). For example, writing in the exercise periodical *Vyayam, the Body Builder* in 1927, Iyer laments, "Will our women bring forth only healthful useful children to save our motherland from this degeneration, from this slavery?" (Iyer 1927: 237). "Physically deficient mothers and devitalized fathers," he goes on, are producing "helpless derelicts and weaklings" (237), and he urges his readers to take up physical culture to forestall this.[9]

Day-to-day activities at Iyer's gymnasium, as well as the popular correspondence courses, were the practical expression of this "blending of the two Systems" of physical culture and yoga (Iyer 1930: 43), offering an integral regime of *sūryanamaskār* (salutations to the sun), "yoga" as medical gymnastics and body-conditioning on the one hand, and state of the art dumbbell work and freehand European bodybuilding techniques on the other. Iyer was not the first to use *sūryanamaskār* as part of a bodybuilding Regimen. The creator of the modern *sūryanamaskār* system, Pratinidhi Pant, the Rajah of Aundh, was himself, like Iyer, a devoted bodybuilder and practitioner of the Sandow method, and he went on to definitively popularize the dynamic sequences of *āsana*s that have become a staple of many postural yoga classes today. As Pant writes in his manual of the *sūryanamaskār* method: "In 1897... we purchased all [Sandow's] apparatus and books, and for fully ten years practised regularly and continuously according to his instructions" (Pratinidhi and Morgan 1938: 90). *Sūryanamaskār*, today fully naturalized in international yoga milieux as a presumed "traditional" technique of Indian yoga, was first conceived by a bodybuilder and then popularized by other bodybuilders, like Iyer and his followers, as a technique of bodybuilding (see Goldberg 2006, forthcoming). Let us stress, however, that at this time, for Pratinidhi, Iyer, and those who practiced and taught their techniques, *sūryanamaskār* was *not yet considered a part of yoga.* We will return to this constellation of *sūryanamaskār*, *yogāsana*, and bodybuilding in more detail in chapter 9.

Iyer's system exemplifies the absorption of postural yoga by physical culturalists as well as the cultural fusion that this could entail between the yogic "saints and Savants of Ancient India" and the mesomorphic athletes and gods of ancient Greece (Iyer, *Suryanamaskar* 1937: 3). Iyer also had a widespread reputation for healing disease through yoga and a special abdominal massage of his own invention. "I will cure your ailments even if they are chronic through yogic therapy," reads one of his advertisements, "and make you *wonderfully muscular and strong* through the most scientific, practical and quickest way possible" (Iyer 1927: 177). Although Iyer's clientèle included an array of influential public figures (such as Babli Maharaja of Andhra Pradesh and the musician Ravi Shankar), his most powerful and famous patient at the time was Krishnarajendra Wadiyar, the Maharaja of Mysore, whom he nursed back to health following a stroke. In gratitude, the Maharaja financed the building of Iyer's Vyāyamśālā and sponsored a Mysore branch in the Jaganmohan Palace, under the direction of Iyer's principal student, Anant Rao (see Goldberg forthcoming). Indeed, Iyer's *Physique and Figure* of 1940 is dedicated to "My Gracious King and Patron, His Highness Sri Bahadur Krishnarajendra Wadiyar G.C.S.I., G.B.E. Maharaja of Mysore," evidencing the ongoing good relations that obtained between the two.

Crucially for the history of the intersection of physical culture and yoga, Iyer not only shared a common patron with one of the founding fathers of modern *āsana* practice, T. Krishnamacharya (the subject of chapter 9 below), but the crucible of today's most popular styles of modern postural yoga—the famed palace *yogaśālā*—was situated only meters away from a modern, Western-style gymnasium, itself offering a synthetic program of bodybuilding and yoga (see Goldberg forthcoming). Yoga and bodybuilding evening classes, moreover, both took place between 5 and 7 p.m. (interview with Krishnamacharya's student T. R. S. Sharma, August 29, 2005, and Iyengar 2000: 53). We will return to this suggestive intersection in chapter 9, but let us note for the time being that this situation is, at the very least, a further indication of the practical and historical proximity of modern yoga and physical culture.

Iyer's student, collaborator, and friend in the yogic physical culture enterprise was one Yogācarya Sundaram. According to Iyer's son, K. V. Karna, whom

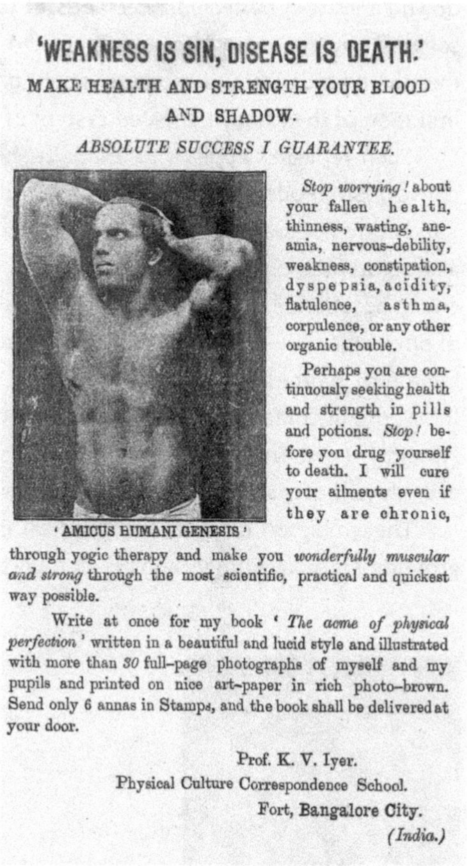
'WEAKNESS IS SIN, DISEASE IS DEATH.'
MAKE HEALTH AND STRENGTH YOUR BLOOD AND SHADOW.
ABSOLUTE SUCCESS I GUARANTEE.
Stop worrying! about your fallen health, thinness, wasting, anaemia, nervous-debility, weakness, constipation, dyspepsia, acidity, flatulence, asthma, corpulence, or any other organic trouble.
Perhaps you are continuously seeking health and strength in pills and potions. Stop! before you drug yourself to death. I will cure your ailments even if they are chronic,
'AMICUS HUMANI GENESIS'
through yogic therapy and make you wonderfully muscular and strong through the most scientific, practical and quickest way possible.
Write at once for my book 'The acme of physical perfection' written in a beautiful and lucid style and illustrated with more than 30 full-page photographs of myself and my pupils and printed on nice art-paper in rich photo-brown. Send only 6 annas in Stamps, and the book shall be delivered at your door.
Prof. K. V. Iyer.
Physical Culture Correspondence School.
Fort, Bangalore City.
(India.)

"I will cure your ailments even if they are chronic, through yogic therapy . . ." Iyer 1927

I interviewed in his home in Bangalore in September 2005, Sundaram ran the "Yogic School of Physical Culture" referred to in Iyer's *Perfect Physique* of 1936, and the two men regularly conducted lecture/demonstration tours together around the country. In his book *Muscle Cult* of 1930, Iyer asserts that the task of "unveiling in detail the how and why and wherfore [*sic*] of Hata-Yoga" shall "be the right only of my pupil" (42). Karna confirms that this is indeed a reference to Sundaram, Iyer's yogic lieutenant (see also Goldberg forthcoming).

In 1928, Sundaram published *Yogic Physical Culture or, the Secret of Happiness* (1989 [1928]), one of the earliest and most successful photographic do-it-yourself books of *haṭha* yoga reconceptualized as gymnastics, hygiene, and bodybuilding. His manual closely and self-consciously rehearses the themes and practices of Western physical culturalists and explicitly pays gratitude to Bernarr Macfadden "and a host or [*sic*] other pioneers in the field of the newly risen Physical Culture creed" who have rendered physical culture into "the real thing it ought to be" (1989 [1928]: 2). In spite of their great advances, however, such innovators are deemed to lag far behind the ancient sages who have handed down "a system perfected thousands of years ago" (1989 [1928]: 3). The message, of course, reenacts a reversal of Orientalist "fulfillment" narratives, such that the ne plus ultra of modern "scientific" physical culture is only an inferior imitation of the wholly perfected system of the ancient Hindu yogins.

Such repeated appeals to antiquity, however, are undermined by the self-consciously modern departures from, and accretions to, tradition enacted by Sundaram. For example, although he acknowledges that yoga was originally used as a spiritual discipline, Sundaram reasons that modern men and women in sedentary occupations, who are not born for saintliness, might "utilise it as a system of physical culture" (1989 [1928]: 4). The sociopolitical situation, moreover, calls for a new synthesis of *āsana* with muscle building, in order that the "sons of India" might "obtain super-strength to make their *Mother* an equal sister among Nations!" (129). In the present situation, asserts Sundaram, "giants of Muscles—even devoid of brain power, are an inevitable necessity!" (129).

The amalgam of yoga and physical culture is also justified on aesthetic grounds since "a human body is not worth looking at without properly devel-

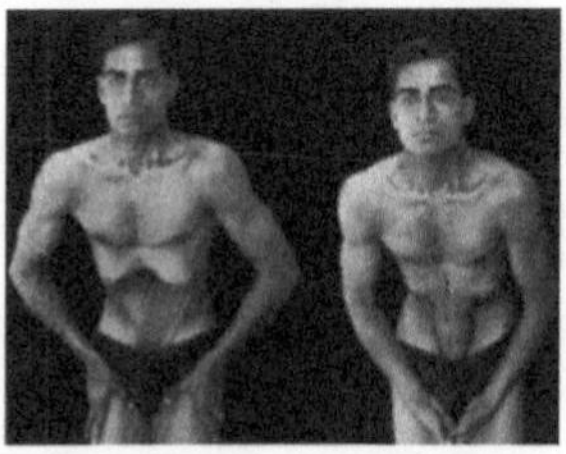

Sundaram, in Iyer's *Muscle Cult* of 1930

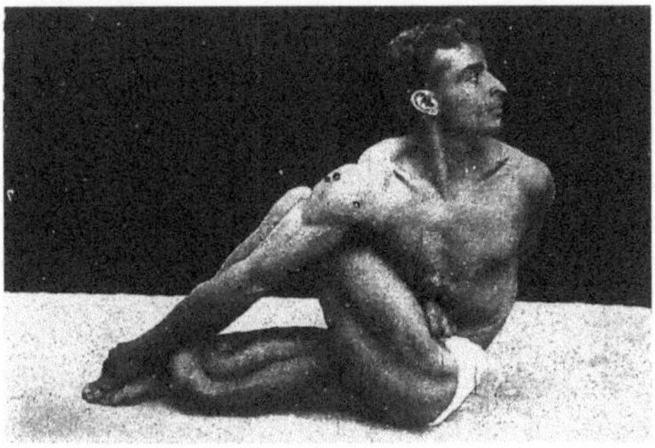

A graduate of Sundaram and Iyer's Yogic School of Physical Culture, in Iyer 1930

oped superficial muscles" (129). *Āsanas* alone, however, are deemed insufficient to furnish such a body and therefore must be combined with conventional physical culture: "Anyone, who wants external muscular cuts and fine super-muscular formations, must do, apart from the Asanas, certain muscular exercises with or without instruments" (135). The emphasis on building a beautiful physique through yogic physical culture and, vitally, the *spectacle* of that physique, is of course perfectly consonant with Iyer's own aesthetic (not to say narcissistic) fixations, as well as the pronounced display culture in the wider, international fitness market. This specular economy, notes Budd, relied on readers' imagined participation in the grand project of physical perfection, so that their very bodies could be sold back to them "as a kind of petrified commodity of the self made whole" (1997: 57).

Sundaram and Iyer's propagation of physicalized yoga as an essentially "spiritual" discipline reflected a path to *religious* wholeness through the aesthetic perfection of the body: a "Physical Culture Religion" (Sundaram 1989 [1928]: 11) in harmony with the aspirations and needs of their modern Hindu clientèle. It is telling that, according to K. V. Karna, every Saturday evening at the *Vyāyamśālā* Iyer would conduct a puja in front of two enormous images of Rām and Hanuman. While this yogic physical culture—presented in contrast to the mechanical Western approach as a "religion for the highest perfection of body to attain the greatest realisation of Self" (12)—is couched in the discourse of the Hindu renaissance, it also plainly reprises Sandow's project for the resacralization of the body through fitness training. As Mosse points out, such linking of body and spirit within physical culture discourse "was basic to the idea of [masculine] beauty and the stereotype it projected" (1996: 24). But that "tinge of religion" (Sundaram 1989 [1928]: 11) that Sundaram infuses into his yogic training is nonetheless the basis on which he distinguishes the merely material West from the spiritual East, thereby reinforcing yoga's religious and physiological superiority.

Mention should also be made here of Ramesh Balsekar's flamboyant experiments with physical culture and yoga many decades prior to his rise to fame as an international *advaita* guru. Balsekar studied in India under Iyer and imbibed his blend of yoga and physical culture. He is pictured in Iyer's 1936 publication *Perfect Physique* with the caption "Every inch of his body perfect and proportionate." In the mid-1930s he was in London and rose to prominence within the British physical culture press as the poster boy of Indian bodybuilding, surpassing even Iyer himself in terms of photographic exposure. Major British physical culture magazines, like *Health and Strength* and *The Superman*, regularly featured pictures of Balsekar during this period. Balsekar studied in England under Lawrence A. Woodford, author of *Physical Idealism and the Art of Posing*, and later became "not only winner of the 'All-India Body Beautiful Competition' in 1938, but also one of *Great Britain's* 'ten most perfectly developed men'" (Budd 1997: 171 n. 28, my emphasis). His book *Streamlines*, of 1940, is a curious combination of instruction in *yogāsana* and *sūryanamaskār*, juxtaposed with a series of glamor shots of the semi- or fully naked author in various heroic postures. The message is clear: through yoga, one can develop a body such as this.

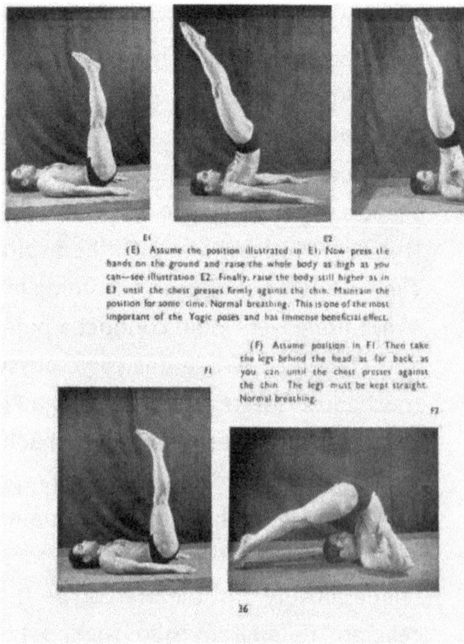

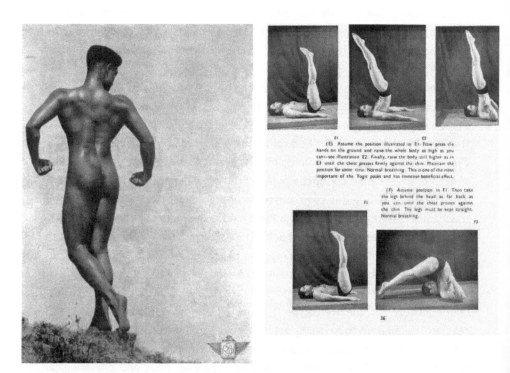

Pictures from Balsekar 1940

Although Iyer, Sundaram, and Balsekar are particularly vivid examples of early experiments with syncretic systems of *āsana* and cosmetic physical culture, they are not isolated cases, and a preoccupation with the aesthetics of the body is common in *yogāsana* manuals through the 1930s. For example, M. R. Jambunathan's *Yoga Asanas, Illustrated* of 1933 promises the reader "a strong and beautiful body" through the practice of yoga (ii). Regular *āsana* practice "will give you a medium appearance nice to look at and will make you happy in all respects. What more do you want?" (ii). Publications such as these purveyed *āsana* as a body-conditioning technique that could deliver happiness through health and aesthetic body perfection.

The New Thought Yogis

> Call his whole performance, if you like, an experiment in self-suggestion.
>
> (William James on an American practitioner of *haṭha* yoga, 1907: 328)

> It took Coué to teach us the virtue of *Japa*, or constant meditation upon a certain idea, or Haddock to instruct us in the importance of will-power, or William James to enlighten us on the significance of mental control. Any one who reads the works of these men even cursorily and compares their teachings with those of ancient Indian sages will not fail to be struck with wonder at the resemblance.
>
> (Pratinidhi, Rajah of Aundh, founder of the modern *sūryanamāskar* system, 1938/1941: 105)

> Always use a mental effort, what is usually called "Christian Science," to keep the body strong. That is all—nothing further of the body.
>
> (Vivekananda, *Raja Yoga* 1992 [1896]: 139)

When the physical postures of yoga were presented in the West as a technique that one *did* (as opposed to a freakish spectacle from which one recoiled), it was largely in the mode of the health and fitness regimes adumbrated by Kuvalayananda, Yogendra, Sundaram, and others. Earlier do-it-yourself yoga books in the West tended to downplay the role of *āsana*, foregrounding instead meditation and deep breathing techniques, sometimes combined with advice on health and hygiene. These earlier manuals illustrate how the popular, para-religious movement known as New Thought permeated thinking about yoga in

India, America, and Europe from the end of the nineteenth century. When the emphasis in transnational yoga began to shift toward the practice of *āsana*, the New Thought influence remained.[10]

Originally a breakaway faction of Mary Eddy Baker's Christian Science, New Thought began in New England in the 1880s as a broad-based, para-Protestant movement preaching the innate divinity of the self and the power of positive thinking to actuate that divinity in the world, usually to the ends of personal affluence and health. It is no exaggeration to say that elements of these popular esoteric doctrines are so uniformly present in practical yoga primers intended for the European and American reading public that it is unusual *not* to find some degree of blending during the first half of the twentieth century. It seems to have been widely taken for granted that positive thinking, auto-suggestion, and the "harmonial," this-worldly belief framework of New Thought was not so much a contribution to yoga as its expression (albeit in optimistic, Americanized accents). Conversely, it was largely assumed that yoga was the perennial, exotic repository of these newly (re-)discovered truths.

Popular yoga writers of the early twentieth century such as Yogi Ramacharaka, O. Hashnu Hara, R. Dimsdale Stocker, and S. D. Ramayandas belong more properly to the distinct "New Thought" subgenre of modern yoga. It was common for authors such as these to also compose books devoted to furthering the widely popular, optimistic, individualistic creed of New Thought. New Thought titles rubbed shoulders with yoga primers in the catalogues of popular esoteric publishers like L. N. Fowler (London) and Fowler and Wells (New York). Yoga manuals were filled with advertisements for New Thought self-help books and vice versa. And in practice, often little distinction was drawn between the two: both are overwhelmingly concerned with health and with the accumulation of personal spiritual power for material well-being.

The many yoga books produced over a twenty-year period by Yogi Ramacharaka are a particularly vivid example of the intersection of New Thought, Nature Cure, and transnational anglophone yoga. Ramacharaka's works represent, in Jackson's words, "the outer limits of New Thought's deep infatuation with India" (Jackson 1975: 537). Ramacharaka was in all likelihood the pen-name of prolific Chicago lawyer and New Thought "guru" William Walker Atkinson (1862–1932), who authored a steady avalanche of esoteric yoga manuals and New Thought self-help books between 1903 and about 1917. As Catherine Albanese has remarked, Atkinson's work expresses "New Thought in its brashest, least Christianized and God-dependent version" (Albanese 2007: 358). The series of manuals and courses that he authored, tremendously popular and with a practical orientation, had a lasting effect on the propagation of modern transnational yoga, and his books are still read by practitioners today, as the recent republications of his books in India, America, and the UK attest.[11]

Ramacharaka's *Hatha Yoga, or the Yogi Philosophy of Physical Well-Being* of 1904 is an early example of *haṭha* yoga reenvisaged as Nature Cure and New Thought, and it is an important precursor to the full-fledged *haṭha* reformulations that began to appear two decades later. Ramacharaka borrows heavily (and sometimes verbatim) from Vivekananda's *Raja Yoga* (1896), a book that was itself deeply imbued with New Thought metaphysics (De Michelis 2004: 168). Having made it clear at the outset that fundamental practices of *haṭha* yoga such as *kriyā* and *āsana* are the circus tricks of fakirs (here as elsewhere echoing Vivekananda's sentiments), Ramacharaka adopts an essentially romantic Nature Cure approach to bodily well-being, recommending the standard prescriptions of sunbathing, fresh air, water bathing, and gentle callisthenic exercise. That these callisthenics are emphatically *not* identified as *āsanas* is important as it suggests both a recognition of the need for physical exercise in modern *haṭha* yoga and the ongoing distrust of the core techniques of the yogins.

Similar to the work of later *haṭha* pioneers, this version of *haṭha* yoga features physical perfectionism strongly; the reader is urged to "form an idea of the Perfect Body" so that the intelligent force of Life can course through the individual frame and *make the body over*: for this creative universal force is not impersonal energy but a beneficent entity "which is anxious to flow through us" (Ramacharaka 1904: 242–43). Success in Ramacharaka's physical system relies on the ability of the student to "[throw] the mind out" into the body. Once this "knack" of sending the mind to the desired part is acquired, then positive messages can be injected into the physical frame to eradicate disease (1904: 192). The author points out that "the auto-suggestions and affirmations of the Western world work in this way" (1904: 144), in reference to the kind of mesmeric incantations that are a hallmark of New Thought. These affirmations are later characterized by Ramacharaka as "mantrams" (1904: 237), an identification that endures up to the present day and thoroughly reconstrues mantra's traditional function in Hinduism as the "mystical sound" of ritual observance and meditation (Eliade 1969: 212).

A number of unaffiliated *Indian* yoga teachers operating in America in the early 1920s (as opposed to Westerners posing as Indians) emulate and expand the kind of New Thought-inspired physical culture that we see in Ramacharaka. The most successful of this small but influential contingent, Paramahaṃsa Yogananda (1893–1952), would later author the bible of mystical India, *Autobiography of a Yogi* (1946), and inspire several generations of Western spiritual seekers. During his early years in America Yogananda taught a version of yogic "muscle control" heavily influenced by New Thought and European bodybuilding. He had "discovered" this method of "muscle recharging through will power" (1946: 374) in 1916 and tested it on students at his school in Ranchi. These students thereafter performed prodigious "feats of strength and endurance" (248). Yogananda's early publications in America promote this auto-suggestive, quick-fix method of apparatus-free gymnastics, which is said to yield "the highest possible degree of *physical, mental and spiritual well-being* at the minimum expenditure of time and effort" (1925b: 10–11). The "Yogoda . . . system of body perfection," trumpets another advertisement, can be practiced anywhere, "puts on or removes fat," and "teaches the spiritualization of the body" (1925a), in an efficient merger of the cosmic and the cosmetic.

Yogananda's principal crowd-puller during these early years, indeed, seems to have been displays of this muscle mastery through willpower. For example, the *Los Angeles Post* of January 28, 1925, declares, "concentration was his subject, demonstrated by physical control over the principal muscles" (in Yogananda 1925b: 44), and the *Boston Post* of Sunday, February 18, 1923, calls Yogananda "the Coué of gymnastics" (44). This refers to Emile Coué's doctrine of positive thought and mental healing which enjoyed an unparalleled vogue in Europe and America in the early years of the twentieth century and which was embraced by positive thinkers and yoga enthusiasts alike, especially on the appearance in English of his two books *My Method* (1923) and *Conscious Auto-suggestion* (1924). While Yogananda's demonstrations of "Body Perfection by Will" (Yogananda 1925b: 7) were by that time common fare in Western vaudeville and bodybuilding milieus, this is perhaps the first time that such muscle manipulation was being sold in America as yoga.

Although, as the journalist intimates, Yogananda's philosophy *was* probably influenced by the teachings of Coué, his physical culture routine appears to be more directly inspired by the techniques of the world-famous bodybuilder Maxick who "astonished audiences in the early part of the century" with the "incredible ability he had to flex and move each muscle of his body almost independently"—performances that in fact gave birth to the common expression "rippling muscles" (n.a. 1933: 124). Maxick's *Muscle Control; or Body Development by Will Power* (1913) and *Great Strength by Muscle Control* (1914) were enormously popular among physical culturalists and went through numerous reprints well into the 1950s. Yogananda's early teachings not only echo the phraseology of Maxick's work but also duplicate an established tradition of New Thought–influenced bodybuilding in the name of yoga.[12]

Yogananda's younger brother, the internationally renowned bodybuilder and modern *haṭha* yogi, B. C. Ghosh, is also an important figure in this regard.

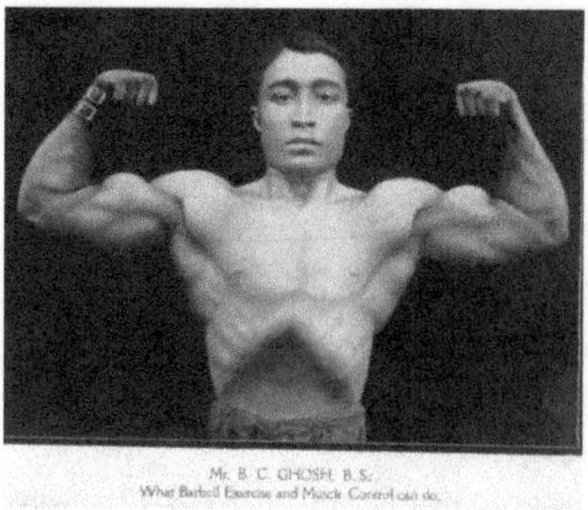

B.C. Ghosh pictured in his *Muscle Control* of 1930

According to a history of Yogananda's life and family published in 1980 (by S. L. Ghosh), he was not only "the first and only Indian judge in a Mr. Universe contest," but also.

> the first Indian of contemporary times to introduce and make popular a system of *Hatha Yoga* that appealed greatly to the general public. He brought the ancient science of *Hatha Yoga* out of the hermitages and into the courtyards of homes and the fields of villages.... He was a devotee of God, as well as a genius in the field of *Hatha Yoga* and physical culture... and will ever be remembered for introducing yoga exercises to the masses. (Ghosh 1980: xvii)

This new, popular *haṭha* yoga was a fusion of *āsanas*, physical culture, and the muscle manipulation techniques that Ghosh had first learned from his brother (Ghosh 1980: 249; Ghosh and Sen Gupta 1930: 52). Significantly, these techniques are referred to as "yoga" by Ghosh in 1930, but fifty years later in the Yogananda biopic have become "yoga exercises." Ghosh's 1930 photographic book *Muscle Control* (dedicated to the nationalist, free-thinking movement "Young Bengal") is a weights-free method of physical training through will-power, strikingly similar in format and content to Maxick's identically titled manual of 1913. Indeed, many of the exercises and poses in Ghosh's book are straight copies from the earlier publication and indicate the extent to which Maxick's system influenced the future *haṭha* yogin. The feats of abdominal muscle isolation that appear in both books are particularly interesting from the point of view of modern yoga and bodybuilding. Immediately recognizable on the one hand as the purificatory *haṭha* yoga exercise *nauli*,[13] this position was also the emblem of muscle-control showmanship in Europe and India, where it was known as the "Maxalding H," in honor of the bodybuilding luminary who popularized it. These two images encapsulate a kind of semiotic porosity

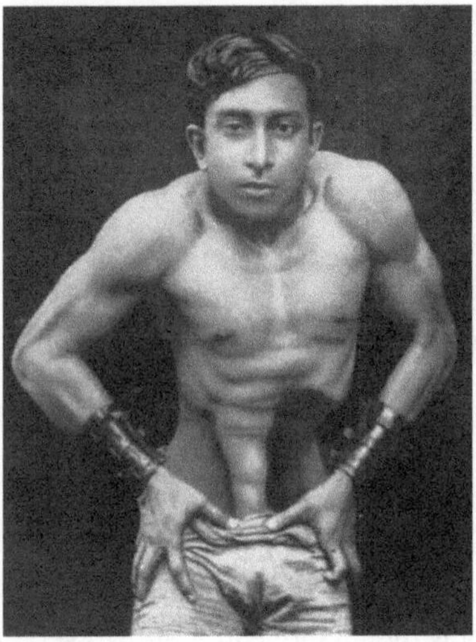

A student performing abdominal isolation, in Ghosh and Sen Gupta 1930

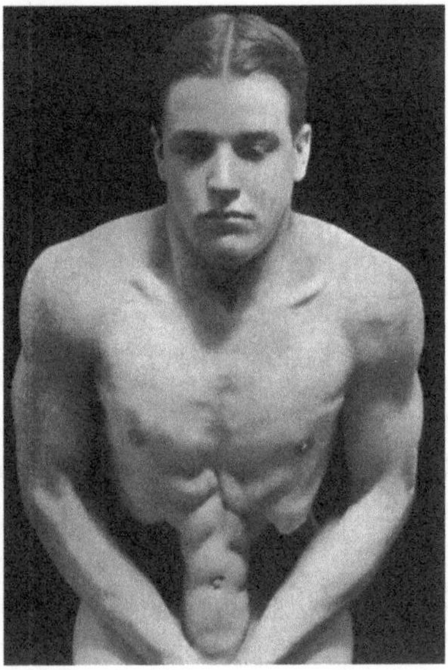

A student performing abdominal isolation, in Maxick 1913

between *haṭha* yoga and bodybuilding at the time and probably also give a good picture of the kinds of performances Yogananda was using to wow audiences in America.

Ghosh opened his College of Physical Education in Calcutta in 1923 and taught a melange of bodybuilding techniques that included *āsana*. It was here that he trained Bikram Choudhury, who would establish what is perhaps the most profitable of today's transnational yoga empires—Bikram Yoga—on the basis of an arduous, athletic sequence of *āsanas* taught to him by Ghosh (see "Concluding Reflections," chapter 9). As we have seen, Ghosh was also propagating such yoga regimes at a grassroots, community level in India. An intriguing addition to this picture of Ghosh's activities is the claim by Tony Sanchez, founding director of the U.S. Yoga Association and a graduate of Ghosh's college, that Ghosh "worked with Swami Sivananda to develop a system of hatha yoga asanas for health and fitness, based on the original classic 84 postures" (Sanchez 2004). While I have been able to find no further evidence to corroborate this, it is far from improbable that Ghosh collaborated in the construction of Sivananda's *āsana* program, which has had a profound effect on the development of the new postural yoga (see Strauss 2005).[14] As an ardent nationalist, one of Bengal's foremost physical culturists, and (to top it all) brother of a yogin who was an international celebrity, he certainly possessed good credentials for the task.

New Thought and the Body

Yogananda's (and to a lesser extent Ghosh's) method of yogic physical culture stems, it seems clear, from New Thought techniques of auto-suggestive body cultivation, such as those we saw earlier with Ramacharaka. The most influential figure in this loose school of thought was Jules Payot, who published his immensely popular *The Education of the Will* in 1893, the same year that Vivekananda arrived in America. Within thirteen years, it had been "translated into most European tongues" and had gone through twenty-seven editions (Payot 1909: ix). For Payot, as for later New Thoughters, the body held the secret of spiritual advancement, and it was through developing the "healthy animal" (247) that the god in man would be revealed. The "physiological conditions of self-mastery" (247) were to be attained through a regime of muscular exercise and "respiratory gymnastics" (259) that would function as "a primary school for the will" (265).

Payot's ideas and methods were taken up by the New Thought movement (Griffith 2001) and developed in the writings of such figures as Frank Channing Haddock, whose "Power Book Library" series represents a momentous event in twentieth-century New Thought history. Haddock draws heavily on Payot's work in his *Power of the Will* of 1909. The physical exercises he describes therein are based, as for Payot, on the exertion of the will—not for physical gains but for the training of the will itself and for the moral and spiritual benefit to be derived from this training. During the exercises, one repeatedly affirms "I am receiving helpful forces! . . . Streams of power for body and mind are flowing in!" (Haddock 1909: 162). One should send such affirmations into the body itself—rather than outward toward the cosmos—and "throw" the thought "into the limbs and muscles" (162). The exercises in Haddock's book represent a kind of embodied Couéism as affirmations are combined with physical exercise to create the corporeal conditions for cosmic influx. Haddock's teaching is clearly of a piece with the *haṭha* yoga methods of Ramacharaka and the early body-based yoga techniques of Yogananda.

In his 1920 therapeutic synthesis, *Massage and Exercise Combined...A New System of the Characteristic Essentials of Gymnastic and Indian Yogis Concentration Exercises,* Albrecht Jensen asserts that "the few more or less fantastic systems of exercise presented during the last fifty years, which consist mainly in producing an imaginary resistance to the muscles by will power only, originate from the Indian Yogis" (19). His statement signals that well before Yogananda's arrival, the exchange between Payot-influenced physical culture and modern *haṭha* yoga was well under way, and that psycho-physiological methods of muscle control were already being identified as *originally* Indian techniques. While it may be true that analogous techniques were used in premodern Indian yoga, the early twentieth-century identification of muscle control with *haṭha* yoga is more likely to have come about through the close association of yoga with modern "alternative" medicine and New Thought), and the subsequent consolidation of this association by the likes of Vivekananda and Ramacharaka. Indeed, Jensen himself seems to have been prominent among New York's health vanguard and ran "Medical Massage Clinics" at several hospitals around New York (Jensen 1920, frontispiece). His book is moreover endorsed by the illuminati of the American alternative health scene, E. L. and W. A. Kellogg. It is quite possible that Jensen assimilated some of his ideas on yoga from direct contact with Yogendra who, as we have seen, established his Yoga Institute in New York in 1919 and was on familiar terms with members of the Kellogg family.

Yogi Gherwal

This rapprochement of post-Payot physical culture and yoga is evident in other Indian "export gurus" active at the time in the United States, such as the California-based Yogi Rishi Singh Gherwal, who published his *Practical Hatha Yoga, Science of Health* in 1923. The book, based on a lecture-demonstration tour of the previous year, is probably the earliest photographic manual of modern, populist *haṭha* yoga—even predating by one year the launch of Kuvalayananda's *Yoga Mīmāṃsā*. Like Yogananda's publications, it functions in part as an advertisement for Gherwal's "First and Advanced Course of Correspondence." Yoga correspondence lessons, probably modeled on Sandow's phenomenally successful postal courses, were already big business at this time. As well as

Yogananda and Gherwal, many of the other yoga writers and gurus considered here (like Sivananda, Iyer, Sundaram, Yogendra, and Ramacharaka) reached their public via the postal service. This marks a fascinating intermediate phase in transnational anglophone yoga's shift away from an exclusive *guru-śiṣya* model and toward the self-help model that dominates today.[15]

As the very title suggests, Gherwal's book is concerned foremost with "the physiology of these asana postures and their application to therapeutics" (1923: 37) and treats in particular the regeneration of the thyroid gland and the correction of constipation. Whereas the postures in the book are in the main drawn from "classical" *haṭha* yoga texts (unlike many of the manuals under consideration), they are interpreted not only in the language of modern medicine but also through the idiom of modern, "psychologized" New Thought physical culture. Gherwal notes that "one of the outstanding features of the Twentieth Century mode of scientific muscular exercise is that this most valuable *will power* or *soul power* is roused, disciplined and developed to an enviable degree," such that "physical culture comes to be studied from the Yogic point of view" (40).

In effect, it is the converse that occurs: yoga comes to be considered as an Eastern variant of New Thought physical culture. Gherwal's manual is steeped in the rationale of the New Thought mode of physical culture, even down to the admiration for the "auto-suggestions imparted to the muscles and physical tissues" (1923: 44) so favored by Haddock and other New Thought luminaries like

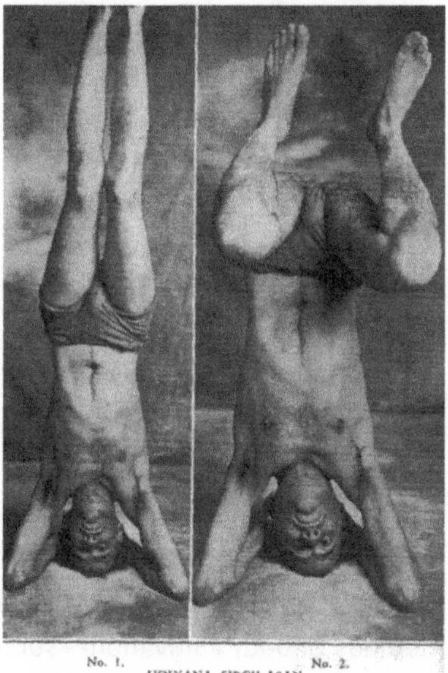

"Udiyan Sirch-Asan," Gherwal 1923

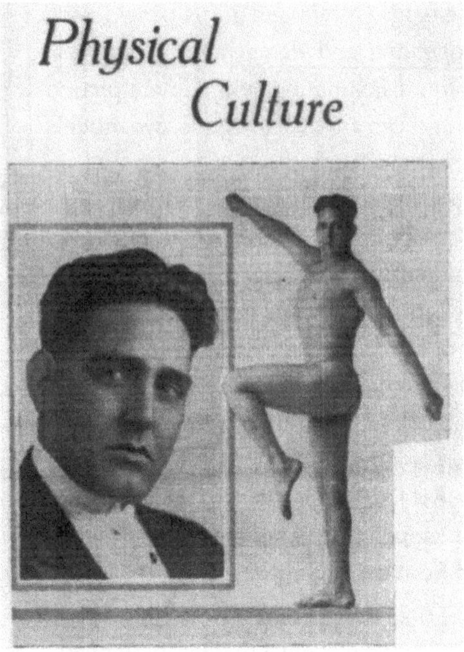

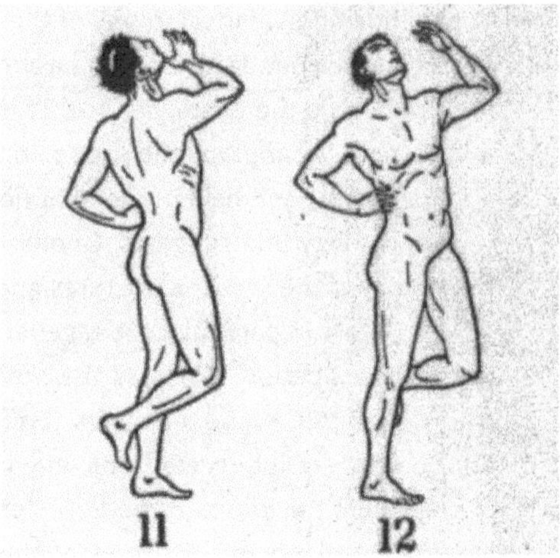

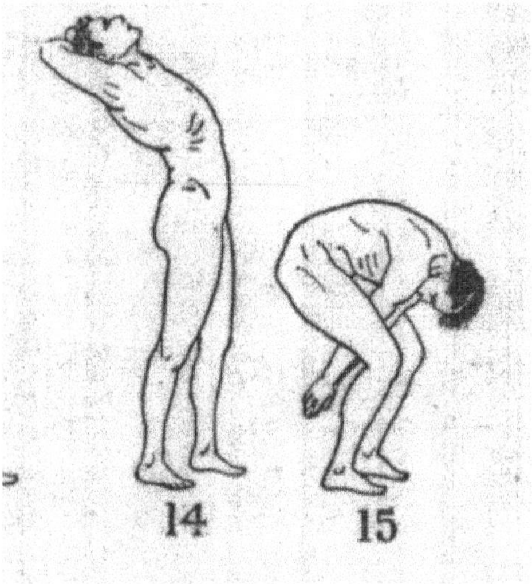

Illustrations from Wassan 1924

Trine (1913). Although the emphasis on body cultivation exceeds that of earlier manuals, it is clear that the system is in keeping with Vivekananda's injunction (see epigraph in "The New Thought Yogis" above) to use "Christian Science" methods of body cultivation—such as those auto-suggestive techniques I have described—as part of a yoga program. Christian Science, of course, was a

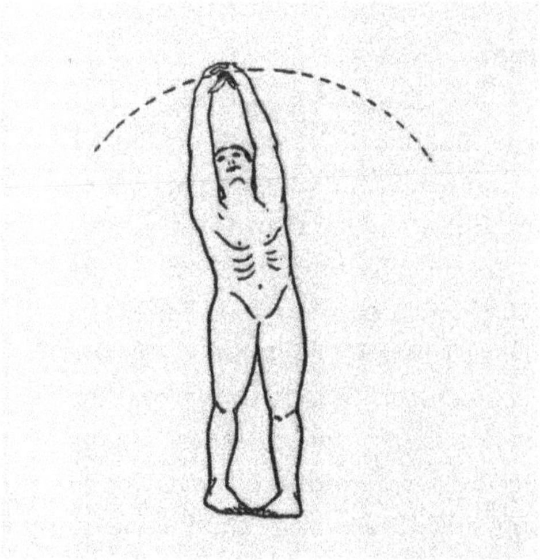

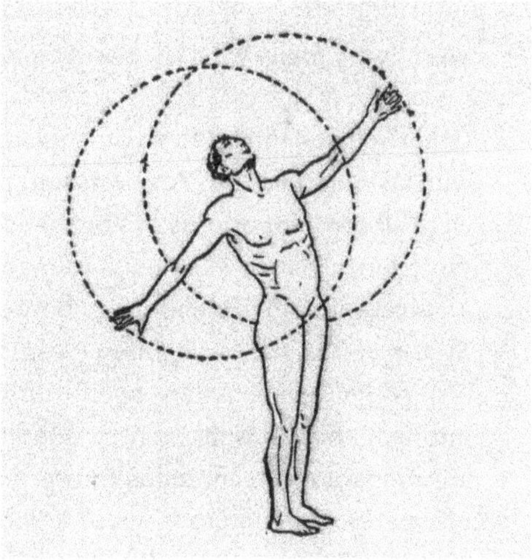

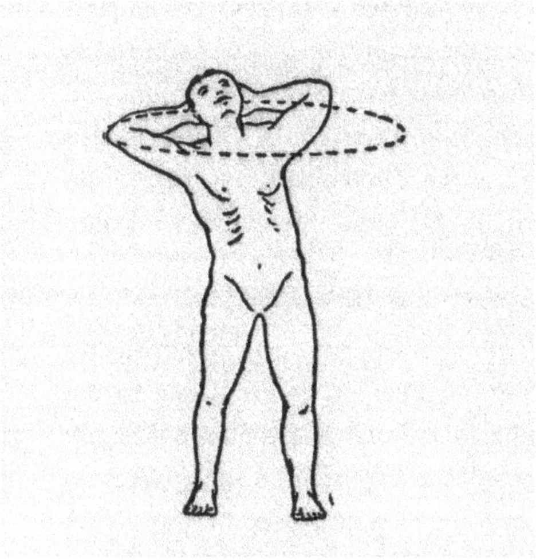

Illustrations from Hari Rama 1926

massively popular system of spiritual health and healing founded by Mary Eddy Baker (1821–1920) and was inspired, like many brands of New Thought (such as that of the Dressers), by the work of New England healer Phineas Parkhurst Quimby (see Meyer 1965; Parker 1973; Jackson 1981). Indeed, for many Americans, movements like Theosophy, Christian Science, New England Transcendentalism, and New Thought functioned as "way stations between participation in the institutional Church and an identification with [neo-] Vedanta" (French 1974: 299). Gherwal's work is exemplary of this process.[16]

West Coast Yogis: Wassan, Hari Rama, Bhagwan Gyanee

Other self-styled Hindu yogins operating in America in the 1920s present us with a similar picture. Yogi Wassan, Yogi Hari Rama, and Bhagwan S. Gyanee were all contemporaries of Yogananda and Gherwal; they all peddled comparable formulae for spiritual and material advancement through nature cure and New Thought religion. The books of the Punjab-born Wassan, *The Hindu System of Health Development* (1924) and his virtually identical *Soroda System of Yoga Philosophy* (1925) open with the ecumenical "Soroda chant" and the intoned, affirmational mantra "Hoon, Young, Young, Young." These chants are preparatory techniques in the therapeutic program of rejuvenation and prosperity designed to teach one "How to Vibrate Brain, Body and Business" (1925: 5). In name, as well as in ideology, Wassan's system is a close match of the Yogoda method of Yogananda and any number of expressions of New Thought nature religion combined with business acumen. "If our vibrations are of the right kind," Wassan tells us, "we have harmony with Nature and we are in perfect health and happiness, peace and poise" (58). There is also an occasional eugenic flavor in Wassan's work, such as in his exhortation that were we only to follow the wisdom of this yoga, "we would become supermen and women" (1925: 60).

His "Hindu System of Physical Culture" (in Wassan 1925: 89–111) consists of a series of exercises derived from contemporary gymnastic regimes like Müller's "My System," which (unlike Gherwal) bear no resemblance to the *āsanas* in *haṭha* yoga texts. The line drawings accompanying the exercises are, instead, the generic, ubiquitous illustrations of the kind seen in 1920s Western physical culture manuals. The very same drawings are also used by Hari Rama for his *Yoga System of Study* (1926: 73–81). Judging from the student testimonials that take up almost half of the book, Wassan traveled all over the United States (in particular the west coast), giving mass lecture demonstrations as well as individual classes, and he was extremely successful as a teacher, especially among "the busy business men and women who have not much time to bother about many things" (Wassan 1925: 40). For thousands of Americans, such regimes of callisthenics, deep breathing, dietics,[17] nature cure, and positive auto-suggestion were the sum of yoga.

Last, Bhagwan S. Gyanee's *Yogi Exercises* of 1931 does not deviate greatly from this pattern and represents an effective imitation of Ramacharaka's *Hatha Yoga* of 1904. Like Ramacharaka, Gyanee authored a plethora of New Thought self-help manuals, with titles such as *Sex, Why Men Fail; Concentration; Creative Wisdom; Pearls of Wisdom* (poems); *The Path to Perfection; Love Marriage and*

Divorce; Foods that Make or Break You; Mysteries and Functions of the Subconscious Mind; The Science of Perpetual Youth; and *Nine Laws of Scientific Living* (titles listed in Gyanee 1931: 1). The movements and positions described (but not illustrated) in *Yoga Exercises* are explicitly presented as yoga's equivalent to the "allied branches" of magnetism, osteopathy, nature cure, and naturopathy (7–10). Although it is implied that they derive from the tradition of eighty-four *āsanas* (9), the "yogic postures" are in fact entirely cognate with common regimes of European weights-free gymnastics such as those we considered in chapter 4.

The *only* posture that one might recognize today as a modern *yogāsana* is Gyanee's "Body Balance" (25), which corresponds to *ardha candrāsana* in Iyengar's nomeclature (Iyengar 1966). This posture, however, is a standard exercise in Western physical culture and is commonly depicted in bodybuilding publications. In one instance it is glossed as "an advantageous nudist exercise" (Buckley 1932: 22). There is good reason to think that its entry into modern yoga was due to its status as a common balancing exercise.

As with many of the new *haṭha* yogic regimes I examine, these international, commercial varieties of postural yoga enact a redefinition of the Indian system to suit local tastes and expectations, much in the same way that Vivekananda's version of *vedānta* "may legitimately be said to represent a degree of strategic, 'glocal' tweaking of received Hindu tradition" (Beckerlegge 2004: 309).[18]

7

Yoga as Physical Culture II: Harmonial Gymnastics and Esoteric Dance

The modern yogic body regimes that I outline in the previous chapter are strikingly congruous to certain forms of unchurched Protestant religiosity that Sidney Ahlstrom has termed *harmonial religion* (1972). New Thought is perhaps the most demotic, practical expression of this diffuse movement, which represents a rejection of the Calvinist denigration of the body in favor of the soul. In this "harmonial" religious model, as Fuller summarizes it, "spiritual composure, physical health, and even economic well-being are understood to flow from a person's rapport with the cosmos" (2001: 51).[1] In terms of the new forms of *haṭha* yoga, one of the most important branches of such practical religion applied to the body is a subtradition I will refer to as "harmonial gymnastics," which is exemplified by the work of two American women: Genevieve Stebbins and Cajzoraṇ Ali. Both were extremely influential in forging esoteric systems of "harmonial" movement associated with yoga that directly prefigure (and enable) the "spiritual stretching," breathing, and relaxation regimes in the popular practice of yoga today. In Britain, practices analogous to many contemporary *yogāsana* forms were promoted by Mollie Bagot Stack of the "Women's League of Health and Beauty" during the 1930s, within a similar "harmonial" framework. Indeed, what is remarkable about regimes such as Stack's, and those prescribed (mainly for women) in the male-dominated physical culture press, is that even though they are not called "yoga," they often resemble today's postural forms far more closely than many of the above-examined gymnastic and bodybuilding forms identified as yoga. The posture-heavy forms of yoga that began to predominate in the West in the latter half of the twentieth century constitute a continuation, in practical, sociological, and demographic terms, of regimes that were already normalized within (secular as well as esoteric) sections of British and American physical culture.

Genevieve Stebbins and American Delsartism

The French teacher of acting and singing, Francois Delsarte (1811–71), became famous in Europe for his theory of aesthetic principles applied to the pedagogy of dramatic expression. His spirito-physical exercises and rules for the coordination of voice and breath with bodily gestures gained popularity not only within theater and opera but also among a wider public.[2] The foremost American exponent of Delsartism was Genevieve Stebbins (1857–c.1915), who began working with Delsarte's student Steele Mackaye in New York in 1876. Mackaye's adapted American regime laid a greater emphasis on gymnastic movement and relaxation than Delsarte's own (Ruyter 1996: 68). Stebbins was also a member of the group Church of Light, "an order of practical occultism" with close links to the influential esoteric group the Hermetic Brotherhood of Luxor (Godwin et al. 1995: ix). She brought these esoteric influences—along with those of Mackaye, Ling gymnastics,[3] *and yoga*—to bear on her interpretation of Delsartism. Stebbins's presentation of Delsarte to American audiences initiated a veritable Delsarte craze, with a flood of imitation Delsarte publications, Delsarte clothes and home designs, and a "Delsarte Club" in "nearly every town in the country" (Williams 2004). The parallels with the yoga craze of the present day are not hard to spot. Stebbins partially trained the famed Ruth St. Denis, who in later years would market herself as a mystical Indian dancer (Srinivasan 2004). The self-appointed historian of American Delsartism, Ted Shawn, established a dance school with St. Denis "which produced a whole generation of [American] Oriental dancers" (Srinivasan 2004; Shawn n.d.). And Stebbins is undoubtedly the godmother of this generation.

The turn-of-the-century "Oriental dance" genre, pioneered by women like St. Denis and Maud Allen, was part of a more generalized assimilation of Asian-inspired techniques such as Transcendentalism, Theosophy, modern Vedānta, and, of course, yoga. The craze for Indian dancing did much to bolster the reputation and self-esteem of "indigenous" artists like Rukmini Devi and Uday Shankar, who (as Erdman 1987 and Srinivasan 2003 demonstrate) adopted many of the innovations of their Western impersonators in an ongoing operation of exchange and translation. Both sides claimed to be teaching and performing the original, authentic dance of India. Much the same can be said for yoga in the modern era, of course. Indeed, the same socioeconomic group of white, mainly Protestant women who lauded Vivekananda and enthusiastically took up the practice of yoga in their own homes (Syman 2003) was also dabbling in mystical dance. It was these women's endorsement of Vivekananda's yoga (which, as De Michelis 2004 has demonstrated, fed back to them a version of their very own esoteric convictions) which was instrumental in establishing Vivekananda as an authoritative spiritual and political voice in his homeland. As Peter van der Veer argues, Vivekananda's cultural nationalist project could not have emerged without his having devised classes on ancient Indian wisdom *for Bostonians*:

> This was one of the first and most important steps in systematizing "Indian spirituality" as a discipline for body and spirit, which has become so important in transnational spiritual movements of Indian origins. Vivekananda's success in the United States did not go unnoticed in India. He returned as a certified saint. (1994: 118)[4]

As is the case with dance, European and American yoga teachers who emerged at the same time claimed to be presenting the original, authentic yoga of India, in spite of many patent innovations. Yoga and Indian dance were in this sense both players in "a drama of appropriation and legitimation within a pan-South Asian framework of nationalist aspiration and cultural regeneration" (Allen 1997: 69) as well as dominant currencies of spiritual and cultural capital in the romanticized Asian marketplaces of the West.

From early on in yoga's "export" phase, American Delsartism was compared with yoga, particularly the *haṭha* variety. For example, in *Raja Yoga*, Vivekananda claims that many of the practices of *haṭha* yoga, "such as placing the body in different postures," are to be found in Delsarte (2001 [Vivekananda 1896]: 138). Ramacharaka—who, we should note, routinely plagiarizes Vivekananda—also affirms that in *haṭha* yoga postures, "there is nothing especially novel or new about their exercise, and they bear a very close resemblance to the calisthenic exercises and Delsarte movements in favor in the West" (1904: 192). Like Vivekananda, he judges such exercise forms negatively (and, as far as Stebbins's synthesis goes, wholly unjustifiably) as purely physical techniques that, unlike yoga, do not "use the mind in connection with the bodily movements" (192). Indeed, Delsarte's Law of Correspondence states that "to each spiritual function responds a function of the body. To each grand function of the body corresponds a spiritual act" (in Ruyter 1988: 63). The Frenchman's system is itself steeped in the embodied spirituality that Stebbins later elaborated to a high degree through

Western esotericism. This of course renders assertions such as Ramacharaka's (that Delsartism is purely physical, in contrast to yoga) wholly inaccurate but nonetheless characteristic of the type of allegation made by yoga writers of the period against Western "gymnastics." Note, finally, that Yogendra also cites Stebbins as an authority on relaxation in his *Yoga Asanas Simplified* of 1928 (156).

Stebbins's *Dynamic Breathing and Harmonic Gymnastics. A Complete System of Psychical, Aesthetic and Physical Culture* (1892) is a combination of callisthenic movement, deep respiration exercises, relaxation, and creative mental imagery within a harmonial religious framework. It is, in Stebbins's words, "a completely rounded system for the development of body, brain and soul; a system of training which shall bring this grand trinity of the human microcosm into one continuous, interacting unison" (57) and remove the "inharmonious mental states" (19) that lead to discord. Stebbins associates her own system of harmonial gymnastics with "the higher rhythmic gymnastics of the temple and sanctuary where magnetic power, personal grace and intellectual greatness were the chief objects sought" (21), and she presents her techniques as belonging to these primordial traditions of "religious training" (21). She combines Ling (sadly now "a purely physical training"), Delsarte, and influences "occult and mystic in their nature" (such as "oriental dance" and prayer) to produce "a life-giving, stimulating ecstasy upon the soul" (58). The gymnastics she describes in the book include, unsurprisingly, a good deal of Ling (such as lunging and weight distribution exercises), with an emphasis on spiraling motions and dance-like sequences. Although she makes reference to "several other exercises in use by the Brahmans of India and the dervishes of Arabia for energizing," she is of the opinion that they are too intricate to describe and should be learned directly from a teacher (133). A significant portion of the gymnastics section is given to "stretching exercises" (123–33) but, significantly, they are not explicitly linked by her to *yogāsana*.

Certain of her deep breathing techniques are, however, directly connected to *prāṇāyāma*, in particular "concentrated-will breathing" or "Yoga Breathing"—"so called because it is used by the Brahmins and Yogis of India" (Stebbins 1892: 86)—which involves imagining cosmic energy flowing into the hollow limbs of the body with the breath, "in one grand surging influx of dynamic life" (86). Although I am concerned principally here with posture, mystical breathing techniques are often inseparable from callisthenic exercise in the "harmonial gymnastics" model. It is therefore worth noting briefly (perhaps as a bookmark for future work) that Stebbins's popular system of "rhythmic breathing" is an important site of exchange for American harmonial beliefs and *haṭha* yoga *prāṇāyāma*. For example, what De Michelis (2004) refers to as

Vivekananda's "prāṇa model" in *Raja Yoga*—itself composed, it should be noted, at the geographical and chronological epicenter of the Delsarte craze—bears an arresting similarity to the diction and context of Stebbins's system. Vivekananda's American readers, that is to say, would have had a ready-made frame of reference with which to understand these esoteric "Indian" notions about the breath and its relationship to the cosmos. As B. Patra notes in his curious manual of esoterica and yoga of 1924, *The Mysteries of Nature*, deep breathing akin to *prāṇāyāma* had long been a "tried maxim" for "the spiritualists of America" (9): it is therefore hardly surprising that Vivekananda would adopt the diction of such enthusiasts in his explanation of *haṭha* yoga. I will go no further into this question at present. Suffice it to say that a mapping of "spiritualist" breathing techniques (in particular, "rhythmic breathing") and their relationship to *prāṇāyāma* within modern yoga, beginning with Vivekananda's model in *Raja Yoga*, would make a fascinating study of its own.[5]

Stebbins's "American Delsartean training regimen" included the following elements: relaxation exercises, posture work and "harmonic poise," breathing exercises, and "exercises for freedom of joints and spine" (Ruyter 1996: 71) and thus closely coincides with the elements of a standard postural yoga class in the West today. Stebbins's 1898 book *The Genevieve Stebbins System of Physical Training* is the first in which she focuses fully on movement. It includes dance-like flows and transitions between poses that are perhaps prototypical of the kind of "flow yoga" classes popular especially in the United States today. Prominent contemporary American yoga teacher Shiva Rea's extraordinary fusions of *āsana* and dance might well be considered late heirs of Stebbins's forms (see Rea 2006).

Stebbins's work spawned a number of similar systems, such as Annie Payson Call's course of mystical breath-work, "relaxationism," and gentle gymnastics of 1893. Although Stebbins is not acknowledged as the inspiration behind the content, Call's title, *Power through Repose*, is actually a phrase from Stebbins's book of the previous year (1892: 78), and the material differs little in content and exposition. Call's method, summarizes one commentator, is "mainly based on stretching and balancing movements which induce freedom from deep-seated and habitual tensions" (Caton 1936: xiv). I have written on Call at greater length elsewhere (Singleton 2005), but it is worth again mentioning the thesis I elaborated there: systems such as Call's and Stebbins's, based as they are on the principle of breath-work and muscular extension as a preparation for "spiritual" relaxation, were instrumental in paving the way for the popular conception of yoga as another means to *stretch and relax*.[6]

Glands for God: Cajzoran Ali

Writing and teaching in the generation after Stebbins, the self-styled American yoginī Cajzoran Ali (pseud.) is very much a product of the same harmonial gymnastic tradition within esoteric Protestantism. Born in 1903 in Memphis, according to Descamps (2004) she spent much of her youth in a wheelchair until she succeeded in curing herself through a system of posture training and prayer of her own devising. Descamps, who learned Ali's system from one of her original students near Toulouse in 1943, claims that she was not only the first person to teach yoga postures in the United States (in 1928) but also the first in France (in 1935). While such claims are overstated (this honor probably goes to Shri Yogendra who was demonstrating *āsana* in America from 1921), it is clear that Ali did exert a significant influence on the practice and theory of postural yoga in both countries. In her history of yoga in France, Sylvia Ceccomori notes that from 1935 Ali authored numerous articles on *haṭha* yoga in the various esoteric journals launched by the immensely prolific novelist, ethnographer, and psychoanalyst Maryse Choisy (1903–1979).[7] Ali's writings in these journals were generally accompanied (perhaps unsurprisingly) by photographs of *dancers* performing the postures (2001: 83).

Cajzoran Ali's method, as set out in her *Divine Posture Influence upon Endocrine Glands* of 1928,[8] locates the key to the ultimate spiritual truth of

FIFTH POSTURE

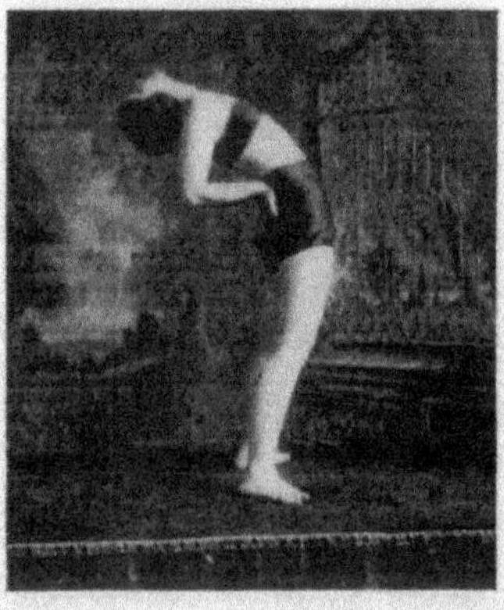

In taking this Posture you are to bend back slowly, keeping the knees firm, supporting the small of the back with palms of hands as illustrated and stretching throat, abdomen and thigh muscles as much as they will give. A wonderful posture for obesity and double chin.

Do not force your body to the point at any time. With faithful practice you will arrive there and feel greatly benefited by doing so. Never be in a hurry.

Fifth Posture from Cajzoran Ali 1928

yoga—and also, disconcertingly, of the biblical Apocalypse—in the individual body. In particular, the "ductless glands" are conceived as "the agents through which changes in our spiritual bodies are brought about" (1928: 7) and are identified simultaneously with the "lotuses" (i.e., *cakras*) of yoga, the anatomical glands, and the "seals" of the Apocalypse.

Her course of posture training and "Breath Culture" is designed to align these "seals" and thereby to bring one into harmony with the God who is "individualised within you" (15). This "harmonial" *haṭha* model is an important early precursor of New Age versions of (postural) yoga that emerged in the West from the 1970s onward (De Michelis 2004: 184–86). Ali's focus on women's health, aesthetic appearance, and spiritual advancement also situates it firmly

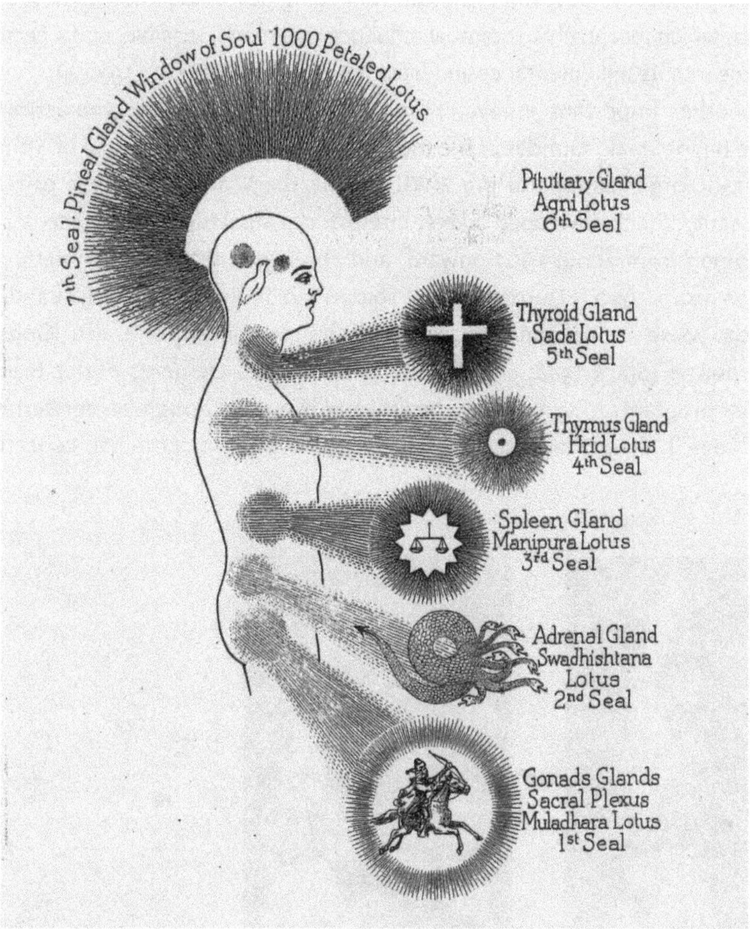

Cakras and Seals, Cajzoran Ali 1928

within the dominant discourse of women's gymnastics of the time (discussed further below).

Harmonial Gymnastics in Britain

Breath-work and gymnastics in the harmonial mode of Stebbins, Call, and Ali also gained popularity in Britain thanks to the efforts of influential advocates like Frances Archer, who studied directly with Call in the 1890s and subsequently (from about 1910 onward) promoted her brand of stretching, balancing, and relaxing for spiritual benefit. The wife of prominent Bloomsbury translator and indo-phobe William Archer (see Archer 1918), Frances was well placed to disseminate the technique learned from Call in the 1890s. Like Call, she did not consider the exercises mere medical gymnastics but rather "a means of finding peace and freedom of soul and body by which receptivity to spiritual influence was made possible, and a personality came into its full inheritance and became a 'channel'" (Caton 1936: 5).

Another important innovator in the field of harmonial gymnastics was Mollie Bagot Stack, founder of the most far-reaching and influential of women's gymnastic organizations in pre-WWII Britain, the Women's League of Health and Beauty. Stack developed a keen interest in gymnastic and hygiene regimes for women from about 1907 onward, and she began teaching her methods in London from 1920.[9] During a 1912 sojourn in India with her husband, she learned some *āsanas* and relaxation techniques from one Mr. Gopal in Landsdowne (Stack 1988: 68) and later incorporated elements of this teaching into her programs of gymnastics, health, and hygiene (though never referring to it as "yoga"). Stack's agenda, like Stebbins's, evinces a combined concern for

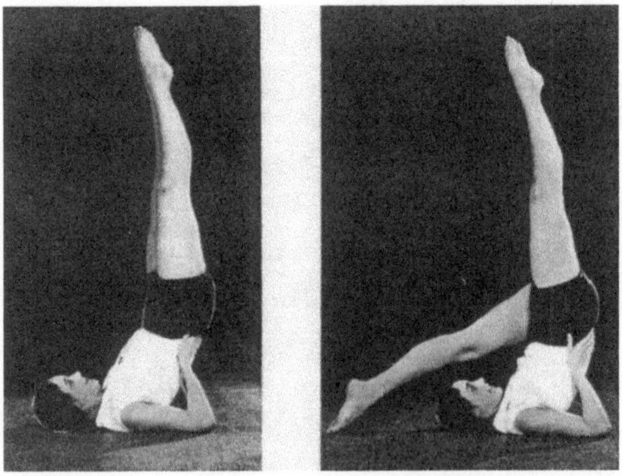

"Legs in Air," from Stack 1931

body aesthetics, health, and embodied spiritual growth. Her 1931 book *Building the Body Beautiful, The Bagot Stack Stretch-and-Swing System* places a marked emphasis on the method's cosmetic value since, as she puts it, "in her heart of hearts, this slim-through-look is instinctively and quite rightly desired by every normal woman" (Stack 1931: 12). Alongside the promise of vibrant health and conventional physical attractiveness, though, Stack stresses the mystical purpose of the exercises, which are deemed to induce equilibrium between body, mind, and universe. By carefully following the regime prescribed, she asserts, a woman "can bring herself into harmony with the great mysterious forces around her, and acquire an inner power which will carry her triumphantly through the rough places of life" (2). The more the body is trained in accord with Nature, she continues, "the more shall we set free the body's dormant powers of expressing

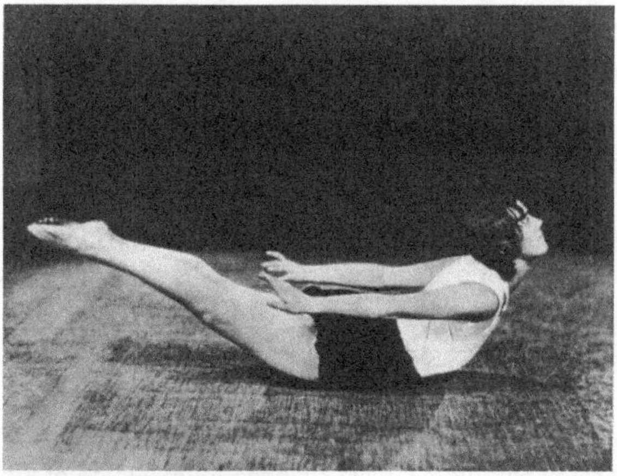

"Seal," from Stack 1931

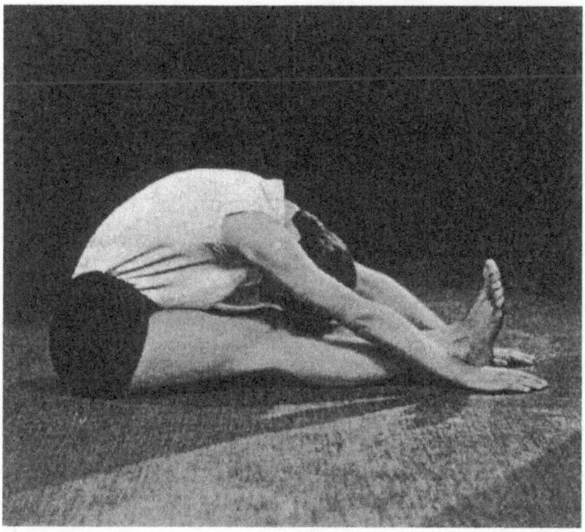

"Swing Forward," from Stack 1931[10]

in itself the rhythm of the Universe which welds all nature, and that includes human nature, into one beautiful whole" (4). This rhythm, moreover, "is the secret of personal magnetism" (3). The diction as well as the message is that of Stebbins and Call, and more generally of mesmeric-influenced nature religion and the Protestant harmonialism identified by Ahlstrom.

What seems clear is that the breathing, stretching, and relaxation classes attended every week by thousands of twenty-first-century Londoners *as yoga* recapitulate the spiritualized gymnastics undertaken by their grandmothers and great-grandmothers in the 1930s. There can be no doubt that Stack's incorporation of *āsanas* into a combined program of dynamic stretches, rhythmic breathing, and relaxation within a "harmonial" context closely mirrors the creative modulations of many of today's "hatha yoga" classes. As already noted, the term "hatha yoga" is routinely used among London's postural yoga teachers and practitioners today to indicate a generic, nondenominational, and eclectic system of *gentle* postural practice and to distinguish it from "named" brands like Iyengar, Ashtanga, or Sivananda. Postural yoga teachers who profess to teach "hatha yoga" will usually creatively combine postures, sometimes in flowing sequences, and invent poses of their own (a far less common occurrence in the "branded" forms like Iyengar). As contemporary posture teacher Dharma Mitra puts it, "even today dozens of new poses are created each year by true yogis all over the world" (2003: 13). A compelling explanation of the often radical dissimilarity of such systems from "classical" *haṭha* yoga is that they stem, to a large extent, from "modern traditions" such as Stack's.

League women did not consider themselves to be doing yoga, but the form and purpose of today's practices—still commonly conceived within a health and beauty paradigm—have changed little, a state of affairs that may go some way to explaining why "hatha" yoga in the West tends to attract predominantly female students. The fitness-oriented yoga available in virtually every health club in London today, that is to say, may represent a direct historical succession from those regimes of New Age,[11] quasi-mystical body conditioning and callisthenics devised exclusively for women in the first half of the twentieth century. Although these regimes generally lacked the trappings of "spiritual India" that we find today, the form and content remain strikingly similar.

German Gymnastik and the Somatics Movement

Brief reference should also be made here to the extensive field of "somatics" which, according to Jeffrey Kripal, draws its *philosophical* rationale from European phenomenology but which has deeper *historical* roots in the turn-of-the-century

German *Gymnastik* movement (2007: 229). This largely female movement is germane to what I call the harmonial gymnastics tradition of America and Britain (it is no coincidence, for example, that one of the figures most closely associated with *Gymnastik*, Hede Kallmeyer, was, like Stebbins, trained by François Delsarte [229]). *Gymnastik* offered an alternative to the macho, militaristic physical education that predominated in schools and "prized awareness and consciousness above all else" (229). It offered a holistic worldview centered on "the spiritualization of the flesh" and "the union of 'body' and 'soul' as the most reliable source of wholeness and health" (229). Like most forms of Somatics, it invoked the "models of subtle life-energy that bridge or, perhaps better, violate the usual boundaries between what we today call *religion* and *science* or, alternately, *spirituality* and *medicine*" (229). These models have their roots in European Mesmerism and have, as De Michelis (2004) demonstrates, substantially influenced the shape of "Modern Yoga" via Vivekananda's "*prāṇa* model" of yoga practice.

While it takes us beyond the historical parameters of this study, we might also briefly note that Somatics continued to interact with twentieth-century international yoga through the development of psychoanalytic bodywork in the tradition of Wilhelm Reich (1897–1957) by way of disciples such as Alexander Lowen. While Reich himself was dismissive of yoga,[12] Lowen explicitly incorporated *āsana* and *prāṇāyāma* into his therapeutic work. For example, the practical exercises in Lowen and Lowen (1977) are explicitly derived from *āsana* and *prāṇāyāma*, with many of them identical to the prop-assisted postures of Iyengar yoga. Bodywork discourses stemming from Reich and Lowen are today extremely pervasive in international postural yoga, often thanks to the contributions of post-hippie era teachers such as Tony Crisp. A 1971 review of Crisp's popular book *Yoga and Relaxation* (Crisp 1970), for instance, states that it is "the first book that has related the importance of the findings of Wilhelm Reich's psycho-analytic research to Yoga and his techniques of relaxation" (n.a.).[13] Thirty-five years later, conflations of Reichianism with yoga are commonplace, and notions of their shared function in human development are rarely challenged. The clearest example of Reichian procedures in postural yoga today is the "Phoenix Rising" style of psychoanalytic *āsana* work, in which clients dialogue with the analyst/teacher while holding supported yoga postures (Lee 2005).[14]

Yoga in Mainstream Western Physical Culture

> The motto of the "Health and Strength" League, "sacred thy Body even as thy Soul," might well be the first lesson in *Hatha Yoga*.
>
> (Hannah 1933a: 153)

> Yogic physical culture is now no longer esoteric. Instead of being exclusively practised by Yogis it has become popular among persons with no particular spiritual aims. Formerly it used to be practised as the first step and fundamental part of spiritual life.... But in modern times Yogic physical culture has escaped from the cloistered boundaries of the hermitage into the larger world.
>
> (Muzumdar 1937a: 861)

The ground was prepared in the West for the reinterpretation of yoga as physical culture by regimens of exercise and breath-work that overlapped to varying extents with *āsana* and *prāṇāyāma*. Into the cultural space carved by harmonial bodywork and the various permutations of post-Lingian medical gymnastics came the new model of yoga, developed in earnest from 1920 onward by Yogendra, Kuvalayananda, and the other *āsana* pioneers examined in this and the previous chapter. Modern *āsana* practice emerged in a dialectical relationship to physical culture and harmonial gymnastics: it absorbed many of these teachings, claimed them as its own, and sold them back to the Western readership as the purest expression of Indian physical culture. In this final section I wish to consider on the one hand the reception and interpretation of yoga, and on the other the various exercise regimes designated specifically for women in the most popular pre-WWII British physical culture magazine, *Health and Strength* (hereafter H&S), the mouthpiece of the national Health and Strength League.[15]

My intention is to demonstrate that what appears in H&S during the 1930s under the name of "yoga" actually resembles the "stretch-and-relax" modalities of postural modern yoga today far less than the *standard, secular women's gymnastics* of the time (also regularly represented in the magazine). Importantly, these women's gymnastics are never identified as yoga: what would be a nigh self-evident association for today's "hatha" practitioners is simply not made in the 1930s. This supports the hypothesis that postural modern yoga displaced—or was the cultural successor of—the established methods of stretching and relaxing that had already become commonplace in the West, through harmonial gymnastics and female physical culture. Indeed, one might expect that a periodical whose primary concern was bodybuilding and gymnastics would immediately latch onto the acrobatic and gymnastic potential of yoga and highlight this above other aspects. The fact that it doesn't suggests that during the 1920s and 1930s the genre of athletic *āsana* was not yet "export-ready." Remember that modern *āsana* was, at this stage, still very much in its infancy—for instance, the man behind some of the most influential forms of international postural yoga today, T. Krishnamacharya, was just beginning to teach the youngsters, like

Iyengar and Pattabhi Jois, who would in later decades popularize *āsana* in the West (see chapter 9).

Let us first consider discussion of yoga in H&S during the 1930s. When the topic does arise, yoga is generally treated with respect and credulity. Senior editor and in-house arbiter of taste T. W. Standwell, for instance, admires the "super-psycho-mental culture" of yoga, which can render men "veritable super beings" (Standwell 1934: 32) and speculates that it should be possible for "any reader to develop powers of which he has scarcely ever yet dreamed, by means of scientifically devised physical culture" (32; see also Physician 1933). Yoga, in other words, can be harnessed to the eugenically inclined project of nationalist man-building. As is predominantly the case in practical yoga manuals, this "physical culture" he refers to is actually *prāṇāyāma*, with the function of posture merely to provide a stable and still basis for this work. To this end, readers are advised to study the seated Buddha statue in the Victoria and Albert Museum in London. Also mentioned positively in this article is the businessman and banker Sir David Yule, who "preferred the company and conversation of Hindus, to those of Europeans" and practiced yoga assiduously (Standwell 1934: 20).

A similar picture is presented by H. Broom's transparently entitled article "Age-Old Physical Culture of the East. Even Modern Physical Culturists Can Learn Not a Little from the Yogis" (1934a). While he does associate the "disciple of the Yoga principle" with the quality of "wonderful suppleness" (738), the distinct impression conveyed by the article is that yoga involves sitting motionless for long periods of time, practicing *prāṇāyāma* and meditation. The most sustained considerations of the topic in the magazine during the 1930s is Cameron Hannah's series of five articles on *haṭha* yoga entitled "Health Wisdom of the East" (1933a–e). This highly medicalized vision of yoga similarly pays scant attention to *āsana*. The five articles comprise (1) a general introduction, (2) a consideration of the importance of *prāṇa* and the breath, (3) food and diet, (5) yogic principles of exercise and their application "in combination with the methods of our own physical culturists" (239), and (6) a sermon on sexual mores. In substance, they are of a piece with the magazine's staple weekly advice on holistic health, hygiene, and personal morality, and (as the epigraph to this section suggests) effect an explicit rapprochement between yoga and the general ideological League goal. The asseverations on sex, for example, are entirely in keeping with magazine's general moral policy on the matter. "The return of decent 'home life' would," asserts Hannah, "do much to destroy the canker of sex" (1933e: 269). Yoga can help to "sweep away the sex fetishism which has of late years engulfed the Western hemisphere" (269). Moral pronouncements such as these (which can go so far as recommending that mothers inculcate in their daughters a sense of shame for their genitals—Partington

1933) are ambiguously juxtaposed in the pages of H&S with undeniably erotic photographs of naked men and women, often in the form of advertisements for the naturist sister magazine *Health and Efficiency*. As Foucault (1979) has demonstrated, Victorian and post-Victorian public condemnations of sex mask society's private fascination with and indulgence in it, and such is clearly the case here.

Much of the teaching of *haṭha* yoga, adjudges Hannah, "is impractical and, indeed, impossible to the Western" (Hannah 1933a: 153), and his is an explicitly tailored version of it. In the fourth article, on yogic exercise, Hannah points out that "while there are no exercises in Hatha Yoga intended for physical development alone, there are *principles* which, when applied in combination with the methods of our own physical culturists, yield very definite results" (Hannah 1933d: 239). Like Sundaram and Iyer, Hannah culls what is useful in yoga and recontextualizes it within physical culture. As one might expect, he first describes some free-standing Ling-type gymnastics and callisthenics and then outlines weights-free "muscle growing" techniques of the kind commonly encountered in H&S (e.g., L. E. Eubanks, "Mind and Muscle" of April 1934) and which derive from the tradition of the early mind/body muscle techniques of Maxick and Haddock examined above.

Hannah accounts for the sense of déjà-vu that many readers may experience at this point by what should by now be a familiar story: "there is more Hatha Yoga in some of our western systems than you might imagine" and many Western physical culture exercises actually "originated in the East" (239). This account of the Asian origin of Western physical culture is of course a pervasive narrative in Indian physical culture, as we saw with K. Ramamurthy (chapter 5 above), but it is significant that it also makes its appearance in the mainstream British physical culture media. It is reiterated frequently in the pages of H&S, such as in the promotional articles on Indian yoga, wrestling, and bodybuilding written by Kuvalayananda disciple and physical culture commentator S. Muzumdar (see Muzumdar 1937a, b, c, and "Scandinavian Gymnastics" in chapter 4 above).

While parallels and overlaps with "classical" yoga procedures are certainly present,[16] Hannah's is a version of yoga radically adapted for a bodybuilding, fitness-conscious readership on the lookout for new ways of improving their physiques. For example, the stylized pose of the naked, oiled, and muscular Moti R. Patel of Secundarabad, which graces Hannah's introductory article (captioned "The Result of the Scientific Health Culture of the East"), unambiguously foregrounds the use-value of yoga in body conditioning. It also suggests that the message of the new Indian physical culturist yogis was by this stage percolating into Western health regimes *as yoga*. Indeed, this is hardly surprising when one

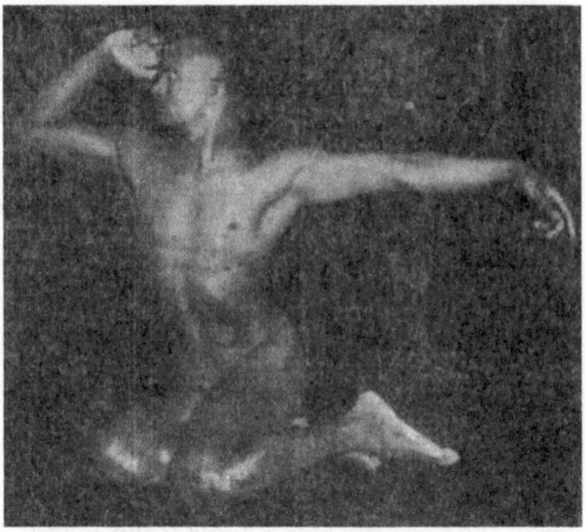

Moti R. Patel, pictured in Hannah 1933a

considers that the international poster boys of "yogic" Indian bodybuilding, Iyer and Balsekar, as well as many lesser known Indian musclemen, are regularly pictured in H&S during this period. India was emerging on the international physical culture scene as a force to be reckoned with, and yoga was often assumed to be a component part of this emergence.

Women's Stretching Regimes

Now, while Hannah, like Broom, notes that *haṭha* yoga "will give you suppleness" as well as a pleasing physique (1933d: 239), the exercises he describes *simply bear no likeness to the stretching regimes of modern postural yoga*. Indeed, among the articles on yoga in H&S (or in its sister magazine *The Superman*) during the 1930s, none outlines a course of bodily extensions of the kind one would expect to find in a modern "hatha yoga" class today: if such articles are to be found, they are scarce. On the other hand, the magazine *is* replete with exercise schema designed exclusively for women and which *are* based to a very large extent on stretching. But these are not designated as, nor associated with, yoga. Bertram Ash's piece in the regular H&S feature "Mainly for the Ladies," entitled "Building the Body Beautiful. S-T-R-E-T-C-H Your Way to Figure Perfection" (1934: 170), is exemplary of the kind of regimens that (male) physical culture journalists usually prescribed for women, in contrast to the acrobatic, balancing, and weight-resistance programs for men. Outlined therein are positions that would be very familiar to modern postural yoga practitioners as part of the modern *āsana* lexicon (e.g., *śalabhāsana, paśchimottanāsana*, and *trikonāsana*, in the nomenclature of Iyengar 1966), but which are conspicuously absent from the yoga articles.

In a revealing polemic of 1937, entitled "The Truth about Suppleness," Frank Miles fulminates against the growing stretching fad, noting that "women are the worst offenders, and are often to be found working painfully through a schedule that consists exclusively of 'suppling exercises'" (572). His article is a good indication of the extent to which stretching dominated the world of women's physical education well prior to the post-WWII *āsana* boom in the West. Indeed, women are almost always pictured in H&S performing stretches while men are more likely to be seen executing acrobatic balances (resembling Iyengar's *adhomukhavṛkṣāsana, pincamayūrāsana*, or *bakāsana*), tumbles, or "classical" muscular poses. The articles dedicated to children's physical education, incidentally, also tend to foreground flexibility, along with vigorous gymnastics similar to those of the Dane Niels Bukh (see Ash 1935 and Gymnast 1934). Ash even uses Bukh's standard commands, such as "prone falling." It will be important to bear this fact in mind in chapter 9, where I suggest that the modern "power yoga" styles that derive from T. Krishnamacharya's innovations in the 1930s are a synthesis of Bukh-inspired children's gymnastics and yoga.

Clayton's 1930 article for H&S, "Eve's Ideal Path to Grace, Health and Fitness," represents women of the "Silver League" performing a number of stretches that correspond closely to modern *haṭha* yoga postures. This regime, he notes, is a mixture of Müller gymnastics and "the ordinary type of Swedish free movements, but each action is combined together to form a sequence of rhythmic movements" (315), a description that would cover most aspects of the "*haṭha* flow" genre of yoga classes taught today, particularly in American health clubs. But again, in H&S the exercises are not associated with yoga in this context.

The co-holder of the title "Best Figure in the British Isles [1930]," Miss Adonia Wallace, to take another (visually arresting) example, claimed to have acquired her prize-winning physique through extreme stretching exercises, such as are pictured. These "exercises" are instantly recognizable as the advanced postures of postural modern yoga (H&S, July 1935). They are, to use Iyengar's (1966) terms, *ekapāda rājakapotāsana I* (top left), *ūrdhva dhanurāsana* (top right), *eka pāda viparīta daṇḍāsana* (lower middle), and two variants of *naṭarājāsana* (lower left and right).

It appears, then, that women during the 1930s commonly engaged in much the same forms of bodily activity that they do today under the name of yoga and that stretching itself has a popular history of its own in the West, entirely independent of yoga. As far back as 1869, indeed, Archibald Maclaren (himself, like Miles, hostile to "excessive" stretching regimes) had noted that suppleness exercises were becoming an established part of British and European physical culture. Although, he observes, it is the French system that lays the greatest emphasis on exercises "propres à l'assouplissement," there is a widespread and

"Exercises Which Gave Me Fame"
Six of the movements used by "the Girl with the Perfect Figure"

Adonia Wallace, "Best Figure in the British Isles," *Health and Strength*, July 1935

growing recognition of "this idea, shared at home as well as abroad, by civilian as well as soldier, of the necessity of suppling a man before strengthening him" (1869: 82). The principle of stretching was an integral part of the modern Western physical culture revival from the mid-nineteenth century onward and became increasingly associated (at least in the early twentieth century) with women's gymnastics. Bickerdike 1934, "The Importance of Correct Posture," and Stanley 1937, "Try Stretching for Strength," are exemplary of this trend. The gender division established at the dawn of modern physical culture between regimens aiming at (masculine) strength and vigor on the one hand and those that sought to cultivate (feminine) grace and ease of movement on the other persists throughout the twentieth century and into the twenty-first. The dichotomy is not always

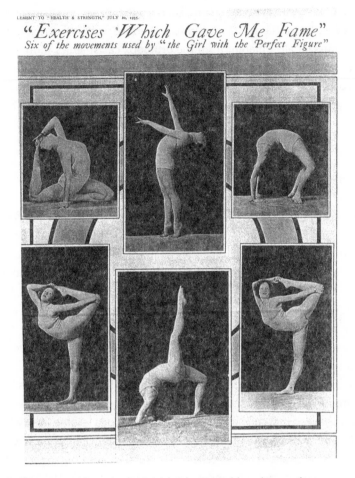

hard and fast: as we have seen, men also engaged in "suppling exercises," and women often broke the gender mold to undertake arduous, strength-building regimes substantially different from the orthodox callisthenics format (particularly interesting here is the case of Dio Lewis. See Todd 1998). However, in spite of these departures, women's exercise came increasingly to signify a program of stretching and rhythmic gymnastics, often with a strong component of "spirituality" of the kind preached by Stebbins, Call, and Stack.

Gendered Yogas?

The dichotomy between men's and women's physical activities in H&S carries forward a gender division formalized in the earliest expressions of modern European gymnastics, in which men are primarily concerned with strength and vigor while women are expected to cultivate physical attractiveness and graceful movement (see Todd 1998: 89). In the early modern Olympics, indeed, the main criteria for the adoption of a women's event were whether the sport was "aesthetically pleasing" and displayed the female body advantageously (Mitchell 1977: 213–14). The women's fitness articles in H&S, inevitably authored by men, exhibit a similar concern.

Insofar as this gendered format of modern sports and gymnastics has been transmitted into international *haṭha* yoga in the twentieth century, we can differentiate between masculinized forms of postural yoga issuing from a "muscular Christian," nationalistic, and martial context (see chapters 4 and 5), and harmonial "stretch and relax" varieties of postural yoga stemming from the synthesis of women's gymnastics and para-Christian mysticism. The former group, which foregrounds strength, classical ideals of manliness, and (often) the religio-patriotic cultivation of brawn, is exemplified by bodybuilders such as Iyer and Ghosh, freedom-fighting yogis such as Tiruka, the early (pre-Pondichery) Aurobindo, and Manick Rao. It is also the dominant form in certain present-day "militant" yoga regimes, such as those of the Hindu cultural nationalist organization, the RSS (see Alter 1994; McDonald 1999).

On the other hand, gentler stretching, deep breathing, and "spiritual" relaxation colloquially known in the West today as "hatha yoga" are best exemplified by the variants of harmonial gymnastics developed by Stebbins, Payson Call, Cajzoran Ali, Stack, and others—as well as the stretching regimes of secular women's physical culture with which they overlap. In practice, however, this is at best a heuristic division, since postural modern yoga forms rarely fit exclusively into one category or the other. It does, however, furnish a framework for thinking through the influences behind varieties of postural styles at large today.

My intention in this chapter has been to demonstrate that there were firmly established exercise traditions in the West that included forms and modes of practice virtually indistinguishable from certain variants of "hatha yoga" now popularly taught in America and Europe. As a result, the sheer number of positions and movements that could be thenceforth classified as *āsana* swelled considerably and continues to do so. For example, both Bühnemann (2007a) and Sjoman (1996) point out the absence of standing postures in premodern *āsana* descriptions. The overlap of standing *āsanas* and modern gymnastics is extensive enough to suggest that virtually all of them are late additions to the yoga canon through postural yoga's dialogical relationship with modern physical culture. The same hypothesis extends beyond the standing poses to the multitude of apparently new *āsana* forms.

Jan Todd argues that "woven throughout the multitude of exercise prescriptions for twentieth-century women can be found most of the basic principles of early nineteenth-century purposive training [i.e., health and fitness regimes]" (Todd 1998: 295). In much the same way, within the regimes that today pass for "hatha yoga" we can discern the thematic and formal persistence of a long and varied tradition of gymnastics, and in particular those systems intended "mainly for the ladies."[17] The genealogy of this exchange interests me less, however, than the way in which the assumptions and associations that cleave to particular postures and exercises superimpose themselves on their "foreign" counterparts. So, for example, a contorted body knot designed to be a component part of the *kuṇḍalinī*-raising project of *haṭha* yoga can, through this superimposition, be reborn as a suppling exercise for health and beauty. In this way corporal postures become "floating signifiers" whose meaning is determined according to context (see Urban [2003: 23–25] on the "floating signifier" of *Tantra*). When the same posture is re-presented in Western postural yoga, the traces of both contexts remain, although typically the *haṭha* context is but vaguely understood (if at all).

The example of the inverted *viparīta karaṇī mudrā* (and the more perpendicular "shoulder stand" pose *sarvaṅgāsana*) is a case in point. There is no doubt that such inversions constitute a component part of medieval *haṭha* yoga. This position, said to be "a secret in all the Tantras" (*sarvatantreṣu gopitā*, *Gheraṇḍa Saṃhitā* 3.32), reverses the flow of the solar and lunar energies of the body such that the endogenous elixir (*amṛta*) that drips from the "moon" (located at the palate) is not consumed by the "sun" (located at the navel), thereby warding off mortal decrepitude. A mirror image of this posture, however, figures prominently in Ling gymnastics and is commonly referred to as "the Swedish Candle." So familiar was this posture to the British reading public of the 1930s that it serves as the line-drawn icon accompanying H&S's "Mainly for the Ladies" features. Although also associated with rejuvenation in this context, what the posture connotes in the *Gheraṇḍa Saṃhitā* and what it means in the pages of H&S are of course radically different. When yoga is presented for Western readers in publications such as these, the poses themselves are wrenched from their *haṭha* orbit by the greater contextual gravity of physical culture and, as S. Muzumdar phrases it with regard to *sarvāṅgāsana* and *śīrṣāsana* (headstand), are "interpreted in the language of modern gymnastics" for the benefit of readers (Muzumdar 1937a: 861). This posture is still referred to in German modern yoga classes as "die Kerze," and in Italy as "la Candela," undoubtedly due to the influence of Swedish gymnastics.

8

The Medium and the Message: Visual Reproduction and the *Āsana* Revival

> When many people from Western countries come to this Yogaśālā funded by the Maharaja, taking photos of *yogāsanas* and exhibiting them in their countries, we can no longer keep quiet and allow *yogāsanas* to be petrified in stone.
>
> (T. Krishnamacharya, *Yogāsanagalu* c. 1941 [in Jacobsen and Sundaram (trans.) 2006: 6])

> For health to be known, it must be seen.
>
> —(Bernarr MacFadden, cited in Whalan 2003: 600)

The phenomenon of international posture-based yoga would not have occurred without the rapid expansion of print technology and the cheap, ready availability of photography. Furthermore, yoga's expression through such media fundamentally changed the perception of the *yoga body* and the perceived function of yoga practice. These propositions rest on the assumption that photography (and the text that accompanies it) is by no means an objective medium reflecting what is simply "there" but an active structuring process through which society and "reality" are themselves endowed with meaning (Barthes and Howard 1981; Burgin, 1982). They are based also on the observation that postural yoga came fully into the public eye only when it was visually represented, most significantly through photography. I take this chronological coincidence less as a process of post factum documentation (i.e., a "transparent" setting down in images of what was already there) than as a *bringing forth* of the modern yoga body. Technologies are never simply inventions people use but means by which they—and their bodies—are reinvented (McLuhan 1962). The yoga body was not an apparition ex nihilo, of course, nor without precursors, but in a very clear way the photographic and *naturalistic* representation of the (generally male) physique performing yoga postures facilitated the creation and popularization of a new kind of body, culturally located within the Hindu renaissance and world physical culturism. Before we consider specific examples of this process within yoga, it will be helpful to briefly survey the function and status of photography in history more generally and the impact that it had not only on perceptions of the body but also on the structuring of subjectivity and reality themselves. I draw my account mainly from John Pultz's *Photography and the Body* (1995).

Pultz argues that photography stands as the very metonym of the empirically driven Enlightenment, which prized sensory evidence as the principal means of understanding human reality. Photography represented "the perfect Enlightenment tool, functioning like human sight to offer empirical knowledge mechanically, objectively, without thought or emotion" (1995: 8). Through photography the world was captured and laid flat, readied for inspection and classification. The popularization of photography—and in particular, portraiture—also brought about a revolution in *social* consciousness, with a whole generation of people seeing, often for the first time, pictorial representations of their own bodies (13). Such images, argues Pultz, radically altered the status of the human body within society and brought a self-conscious, self-observing, and corporeally aware European middle class into existence (17). It is important to remember alongside this that photography was at the same time the "perfect tool" of Empire, serving as an (apparently) objective, expedient method for the ethnographic cataloguing of subject peoples in the interests of "scientific" anthropology. In 1869, for example, the distinguished evolutionary biologist and president of the Ethnological Society, T. H. Huxley, was asked by the Colonial Office of Great Britain to devise instructions for the "formation of a systematic series of photographs of the various races of men comprehended within the British Empire" (Pultz 1995: 24). These photos were to be used to classify and establish fixed racial types, and (often explicitly) to consolidate the superiority of the white European races. Thanks to *commercial* photography, also, postcards of exotic human curios from around the colonial globe—including, of course, the kind of "fakir" snaps considered in chapter 3—became popular in the drawing rooms of Europe from the 1850s onward and were used "for the fetishistic collecting, controlling, and defining of the bodies of native inhabitants of newly colonized lands" (21).

Photography, in brief, was part of the apparatus of commercial and cultural domination that defined Empire. It could operate simultaneously as a mode of control and power over the colonial "other" and as an expression of personal and collective identity set in opposition to that other. As a vital locus of power, then, photography was to become a hotly contested medium for those colonial subjects who would assert their own identities and their own vision of their bodies against the demeaning visual narratives of foreign ethnography and casual voyeurism. As Narayan (1993) puts it, such photographs remind us that what is supposedly objective "in fact derives from a positioned gaze that highlights, circumscribes, and is implicated in a system of power-laden social relations" (485; see also Pinney 2003). In India, one of the key forums in which this struggle took place was the area of physical culture. The international physical culture movement was itself only possible thanks to mass produced, mass circulated images of the predominantly male body. Physical culture in India was no exception. Photography lent an unprecedented primacy to the imaged body, resulting in an overt, widespread concern for its cultivation. The body was brought to the center of public attention to a degree that had not been possible before. In this way, photographs of Indian bodies became powerful documents with which to refute the Western ethnographic case for Indian degeneracy and to assert the powerful, immediate and self-evident spectacle of national strength (see chapter 5). The pages of Indian periodicals such as *Vyayam, the Bodybuilder* and books by physical culture luminaries like Ghose, Bhopatkar, and Ramamurthy are crammed with such images, which bespeak the nationalist project of citizen building. Often, as in Bhopatkar's book of 1928, *yogāsanas* are a component part of this project.

Postural yoga was construed, popularized, and made possible within this visual context. If new *āsana* forms began to gain popularity in the mid-1920s, it was as a result of the representation of Indian bodies in the kind of mass-produced primers and journals that flourished alongside comparable physical culture material. One perhaps rather obvious point to be made here is that modern postural yoga *required* visual representation in a way that more "mental"

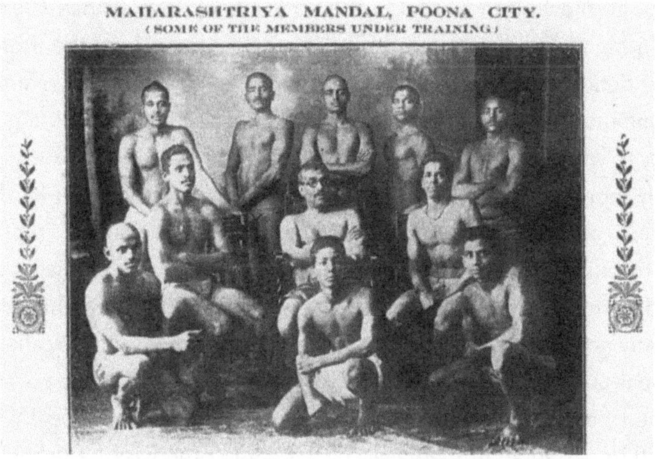

Bhopatkar and His Students, 1928

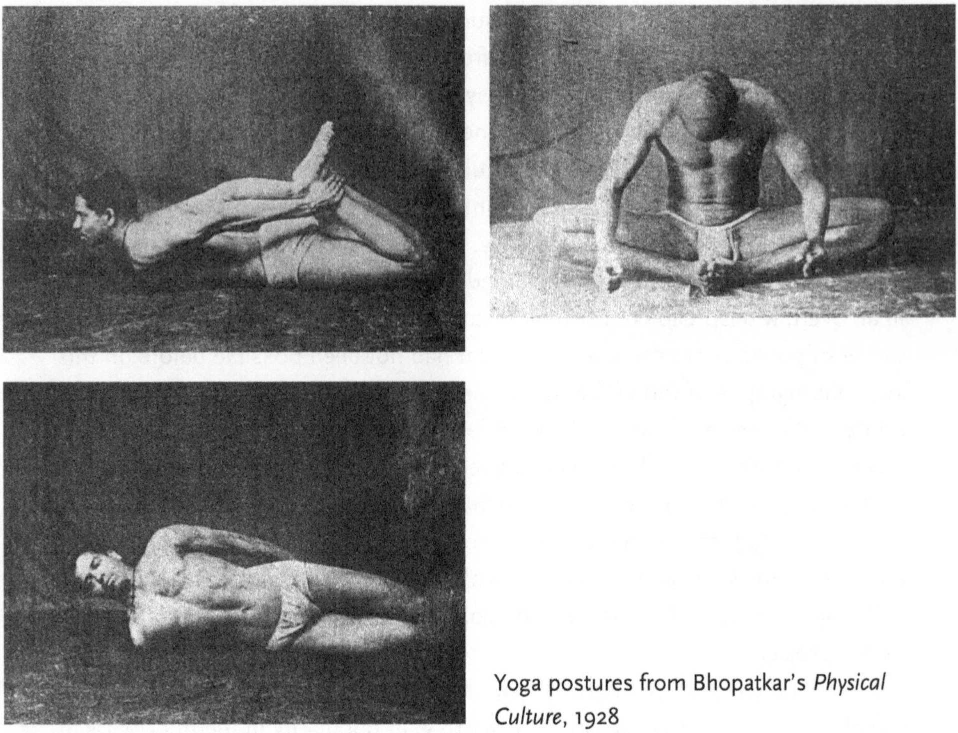

Yoga postures from Bhopatkar's *Physical Culture*, 1928

forms of modern yoga did not. To take but one example: Vivekananda's *Raja Yoga*, which openly shuns *āsanas*, does not lose much from a complete absence of visual images—the message is fairly effectively (if not always cogently) conveyed through the written word. On the other hand, Kuvalayananda's *āsanas* of 1931 would be a far duller, more difficult to follow book were the motions and postures it details not supported with clear, visual, photographic references.

The coda to this point is that, conversely, the new visual culture gave *popular primacy* to what could be represented through images—a book with pictures was simply more appealing (and accessible) than one without. As Partha Mitter emphasizes, print technology and processes of mechanical reproduction effected profound shifts in Indian sensibilities, "turning urban India into a 'visual society,' dominated by the printed image" (1994: 120). Guha-Thakurta (1992: 111) similarly notes the "general preponderance of photographic, realistic values in the visual tastes of the time." One of the main reasons that postural yoga itself gained popularity is the simple fact that it had visual appeal within this society and imparted an immediacy to what could otherwise be (when confined to textual exposition) an opaque, perplexing subject. The yoga body was brought

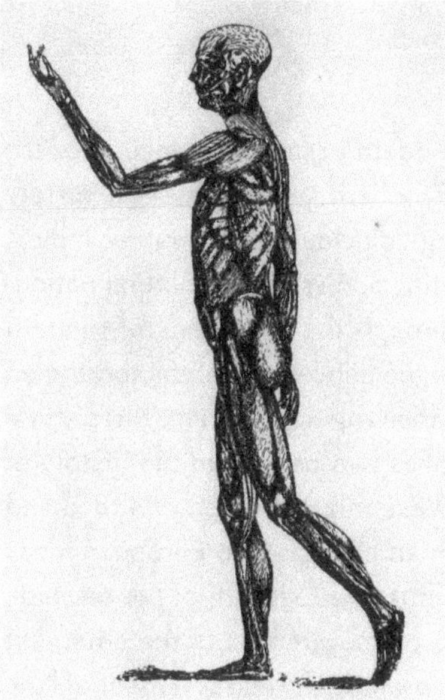

FIG. 2.—The Muscles.

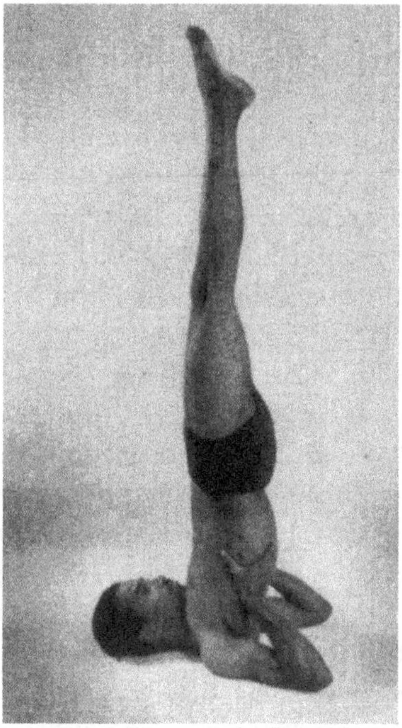

Anatomical Drawing from Kuvalayananda's *Āsanas*(1972) [1931]) (with permission of Kaivalyadhama Institute)
Shoulderstand from Kuvalayananda's *Āsanās* (1972 [1931]) (with permission of Kaivalyadhama Institute)

into the light. These specular representation of yoga postures in mechanically reproduced, modern photographic primers laid the "yoga body" out for objective scrutiny (and emulation) in an unprecedented way. The yogic body, as it shifted from the private into the public sphere, was thus transformed from the conceptual, ritual, "entextualised" body (Flood 2006) of tantric *haṭha* to the perceptual and *naturalistic* body of scientific modern anglophone yoga. Yoga—or rather a particular, modern variant of *haṭha* yoga—began to be charted and documented through photography with something like the "objective stance of the pathologist" (Budd 1997: 59), much in the same way that Dayananda set out to investigate the body of (*haṭha*) yoga through the dissection of a corpse. Both projects start out with the assumption that modern and "traditional" ways of knowing conduce to a single, unitary reality and that the former can therefore be used to prove (or disprove) the validity of the latter. In this way, the rise of the modern, photographic yogic body effected the illusion of continuity with the *haṭha* tradition while in fact constituting an epistemological break from it.

Tradition and Modernity in Indian Art

As the most visually appealing facet of the modern yoga renaissance, modern *āsana* invites comparison with a history of modern Indian art. This history evinces parallels that are not simply engaging coincidences but rather indications of common ideological strategies operating across Hindu cultural nationalism; as such, they may help us to think through the conditions of modern postural yoga's genesis. It is a history of dialogue between Western and Indian ideas and technologies, and of a variegated, wide-ranging search for the cultural values of Hindu identity. Partha Mitter identifies two periods in the history of "colonial" art in India: an era of "optimistic Westernization" between 1850 and 1900, dominated by pro-Western groups with an allegiance to European ideas and sensibilities; and its counterpoint, the cultural nationalism of the *swadeshi* doctrine of art (c.1900–1922), sympathetic to the sovereignty of the emergent Hindu identity (1994: 9). This new orientation prompted a reassessment of "the traditional heritage, from which the elite had recoiled in the first place" (9) and sanctioned long-ignored indigenous modes of artistic expression, which were now seen to be in harmony with modern Indian aspirations. Within this revival, however, art remained permeable to the *technological* advances of the West, which was felt to have the upper hand in the areas of painting and sculpture. In the art schools of India, Mitter notes, "the student was expected to be schizophrenic in his response: he would learn to appreciate Indian design and apply this insight in his work. But when he needed instructions in the "true" principles of drawing, he would turn to the West" (51). Such responses were never wholly expunged from cultural nationalist forms of painting, which mediated their vaunted indigenous authenticity through modernity itself. As in modern Europe, "the historicist revival of an 'authentic tradition' in India was a symptom of its loss. Significantly, the quest for authenticity did not begin in India until traditional art had virtually disappeared" (243). Much in the same way that the category of the "classical" was a symptom and expression of the modernity with which it was contrasted, so too the quest for the authentic tradition was a singularly modernist preoccupation, indicative of an acutely felt disconnection from that tradition.

The situation is illustrative of the cultural and historical impulses that shaped the yoga renaissance. The "optimistic Westernization" in art is mirrored in the assimilation of (Pātañjala) yoga into philosophy from the time of J. R. Ballantyne onward, with Indian scholars and pandits working in close collaboration with Western scholars within the "constructive Orientalist" project (Singleton 2008b). A more markedly "swadeshi" era arrived with Vivekananda, who rescued yoga from the merely philosophical or philological and presented it as the *summum bonum* of the (authentic, practical) Indian spiritual tradition. Largely thanks to his efforts, yoga was refashioned as a cultural symbol, in harmony with the religious and intellectual aspirations of educated Indians—but also, as De Michelis (2004) has shown, shot through with Western influences and standards. Finally, the propagation of an authentic, age-old practice tradition based on the teachings of Patañjali represents the very symptom of its loss, in the sense that Pātañjala yoga was (at least by that time) probably a largely defunct tradition. A similar passage can be traced, indeed, within the history of physical culture in India: from the "Westernized" gymnasia of Maclaren and the Swedish gymnastics of Ling, which dominated in the mid-nineteenth century, to the ardently "swadeshi" revival of "authentic" indigenous exercise in the early years of the twentieth century, which itself incorporated a battery of received expectations and assumptions regarding the purpose of physical culture for the modern Indian citizen.

As we might expect, modern *haṭha* yoga of the colonial period—as a melting pot comprising large doses of physical culture and Vivekananda yoga, as well as other elements—mediated its relationship to the medieval *haṭha* tradition in similar ways and is subject to the same kind of "schizophrenia" that Mitter identifies in Indian colonial art. While scholars studying yoga (viz. Patañjali) during the "optimistic," philosophical period of colonialism mainly recoiled from the figure of the *haṭha* yogin, the cultural nationalists of the late nineteenth century began to look to grassroots ascetic traditions to forge a new ideal of heroism and nobility for the modern Indian. This reworking of spiritual heroism created the conditions that would eventually allow *haṭha* yoga's integration into transnational anglophone yogas, but in greatly modified form. As Sondhi writes half a century later in the Santa Cruz Yoga Institute's journal, within the "renaissance" brought to full flower by the likes of Yogendra, *haṭha* yoga was expected to render "the rationale for what was known in the freedom struggle as the "Swadeshi" movement" (1962: 66). That is to say, as the exemplary Indian body-discipline-elect, the practice of *haṭha* yoga represented the most basic, elemental assertion of self-rule and, some years later, of emancipated and internationally recognized cultural identity. As such, it could reasonably be considered "the physiological basis of other Indian cultural disciplines" (66). However, as with Indian colonial art, the search for "'true' principles" (66) underlying *haṭha* yoga occasioned an extensive project of validation through scientific, medical, and physical culture paradigms that were largely extraneous to the prior tradition, and it is in this sense that we can speak of an ongoing "schizophrenia" within modern *haṭha* yoga, as Mitter does with regard to Indian art.

The Pictorial Postural Yoga Manual

I have been considering these two histories, of postural modern yoga and art, as analogous or parallel expressive forms within the early cultural nationalist project in India. They converge more explicitly, of course, in pictorial representations of *āsana*, where the body becomes *figure* and—in those cases where the functional is eclipsed by the aesthetic—becomes *art*. Gudrun Bühnemann's recent work on an 1830 illustrated manuscript of the *haṭha* text *Jogapradīpakā* (1737) demonstrates that *āsanas* were subject to occasional artistic representation from very early on in the modern period (Bühnemann 2007a, 2007b). According to Losty (1985), these paintings of eighty-four *āsanas* and twenty-four *mūdras* are executed in the Rājput style with elements of the Kangra idiom, and were probably composed in the Punjab. "The artistic quality of the paintings," notes Bühnemann, "is high throughout the manuscript" (157).

What is significant for our consideration of mass-produced, photographic modern yoga primers is the extreme rarity of this text, which remains "quite unique" (Bühnemann 2007a:156) in its visual representation of *āsana*. Indeed, the text and illustrations, warns Bühnemann, should by no means be taken to point toward an ancient *āsana* lineage: "such an ancient tradition of 84 postures," she writes, "is not accessible to us, nor is there any evidence that it ever existed" (160). Neither do these images indicate the beginnings of a popular revival of *āsana* forms in the early nineteenth century. Crucial here is the stylistic gulf that separates these two-dimensional images from the naturalistic representations in modern *āsana* manuals. The most striking difference in this regard is that the shallow figure of the *Jogapradīpakā* is inscribed with representations of the kind of *haṭha* yogic "physiology" (*nādis, cakras*, and *granthis*) outlined in early, premodern texts such as the *Gorakṣaśataka*. It is a *heuristic*, metaphorical model in which realism is not the primary concern (Flood 2006). In later, photographic representation, on the other hand, the emphasis is overwhelmingly on naturalistic representation and outward appearance. As *āsana* was assimilated into modern (often medical) physical culture, aspects of the "subtle" *haṭha* yoga body were selectively dropped, and the naturalistic (or anatomical) body brought to the fore. The photographic medium aided greatly in this progression.

A key transitional moment in the history of the representation of the yogic body is *Yogasopāna Pūrvacatuṣka* (Yogi Ghamande 1905), published by Janardan Mahadev Gurjar of the Niranayasagar Press in Bombay.[1] The book contains illustrations of thirty-seven *āsanas*, six *mūdras*, and five *bandhas* modeled by Ghamande himself, produced using the then-novel method of the "half-tone block" developed in the West around 1885 (Mitter 1994: 121). This "revolution in

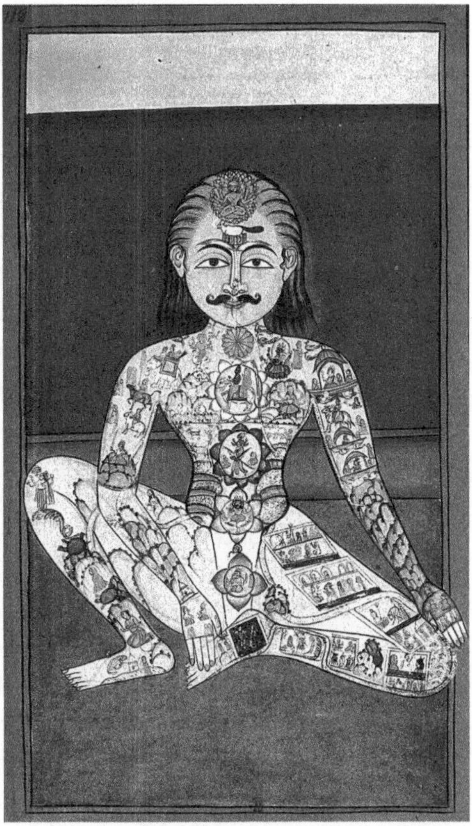

From the 1830 illustrated *Jogapradīpikā* (© British Library Board. All Rights Reserved. Add. 24099, f.118)

reproduction made possible by photography," notes Mitter, "captured the subtle gradations of light and shade essential for a faithful rendering of naturalism" (121), and the *Yogasopāna* (lit. "stairway to yoga") is perhaps the first (and only?) self-help yoga manual to use this reproduction technique. As such, it stands in a technological and chronological interim between the traditionally illustrated *Jogapradīpikā* of 1830 and the full-fledged photographic *āsana* primers that would begin to appear in the 1920s. *Yogasopāna* was conceived as a *work of art* as well as a practical instruction manual.

The blocks were crafted by Puruṣottam Sadāśiv Joshi, chief clerk of A. K. Joshi, agent to the legendary artist Ravi Varma (1848–1906; cf. Ghamande 1905: 11). Varma was a national idol and a cult figure in the world of Indian art, having secured a popular reputation through sales of cheap reproductions of his naturalistic paintings of scenes from Hindu epics. As an "art form that became universally accessible regardless of wealth and class," Varma's mass prints "had a profound impact on society" (Mitter 1994: 174). Varma had a close working relationship with his highly successful agent A. K. Joshi, who procured artisans to assist with this reproduction work (Mitter 1994: 213). It is worth noting that, like Vivekananda, Varma represented India at the 1893 Chicago World's Columbian Exhibition (Mitter 1994: 207), one more instance of the concurrent emergence of modern Indian art and modern Indian yoga onto the international stage. The following suggestive intersection of modern art and modern yoga also deserves mention: the Jaganmohan Palace *Citraśālā* (lit. "picture hall") in Mysore was not only "the first gallery of modern Indian art" and "Ravi Varma's stronghold" (Mitter 1994: 329), but it also housed what we might consider the most influential and enduring "gallery" of modern postural yoga, T. Krishnamacharya's famous *yogaśālā* (see chapter 9).

In its self-consciously modern, naturalistic reproduction of *āsanas*, *Yogasopāna* epitomizes the intersection of modern Indian art and *haṭha* yoga and betokens the transformations undergone by the yogic body through its interaction with modern reproduction technology. If the *Jogapradīpakā* illustrations of 1830 are exemplary of the "conceptual mode of art followed by Indian artists since antiquity," in which an initial, two-dimensional outline drawing or stencil is "coloured in without any significant modification" (Mitter 1994: 30), *Yogasopāna* marks a distinct departure toward the kind of "western perceptual [model]" (30) popularized by Varma. This revolutionary shift at the level of reproduction technology necessarily also effects a "paradigm dislocation" in the understanding of the yogic body—away from the *conceptual*, heuristic tantric body, toward the

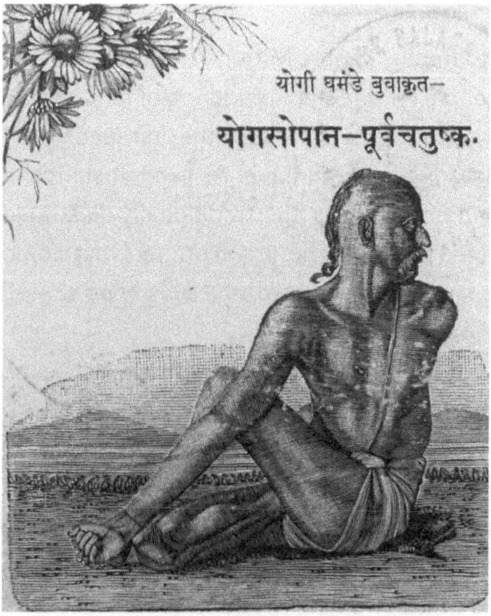

Detail from front cover of *Yogasopāna Pūrvacatuṣka*

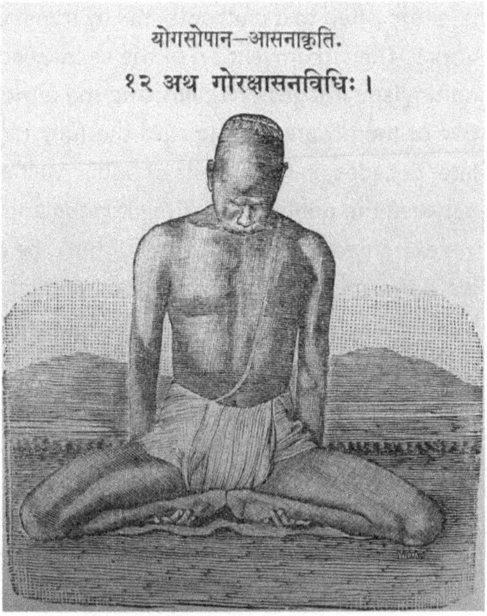

Mūlabandhāsana from *Yogasopāna Pūrvacatuṣka*

perceptual, objective, empirical and realist body of modern *haṭha* yoga. Similarly, just as Varma's paintings of cameos from the Indian epics "reinforced a well-certified notion of India's 'classical' canon" (Guha-Thakurta 1992: 110), so too the rendering of the yoga body into *art* lends Ghamande's postures a "classical" validation that ethnographic fakir snapshots from the same era so patently lack. *Yogasopāna* is, then, not simply analogous to the wider project of Indian art initiated by Varma but part and parcel of it.

The book also marks a transitional phase in the shift away from the secretive transmission of *haṭha* lore from guru to disciple toward an open, public model of dissemination. Ghamande acknowledges the injunctions to secrecy within *haṭha* literature but justifies his exposition in a somewhat sophistic fashion by arguing that "nobody says from whom you have to keep it secret, nor how much you have to hide" (1905: 6). Veronique Bouiller (1997: 19) has written very well on the ambiguous oscillation between secrecy and ostentation in the self-presentation of yogis at the Caughera *maṭha* in the Kathmandu valley. However, it is clear that Ghamande's work represents a different order of unveiling from the "dialectique de l'evident et du caché" (19) of these *Nāth* yogis, insofar as it occurs firmly within the public domain of mass print reproduction.

Students who have doubts about the yoga method presented in *Yogasopāna* are invited to write a letter to Ghamande's house in Taluka (near Pune) or to visit him in person (Ghamande 1905: 10). This may be the earliest example of a proto-correspondence course of *haṭha* yoga, prefiguring the learning format later exploited to its full potential by transnational gurus like Sivananda (Strauss 2005). The circumvention of the secrecy edict; the production of sophisticated, naturalistic images of *āsanas*; and the removal of the guru himself are all indicative of the progression toward the fully formed modern *haṭha* yoga primers of later decades, in their mode of public, self-evident self-help. The two-decade gap between the publication of *Yogasopāna* and these later manuals (some of which are examined in chapter 6) can, I think, be explained by the fact that Indian bodies performing postures were still at that time predominantly represented as freakish fakir-yogis. Although Ghamande's pictures certainly have a dignity that is denied to the "carnival swami," the cultural space in which postural contortions could reclaim a popular appeal as health and fitness regimes would require more time to emerge.

Today, the yoga body has become the centerpiece of a transnational tableau of personalized well-being and quotidian redemption, relentlessly embellished on the pages of glossy publications like *Yoga Journal*. The locus of yoga is no longer at the center of an invisible ground of being, hidden from the gaze of all but the elite initiate or the mystic; instead, the lucent skin of the yoga model becomes the ubiquitous signifier of *spiritual* possibility, the specular projection screen of characteristically modern and democratic religious aspirations. In the yoga body—sold back to a million consumer-practitioners as an irresistible commodity of the holistic, perfectible self—surface and anatomical structure promise ineffable depth and the dream of incarnate transcendence.

9

T. Krishnamacharya and the Mysore *Āsana* Revival

> You may ask, "It may be true for Indians, but what about foreigners who are healthy, long-lived, and do not practice yoga: are they not intelligent? Are they not happy?" You are right, but you should realise that God has created an appropriate system of educational activity for the geographical condition, the quality of the air and the vegetation of the country.... It is not true that the physical exercises practiced by such people are not in conformity with our Yoga system. We don't know what they were practicing in the past, but at present all of you should know for sure that they are practicing the same Yoga *sādhana* as us.
>
> (Krishnamacharya 1935: 22)

> For your own sakes, for the sake of the world in general, and for the sake of the youth of Mysore in particular, I wish you all possible success in your endeavours to give direction to a civilisation that has lost its way. And I suggest that the signposts are to be found... in the simple truths that lie at the base of all religions and in their application, by the aid of the great discoveries of science, to the needs of the present day.
>
> (Maharaja Krishnaraja Wodiyar IV, Opening Address, 1937 YMCA World Conference, Mathews 1937: 90)

The legacy to contemporary transnational yoga of T. Krishnamacharya (1888–1989) is second to none, largely due to the propagation and development of his teachings by well-known students such as K. Pattabhi Jois, B. K. S. Iyengar (brother-in-law), Indra Devi, and T. K. V. Desikachar (son). In recent years Krishnamacharya has posthumously attracted the reverence of thousands of practitioners worldwide and has been the subject of two biographies by his disciple Mala Srivatsan (1997) and his grandson (and son of T. K. V.) Kausthub Desikachar (2005). Also important in this regard is T. K. V. Desikachar's *Health, Healing and Beyond* of 1998, which combines biographical stories with lessons on yoga's healing power. Finally, we must note Kausthub Desikachar's recent "family album" of Krishnamacharya and others, *Masters in Focus* (2009), conceived as a photographic tribute to the major figures of twentieth-century yoga.

Although Krishnamacharya's teaching career spans almost seven decades of the twentieth century, it is the years spent in Mysore, from the early 1930s until the early 1950s, that have arguably had the greatest influence on radically physicalized forms of yoga across the globe. During this period, Krishnamacharya elaborated a system whose central component was a rigorous (and oftentimes aerobic) series of *āsanas*, joined by a repetitive linking sequence. The highly fashionable Ashtanga Vinyasa yoga of Pattabhi Jois is a direct development of this phase of Krishnamacharya's teaching, and the various spin-off forms (like "power yoga," "vinyasa flow" and "power vinyasa") that have burgeoned, particularly in America, since the early 1990s derive often explicit inspiration from these forms. The clearest example may be Beryl Bender Birch's *Power Yoga* of 1995. Birch, along with Larry Schultz (a long-term student of Pattabhi Jois), were two of the earliest innovators of the American power yoga craze. B. K. S. Iyengar, who has perhaps done more than any other individual to popularize a global *āsana*-based yoga in the twentieth century, similarly developed his method as a result of his early contact with Krishnamacharya in Mysore. Although the aerobic component of Iyengar's teaching is greatly diminished, it remains heavily influenced by the *āsana* forms that he learned from his guru.

I have been considering the growth of postural yoga as a function of a worldwide revival of physical culture. Here I focus on a single school of postural yoga—the Jaganmohan Palace *yogaśālā* of T. Krishnamacharya—arguing that *it is only against this broader backdrop of physical education in India that we can fully understand the historical location of Krishnamacharya's* haṭha *yoga method.* The style of *yogāsana* practice that has come to prominence in the West since the late 1980s through Pattabhi Jois's Ashtanga Vinyasa (and its various derivative forms) represents a unique and unrepeated phase of Krishnamacharya's teaching. After he left Mysore in the early 1950s, his methods continued to evolve and adapt to new circumstances, and it is telling in this regard that the teaching style of his later disciples in Chennai (such as son T. K. V. Desikachar and senior student A. G. Mohan) bears little resemblance to the arduous, aerobic sequences taught by Pattabhi Jois. If we are to understand the derivation and function of modern forms of "power yoga" we must first enquire why Krishnamacharya taught this way during his years in Mysore.[1]

Initially, I will look at the circumstances surrounding Krishnamacharya's employment as a yoga teacher in Mysore. Thanks largely to the efforts of the Maharaja Krishnaraja Wodiyar IV, Mysore had, by the time Krishnamacharya arrived, become a pan-Indian hub of physical culture revivalism. Krishnamacharya, working under the personal direction of the Maharaja, was entrusted with the task of popularizing the practice of yoga, and the system he developed was the product of this mandate. Basing my argument on the administrative records of the Jaganmohan Palace where Krishnamacharya opened his *yogaśālā* in 1933, and on oral and textual testimonies of the few surviving students from those years (mainly gathered during the summer of 2005), I contend that this system, which was to become the basis of so many forms of contemporary athletic yoga, is a synthesis of several extant methods of physical training that (prior to this period) would have fallen well outside any definition of yoga. The unique form of yoga practice developed during these years has become a mainstay of postural modern yoga.

Born in Muchukundapuram, Karnataka State, Tirumalai Krishnamacharya was the eldest child of a distinguished Vaiṣṇava Brahmin family. His great-grandfather had been head of the Śrī Parakālamaṭha in Mysore, which was, according to T. K. V. Desikachar, the "first great center of Vaishnavite learning in South India" (1998: 34). From a young age his father began to initiate him into this culture and to instruct him in the bases of yoga. He divided his early studies between Benares and Mysore, mastering several of the orthodox *darśana* (philosophical systems). In 1915, eager to learn more about the practice of yoga, he set out to find one Rāmmohan Brahmacāri who was, according to Krishnamacharya's preceptor in Benares, the only person capable of teaching him the full meaning of Patañjali's *Yoga Sūtras* (Desikachar 2005: 54).[2] After seven years under his tutelage at Lake Mansarovar in Tibet, Krishnamacharya had absorbed "all of the philosophy and mental science of Yoga; its use in diagnosing and treating the ill; and the practice and perfection of *asana* and *pranayama*" (Desikachar 1998: 43). At the end of his apprenticeship, his guru instructed him to go back to India, start a family, and teach yoga. In accordance with these instructions he returned to Mysore in 1925, married a young girl called Namagiriamma, and for the next five years toured the region promoting the message of yoga (Chapelle 1989: 30).

According to Pattabhi Jois, he was sponsored during this period by an influential Mysore official, N. S. Subbarao, who paid Krishnamacharya to lecture on yoga in the various districts of the state (interview, Pattabhi Jois, September 25, 2005). Then in 1931 he was invited by the Maharaja to teach at the Sanskrit Pāṭhaśālā in Mysore, and two years later he was given a wing of the Jaganmohan Palace for a *yogaśālā*. It was during this time that two of his most influential disciples, B. K. S. Iyengar and Pattabhi Jois, studied under him. Patronage, however, came to an end soon after Independence and the *yogaśālā* closed forever. In 1952 he was invited to Chennai by a leading jurist and took over the evening yoga classes at the Vivekananda College there (Chapelle 1989: 31). He would remain in Chennai until his death in 1989. In 1976 his son T. K. V. Desikachar established the Krishnamacharya Yoga Mandiram in his honor, and it remains the principal organ for the dissemination of Desikachar's vision of his father's teaching.

The Maharaja and the Mysore Physical Culture Movement

The Maharaja Krishnaraja Wodiyar IV (1884–1940), ruled the state and city of Mysore from 1902 until his death and was "by all accounts a gentle person, a reflective man of great sensitivity who lived a reclusive life within his palaces" (Manor 1977: 14). In spite of his naturally introverted nature, however, during his thirty-eight-year rule he tirelessly promoted a wide range of cultural innovations, financed scientific and technological experimentation, revolutionized education in the region, and implemented an array of political reforms, including early experiments with democracy. His reign is remembered by many as "the best and most significant period in the history of Mysore" (Ahmed 1988: 4).

One of the principal arenas of revitalization during his reign was physical education, a subject close to the Maharaja's heart. Throughout his life he promoted physical culturalism in various ways, such as his hosting in January 1937 "the first and only World Conference in the hundred year history of the Indian YMCA" and giving a large parcel of land for the new Bangalore YMCA (David 1992: 306; Matthews 1937). Always a champion of Indian cultural and religious expression, Krishnaraja Wodiyar was nonetheless enthusiastic in embracing positive innovations from abroad and incorporating them into his programs of social betterment. As John R. Mott—World Committee president and later Nobel Peace laureate—puts it in his opening address to the conference, the Maharaja was a man with

> reverential regard for the great traditions of ancient India, and yet with up-to-date contacts with modern progress the world over, and responsiveness to new visions and plans; one, therefore, who has successfully blended the priceless heritage of the East with much that is best in the Western world. (Mathews 1937: 90).

We will remember that the Indian YMCA sought to revitalize the moral mettle of the populace through indigenous and foreign physical culture, and that *yogāsana* was one of the components of this project. It is significant for what follows, indeed, that B. K. S. Iyengar recalls demonstrating *āsana* before the Maharaja and the YMCA delegates (1987 [1978]).

The Maharaja was an early advocate of the YMCA's mission; the Mysore government was "the first to take up the cause of indigenous physical culture as early as 1919,"[3] with a full-time organizer, Professor M. V. Krishna Rao, appointed to oversee its development (Kamath 1933: 27). Rao's mission was to popularize Indian exercise and games throughout the state and "was of great value in resuscitating the indigenous system" (27). Importantly, as we saw in chapter 5, Rao is also credited with being one of the early proponents of the synthesis of physical culture and *āsana* (Ghose 1925: 25). As a result of his efforts, "the message of the indigenous system had spread far and wide and public interest was effectively enlisted in its cause and several institutions of a similar nature have grown up in Bangalore under Prof. K. V. Iyer, Prof. Sundaram and others." (Ghose 1925: 25)

The Maharaja actively fostered a climate of eclectic, creative physical culture in Mysore State, establishing the material and ideological conditions that would directly facilitate the synthetic *haṭha* experiments of his beneficiary Iyer, Iyer's student and collaborator Sundaram, and others (see chapter 6). The vital point here is that physical culture in Mysore during the 1920s and 1930s was based on a spirit of radical fusion and innovation promulgated by the Maharaja (via Krishna Rao) and in which *yogāsana* played a major role. As Manor points out, the Maharaja's authority over government exceeded that of any official of British India and "was essentially *personal* in nature" with "ultimate power flowing from the Maharaja himself" (1977: 15). The physical culture experiments that burgeoned in the state during this period should therefore be understood as being in accord with his wishes and with the combined expertise in *āsana* and physical culture of lieutenants like Krishna Rao. It was within this milieu that another of the Maharaja's donees, Krishnamacharya, would develop his own system of *haṭha* yoga, rooted in brahminical tradition but molded by the eclectic physical culture zeitgeist.

Sūryanamaskār and Palace Physical Education

The administrative reports of the Jaganmohan Palace, where Krishnamacharaya was to open his *yogaśālā* on August 11, 1933 (Krishnamacharya c. 1941, Introduction), show a marked emphasis on physical attainment. Gymnastics, military exercises, and all manner of Western sports and games were a major part of the daily life of the royal guards and the extended maternal royal family, the Arasus (or "Ursus" as the name appears in the records). The first reference to Krishnamacharya in these reports comes in the year 1932–1933, when he is mentioned as an instructor at the palace boy's school:" The Physical Instruction Class was under Mr. V. D. S. Naidu, and during the latter part of the year Mr. Krishnamachar was appointed to teach the Yogic System of exercises to the Prince" (n.a. 1931–1947, Year 1932–1933: 33).

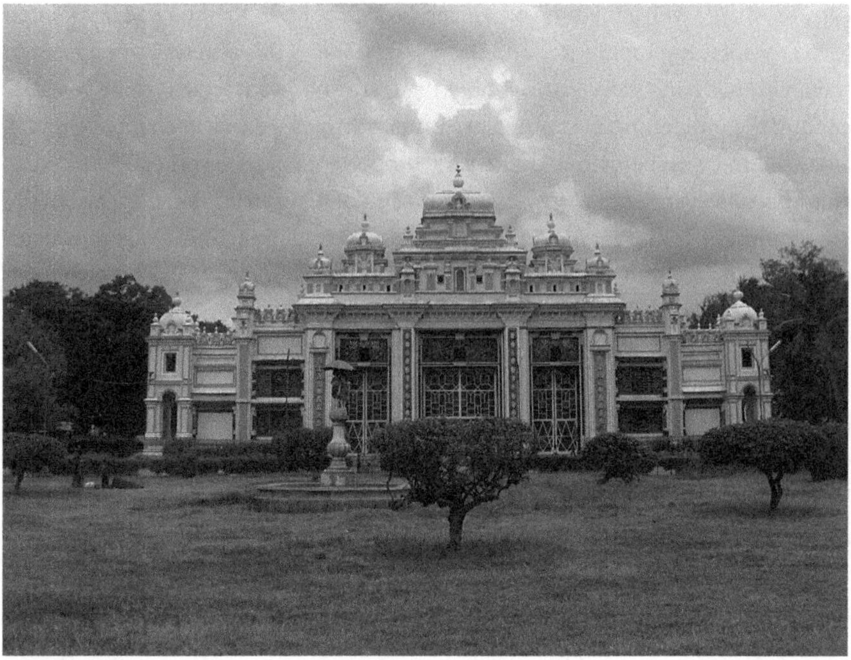

Jaganmohan Palace, Mysore (photo by author)

Throughout these palace records, Krishnamacharya's yoga classes are categorized as "physical culture" or "exercise" and are often mentioned in conjunction, as they are here, alongside other, non-yogic physical activities, such as those of his colleague V. D. S. Naidu. In the 1934–1935 school report, for example, we read under the heading "Physical Culture" that "thirty-two boys attended the Yogasana Classes and a large number of boys attended the Suryanamaskar Classes" (n.a. 1931–1947, Year 1934–35: 10). The entry is also significant as it suggests (once again) that at this time *sūryanamaskār* was not yet considered part of *yogāsana*. Krishnamacharya was to make the flowing movements of *sūryanamaskār* the basis of his Mysore yoga style, and Pattabhi Jois still claims that the exact stages of the sequences ("A" and "B"), as taught by his guru, are enumerated in the Vedas. As noted in the introduction, this last claim is difficult to substantiate.[4] What is important for our purposes, however, is that in those days it was far from obvious that *sūryanamaskār* and yoga were, or should be, part of the same body of knowledge or practice. As Shri Yogendra insists, "*sūryanamaskāras* or prostrations to the sun—a form of gymnastics attached to the sun worship in India—indiscriminately mixed up with the yoga physical training by the ill-informed are definitely prohibited by the authorities" (Yogendra 1989 [1928]).[5]

Goldberg (2006) believes that that *sūryanamaskār* became a part of Krishnamacharya's yoga system during these years due to the influence of K. V. Iyer and his senior student Anant Rao, who taught Iyer's method only meters away from Krishnamacharya's *yogaśālā*. T. R. S. Sharma who, as a boy, was a student at the *śālā*, confirms the close proximity of the venues and adds that these bodybuilding classes happened at the same hour as Krishnamacharya's evening classes (interview, T. R. S. Sharma, August 29, 2005). K. V. Iyer's son, K. V. Karna in fact stated to me that Iyer and Krishnamacharya would occasionally meet socially, and that Iyer, as a nationally admired physical culture celebrity and favorite of the Maharaja, would offer the yoga teacher advice on his classes at the palace (interview, K. V. Karna, September 17, 2005; Goldberg (2006) uses Karna's assertion in this interview as evidence that Krishnamacharya introduced *sūryanamaskār* under Iyer's influence. While this may be possible, it should probably be taken with a grain of salt. A sounder and more compelling explanation may be that Krishnamacharya's addition of *sūryanamaskār* to his *yogāsana* sequences was simply in keeping with a growing trend within postural modern yoga as a whole (as evidenced by Yogendra's admonition, above).

The 1933–1934 Palace report, under the heading "Farashkhana Department," announces the opening of a new *yogaśālā* "(in one of the rooms attached to the departments) under the guidance of Br. Sri Krishnamachari" (n. a. 1931–1947, Year 1933–34: 24). Each year thereafter, until 1947 when the records end, a brief note is made of its good progress.[6] The report makes explicit that the *śālā* has been established "to promote the physical well-being of Ursu Boys" (24). These boys were pupils at the Sri Chamrajendra Ursu Boarding School and seem to have trained with Krishnamacharya and his assistants at the *yogaśālā* as part of their physical education program, with certificates being awarded for achievement in *āsana* (n. a. 1931–1947, Year 1934–1935: 20). This is confirmed by T. R. S. Sharma, who was himself awarded such a certificate (interview, Sharma, August 29, 2005). In the palace report of 1938–1939, for example, we read, "Sports, games and scouting continued to receive considerable attention. The boys entered for the Dasara and other athletic Tournaments. A batch of students attended the "Palace Yogasala" (n. a. 1931–1947, Year 1938–1939: 9).

These reports strongly suggest that the *yogaśālā* was principally conceived as a forum for developing the physical capacities of the young royals, with Krishnamacharya's classes seemingly functioning as an optional counterpart to physical education lessons. This conceptual melding of *āsana* and exercise was not confined to the royal classrooms of the Jaganmohan Palace, however, but was widespread in the schooling systems across Mysore State: we will examine the particularities of this in more detail below. Suffice it to note for now that

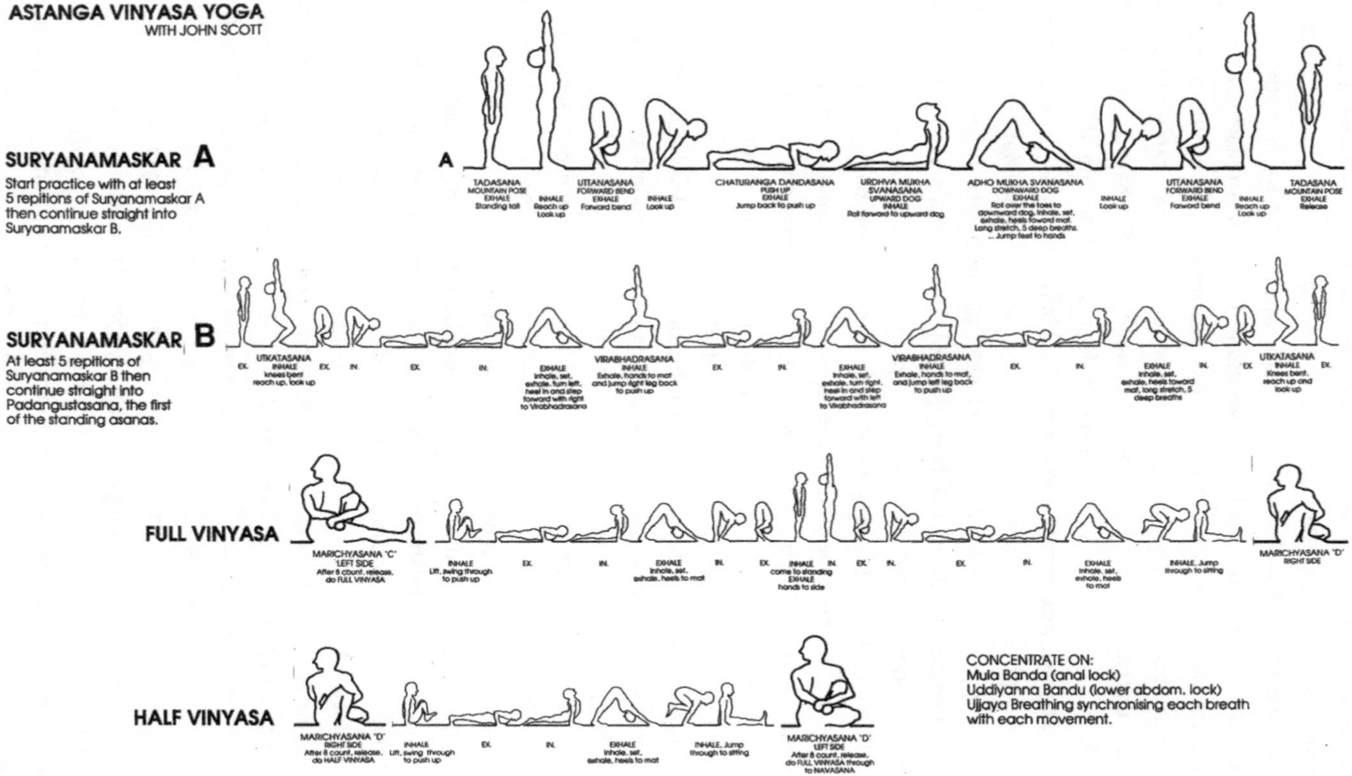
ASTANGA VINYASA YOGA
WITH JOHN SCOTT
SURYANAMASKAR A
Start practice with at least 5 repitions of Suryanamaskar A then continue straight into Suryanamaskar B.
A
TADASANA
MOUNTAIN POSE
EXHALE
Standing tall
INHALE
Reach up
Look up
UTTANASANA
FORWARD BEND
EXHALE
Forward bend
INHALE
Look up
CHATURANGA DANDASANA
PUSH UP
EXHALE
Jump back to push up
URDHVA MUKHA
SVANASANA
UPWARD DOG
INHALE
Roll forward to upward dog
ADHO MUKHA SVANASANA
DOWNWARD DOG
EXHALE
Roll over the toes to downward dog. Inhale, set, exhale, heels toward mat. Long stretch, 5 deep breaths. ... Jump feet to hands
INHALE
Look up
UTTANASANA
FORWARD BEND
EXHALE
Forward bend
INHALE
Reach up
Look up
TADASANA
MOUNTAIN POSE
EXHALE
Release
SURYANAMASKAR B
At least 5 repitions of Suryanamaskar B then continue straight into Padangustasana, the first of the standing asanas.
UTKATASANA
INHALE
knees bent
reach up, look up
VIRABHADRASANA
INHALE
Exhale, hands to mat and jump right leg back to push up
VIRABHADRASANA
INHALE
Exhale, hands to mat, and jump left leg back to push up
UTKATASANA
INHALE
Knees bent, reach up and look up
FULL VINYASA
MARICHYASANA 'C'
LEFT SIDE
After 8 count, release, do FULL VINYASA
INHALE
Lift, swing through to push up
EXHALE
Inhale, set, exhale, heels to mat
INHALE
come to standing
EXHALE
hands to side
INHALE, Jump through to sitting
MARICHYASANA 'D'
RIGHT SIDE
HALF VINYASA
MARICHYASANA 'D'
RIGHT SIDE
After 8 count, release, do HALF VINYASA
INHALE
Lift, swing through to push up
EXHALE
Inhale, set, exhale, heels to mat
INHALE, Jump through to sitting
MARICHYASANA 'D'
LEFT SIDE
After 8 count, release, do FULL VINYASA through to NAVASANA
CONCENTRATE ON:
Mula Banda (anal lock)
Uddiyanna Bandu (lower abdom. lock)
Ujjaya Breathing synchronising each breath with each movement.

Sūryanamaskārs A and B, and *Vinyāsa* sequences of Ashtanga Vinyasa Yoga (drawings reproduced with permission of John Scott)

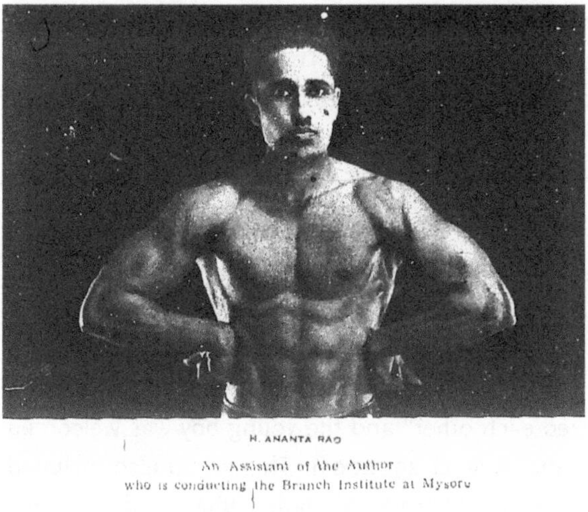
H. ANANTA RAO
An Assistant of the Author
who is conducting the Branch Institute at Mysore

Anant Rao in K. V. Iyer's *Perfect Physique* of 1936

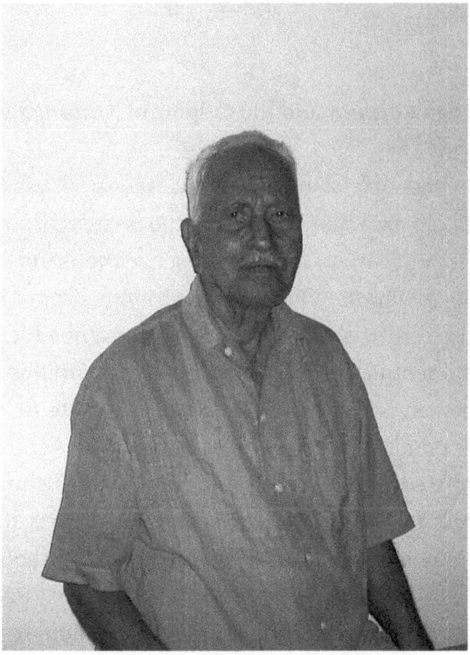

Anant Rao in 2005, aged 100 (photo by author)

Krishnamacharya's teaching seems to have been based on certain of the predominant popular styles of children's physical education in 1930s India, with significant personal innovations and synthesis.

We should also note that, at least in the early years, there were but a handful of nonroyal students at the *yogaśālā*. As B.K.S. Iyengar notes:

> The *Yoga Shala* was meant only for the members of the Royal Family. Outsiders were permitted on special requests. Therefore, it was a formidable task for an outsider to get entry into the *Yoga Shala*. *Guruji* used to have only a few select outsiders with him apart from the Royal Family. (B. K. S. Iyengar, in Desikachar 2005: 188; see also Iyengar 2000: 53)

Some of these outsiders, like Pattabhi Jois, came from the Sanskrit Pāṭhaśālā where Krishnamacharya also taught *āsana*. T. R. S. Sharma attributes his membership in this closed circle to the intercession of his father, who was, like Krishnamacharya, a Vaiṣṇava Brahmin: on seeing each other's religious markings, the two men "recognized each other" and the young boy was welcomed into the *śālā* (interview, Sharma, August 29, 2005). This group also included T. R. S. Sharma's cousin Narayan Sharma, Mahadev Bhat, and Śrīnivāsa Rangācar (see section "Dissent" below).

Yoga Kurunta and the Origins of *Ashtanga Vinyasa*

In the official history of Ashtanga Vinyasa (as sanctioned by Pattabhi Jois), Krishnamacharya learned the system from his Himalayan guru Rāmmohan Brahmacāri on the basis of a five-thousand-year-old text by Vamana Rishi, called *Yoga Kurunta*. On his return to India from Tibet, Krishnamacharya "discovered" the text in a Calcutta library, transcribed it, and then taught it verbatim to his student Pattabhi Jois (for an account of this story by one of Pattabhi Jois's most senior Western students, see Eddie Sterne's introduction in Jois 1999: xv–xvi). According to some older students of Ashtanga Vinyasa, Pattabhi Jois has also related that he was in Calcutta with Krishnamacharya when he discovered the text (author's fieldwork data). He insists that the text describes in full all the *āsanas* and *vinyāsas* (or steps) of the sequences and treats of nothing other than the Ashtanga system (interview, Pattabhi Jois, September 25, 2005). Unfortunately, the text of the *Yoga Kurunta* is said to have been eaten by ants, and no extant copy appears to exist, so it is difficult to verify the truth of such assertions. It is, however, surprising that the text does not seem to have been transcribed by Pattabhi Jois (or another close disciple of Krishnamacharya), nor passed on to a disciple, as the traditional brahminical oral transmission would require. It is also surprising that the text is not (even partially) recorded in either of Krishnamacharya's books of this period—*Yoga Makaranda* (1935) and *Yogāsanagalu* (c. 1941)—nor as far as I know in any other of his writings. It does not even feature among the twenty-seven cited sources for *Yoga Makaranda*.[7]

Whether the text ever did exist is a topic of much controversy among Jois's students.

Yoga Kurunta is one of a number of "lost" texts that became central to Krishnamacharya's teaching; Śrī Nāthamuni's *Yoga Rahasya*, which Krishnamacharya received in a vision at the age of sixteen, is another. Some scholars are of the opinion that the verses of *Yoga Rahasya* are a patchwork of other, better-known texts plus Krishnamacharya's own additions (Somdeva Vasudeva, personal communication, March 20, 2005), while even certain students of Krishnamacharya have cast doubt on the derivation of this work. For instance, Srivatsa Ramaswami, who studied with Krishnamacharya for thirty-three years until the latter's death in 1989, recalls that when he asked his teacher where he might procure the text of the *Yoga Rahasya*, he was instructed "with a chuckle" to contact the Saraswati Mahal library in Tanjore (Ramaswami 2000: 18). The library replied that no such text existed, and Ramaswami, noticing that the *Ślokas* recited by Krishnamacharya were subject to constant variation, concluded that the work was "the masterpiece of [his] own guru" (18). It is entirely possible that the *Yoga Kurunta* was a similarly "inspired" text, attributed to a legendary ancient sage to lend it the authority of tradition.

Moreover, Krishnamacharya's grandson, Kausthub Desikachar, refers to writings by his grandfather that "contradict the popularly held notion that the *Yoga Kuranta* [*sic*] was the basis for *Astanga Vinyasa Yoga*" (Desikachar 2005: 60). Since nobody has seen this text, such statements can be more profitably interpreted as an indication that the "content" of the work changed as Krishnamacharya's teaching changed (and perhaps also as another symptom of the struggles to manage the memory and heritage of Krishnamacharya). That is to say, during his time in Mysore with Pattabhi Jois, Krishnamacharya may have invoked the text to legitimize the sequences that became Ashtanga yoga, but in later life he used it to authorize a wider set of practices.

The elusive manual is also today commonly elicited as a practical elaboration of Patañjali. In one version of Krishnamacharya's biography, the *Yogakurunta* is said to have combined in one volume Vamana's "jumping" system of Ashtanga yoga and the *Yogasūtras* with Vyāsa's *Bhāṣya*, and is therefore taken to represent one of the few "authentic representations of Patanjali's sutra that is still alive" (Maehle 2006: 1). Hastam (1989) attributes a similar view to Krishnamacharya himself. As I argue elsewhere (Singleton 2008a), such assertions can be better considered as symptomatic of the post hoc grafting of modern *āsana* practice onto the perceived "Pātañjala tradition" (as it was constituted through Orientalist scholarship and the modern Indian yoga renaissance) rather than as historical indications of the ancient roots of a dynamic postural system called Ashtanga Yoga. In accounts such as these, a talismanic Patañjali provides the source authority and legitimation for the radically gymnastic *āsana* practices that predominate in modern yoga today. Indeed, it is telling that according to one Mysore resident who studied these practices with Pattabhi Jois in the 1960s (and who preferred to remain anonymous), the name "Ashtanga Vinyasa" was applied to the system only after the arrival of the first American students in the 1970s. Prior to this, Jois had simply referred to his teaching as "*āsana*."

Krishnamacharya, then, was a major player in the modern merging of gymnastic-style *āsana* practice and the Pātañjala tradition. Peter Schreiner (2003) has suggested that for Krishnamacharya, "the *Yogasūtras* are an authority which overrules the textual tradition of Haṭhayoga" and that it is for this reason he could countenance the practice of *āsana* (even in radically modernized form), but did not generally teach *haṭhayogic* techniques such as the *ṣaṭkarmas* (see chapter 1). As we read in Krishnamacharya's *Yogāsanagalu* of c. 1941,

> A number of people think that the *yogakriyās* [i. e. the *ṣarkarmāṇi*] are part of yoga, and they will argue as such. But the main source for yoga, Patañjali Darśana [viz. the *Yogasūtras*] does not include them... It is gravely disappointing that they defile the name of yoga. (Jacobsen and Sundaram [trans.] 2006: 18)

Given Krishnamacharya's commitment to the "Pātañjala tradition," and his uncompromising rejection of the *ṣaṭkarmas* because they do not appear in the *Yogasūtras*, it may seem quite a stretch to promote a form of aerobic *āsana* practice that has such a tenuous link to this tradition. Ultimately, Krishnamacharya's sublimation of twentieth-century gymnastic forms into the Pātañjala tradition is less an indication of a historically traceable "classical" *āsana* lineage than of the modern project of grafting gymnastic or aerobic *āsana* practice onto the *Yogasūtras*, and the creation of a new tradition.

Skilful Means: Pragmatism in Krishnamacharya's Yoga

In his introduction to Krishnamacharya's *Yoga Makaranda* of 1935, the de facto "Reader in Philosophy" to the Maharaja of Mysore, V. Subhramanya Iyer (cf. Wadia 1951) states that the book is "a result of the many tests conducted under the special orders of the Maharaja of Mysore" (Krishnamacharya 1935: v). As well as indicating the keen interest that the Maharaja took in *yogaśālā* activities and his ultimate authority in its affairs, Iyer's statement also suggests the "pilot" status of the work conducted there: Krishnamacharya's teaching was intended to be, and in practice was, *experimental*. This is confirmed by

T. R. S. Sharma, one of a group of students at the *yogaśālā* not of royal descent. Sharma affirms that during the yoga classes, Krishnamacharya

> was innovating all the time in response to his students. He would make up variations of the postures when he saw that some of his students could do them easily. "Try this, try putting this here, and this here." He was inventing and innovating. Krishnamacharya never emphasized a particular order of poses, there was nothing sacrosanct about observing order with him. He would tell me "practice as many as you can." (interview, T. R. S. Sharma, September 28, 2005)

Sharma is emphatic that Krishnamacharya's teaching did not necessarily conform to a fixed or rigid order of postures but was undertaken in a spirit of innovation and investigation—an assessment that clearly contradicts Pattabhi Jois's presentation of these years but which corroborates T. K. V. Desikachar's

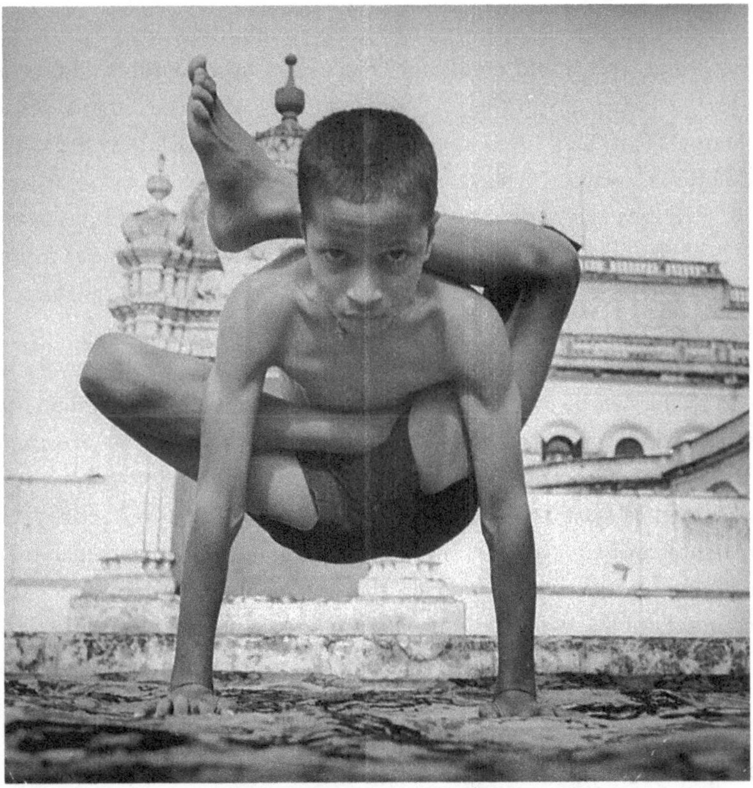

A young T. R. S. Sharma performing Vīrancyāsana outside the Mysore Palace (*Life Magazine*, Kirkland 1941, ©Getty Images)

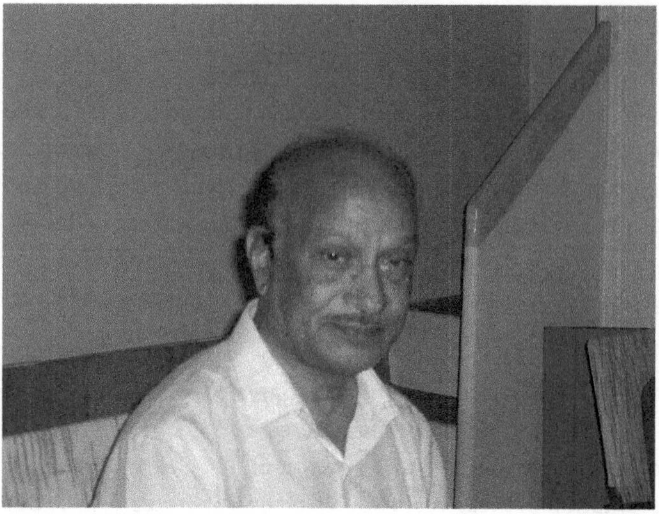

T. R. S. Sharma in 2005 (photo by author)

observation that at this time Krishnamacharya would modify postures to suit the individual, and would create (or "discover") new postures when needed (Desikachar 1982 :32). In the mid-1950s, after Krishnamacharya's departure for Chennai, T. R. S. Sharma spent two more years studying with the already world-famous Swami Kuvalayananda in Lonavla (where he also participated in J. B. S. Haldane's experiments on the physiological effects of yoga practice).[8] Significantly, he found the instruction at Kaivalyadhama far more systematized and ordered than Krishnamacharya's "rough-hewn" teaching at the Mysore *yogaśālā* (interview, T. R. S. Sharma, September 28, 2005).

Although Krishnamacharya did eventually systematize his Mysore teaching—as evidenced by his book *Yogāsanagalu* (c. 1941), which contains tables of *āsana* and *vinyāsa* comparable to Pattabhi Jois's system—it seems clear that the kind of "jumping" yoga propagated at the Jaganmohan Palace was in a near constant state of flux and adaptation. This conforms, indeed, to the fundamental principle of Krishnamacharya's long teaching career that the yoga practice must be adapted to suit the period, location, and specific requirements of the individual (Desikachar 1982: 10). The age and the constitution of the students (*deha*), their vocation (*vṛttibheda*), capability (*śakti*), and the path to which they feel drawn (*mārga*) all dictate the shape of a yoga practice (ibid.). This, continues Desikachar, "is the basis of [Krishnamacharya's] teaching" (1982: 13).

Similarly, another senior Mysore resident who was personally acquainted with early yogaśālā students Śrīnivāsa Rangācar, Mahadev Bhat, Keshavamurthy,

Pattabhi Jois and others, insists that even at that time Krishnamacharya's teaching was "based on the constitution" of the particular student, and that,

> ...there was no such concept as the Primary Series, etcetera. If [Krishnamacharya] saw that a student had good backbends, he used to teach some backward bending postures. If he saw the body was stiff, he would teach *mayūrāsana*... there was no such series. (Anonymous interviewee, September 2005)

The various sequences of Ashtanga Vinyasa are, he asserts, the innovation of Pattabhi Jois, and do not reflect how Krishnamacharya was teaching at this time. In his opinion Pattabhi Jois' system may even prove harmful in so far as it "continues without any consideration of the constitution [of the individual]."

Now, while this certainly supports T.R.S. Sharma's memories of the *yogaśālā* style of teaching, the ascription of the Ashtanga Vinyasa series to Pattabhi Jois is probably mistaken, not least because Krishnamacharya published a list of the series in *Yogāsanagalu*. Furthermore, according to B. K. S. Iyengar, Pattabhi Jois was deputed by Krishnamacharya to teach *āsana* at the Sanskrit Pāṭhaśālā when the *yogaśālā* was opened in 1933, and so was actually "never a regular student" there (Iyengar 2000: 53). This in itself would account for why Jois's system differs from what Krishnamacharya appears to have taught to others at this time. It may well be the case, then, that the aerobic sequences which now form the basis of Ashtanga Vinyasa yoga represent a particularized method of practice conveyed by Krishnamacharya to Pattabhi Jois, but are not representative of Krishnamacharya's overall yogic pedagogy, even during this early period.

It also seems likely, given Krishnamacharya's commitment to the principle of adaptation to individual constitution, that these sequences were designed for Pattabhi Jois himself and other young men like him. Since Pattabhi Jois's duties at the Pāṭhaśālā prevented him from being exposed to the kind of instruction in *āsana* given to T.R.S. Sharma and others, his teaching remained confined to the powerful, aerobic series of *āsana* formulated for him and his cohort by Krishnamacharya. These series would eventually form the basis of today's Ashtanga Vinyasa yoga. What is more, a prescribed sequence where each *āsana* is part of an unchanging order, performed to a counted drill, would have offered a convenient and uncomplicated method for a novice teacher like Jois (who was then eighteen years old). Such a schema would have avoided the considerable complexities inherent in designing tailored sequences according to an individual's *deha, vṛttibheda*, and *mārga* etc. and would have provided a serviceable teaching format for large groups of boys. While this last reflection is partly supposition, it does offer a plausible explanation of the relative lack of attention to individual constitution in Jois's system (at least in comparison to the teachings of T.K.V. Desikachar, and other Krishnamacharya disciples such as A.G. Mohan and Srivatsa Ramaswami) and is certainly consistent with the perceived advantages of nineteenth-century drill gymnastics with which Ashtanga arguably has a close genealogical affiliation (of which more below).

Indeed, Krishnamacharya himself indicated to Ramaswami that such dynamic sequencing, called "vṛddhi" (lit. *growth, increase*) or "śruṣṭikrama" (from *śruṣṭim-kṛ*, lit. *to obey*), is "the method of practice for youngsters," and is particularly suited to group situations (Ramaswami 2000: 15). In such a system, "one will be able to pick and choose some of the appropriate *vinyāsas* and string them together" (ibid.). Could it be that what has come to be known since the 1970s as "Ashtanga Vinyasa" represents the institutionalization in transnational anglophone yoga of a specific and localized *vinyāsa* bricolage designed by Krishnamacharya in the 1930s for South Indian youths, but transmitted subsequently by Pattabhi Jois to (mainly Western) students as the ancient, orthopractic form for *āsana* practice, delineated in the Vedas and the lost *Yoga Kurunta*?

Clearly a lot hangs on the usage of the term "*vinyāsa*." In Pattabhi Jois's system, it is used to indicate the repeated sequence of "jump back," partial or complete *sūryanamaskār* (viz. "half" or "full" *vinyāsa*), and "jump forward" which link the postures of each series. In Krishnamacharya's later teachings, however, the term simply designates an appropriately formulated sequence of steps (*krama*) for approaching a given posture, and not necessarily the fixed, repetitive schema of Ashtanga Vinyasa. T.K.V. Desikachar writes "In the beginning of [Krishnamacharya's] teaching, around 1932, he evolved a list of postures leading towards a particular posture, and coming away from it" (1982: 33), initial experiments in sequencing which are at the origin of Pattabhi Jois's system. The narrowing of the semantic range of the term *vinyāsa* to refer exclusively to the repetitious linking movements of Ashtanga Vinyasa once again suggests the particularity of this approach to *āsana* practice, as well as the preliminary and marginal nature of Ashtanga in terms of the fuller evolution of Krishnamacharya's teaching.

The question remains, however, as to the specific historical reasons that Krishnamacharya developed the repetitive, aerobic jumping sequences of Ashtanga *vinyāsa*, and the unique "count" format of the modern "Mysore class." This will be considered in more detail below.

Demonstrations: Yoga as Spectacle

> Watching Norman do his practice was like watching an Olympic gymnast work out.
>
> (Beryl Bender Birch on first witnessing Ashtanga Vinyasa yoga, Birch 1995: 19)

> The purely spiritual achievements of the man devoted to Yoga, or Yogin, present no features of interest to the gazer or the tourist photographer. On the other hand, the more obvious outward manifestations of Yoga-practice are so striking and often so sensational, that they have attracted the notice of the casual observer, from the days of Alexander even to our own.
>
> —(Lanman 1917: 136)

The rhythm and fluidity of Ashtanga yoga's advanced contortions carries an undeniably aesthetic appeal. The smoothly executed movements of accomplished practitioners appear to defy gravity and suggest the physical mastery of a professional gymnast. In 1930s India, however, yoga lacked the celebrity luster that it enjoys in the West today and was subject to ridicule and scorn (Iyengar 2000: 60). T. R. S. Sharma relates that while it was fashionable among Mysore youth to attend K. V. Iyer's gymnasium a little farther along the palace corridor (directed by Anant Rao), Krishnamacharya's *yogaśālā* was considered distinctly *démodé*. Sharma recalls being made fun of by a friend who was a bodybuilding student there: yoga was for weaklings, a feminizing force in contrast to Iyer's manly muscle building, and was moreover the preserve of Brahmins (interview September 29, 2005). It was considered "the poor man's physical culture because it was available free of cost" and some of the young boys would "feel even apologetic that we took to *yogāsana* rather than K. V. Iyer's bodybuilding" (personal communication, T. R. S. Sharma, January 3, 2006). Alter notes that "yoga's association with asceticism and world renunciation, as well its primary concern with restraint, can easily be interpreted as effete and the very antithesis of muscular masculinity" (2007: 22). Sharma's account illustrates how such a state of affairs still obtained in 1930s Mysore. Sharma qualifies his statements by noting that the brahminical and vedic associations of yoga were in fact a draw to the more tradition-minded youth (personal communication, January 3, 2006).

Indeed, some of Krishnamacharya's yoga students at this time appear to have studied concurrently with K. V. Iyer. B. N. S. Iyengar, for example, was among the last batch of Krishnamacharya's Mysore students in the early 1950s and still teaches *vinyāsa* yoga in a room of the Parakālamaṭha once frequented by his guru. He recalls traveling to Iyer's gymnasium in Bangalore to learn dumbbells and barbells with the famous bodybuilder, but in the end he chose yoga "because it is more cultural" (interview, B. N. S. Iyengar, September 23, 2005), echoing Professor K. Ramamurthy's early appeal to reshape Indian physical culture along "cultural lines" (chapter 5). For a young man in Mysore, Krishnamacharya's yoga represented an alternative to Western bodybuilding and gymnastics but had the advantage of being an indigenous, "cultural" form of exercise.

It is intriguing that in the English preface to Krishnamacharya's *āsana* primer *Yogāsanagalu*, commissioned for use by students at Mysore University, T. Singaravelu Mudaliar makes reference to an article in Bernarr Macfadden's *New Physical Culture Magazine* that "describes how the famous Film Star Acquanetta of Hollywood practices Yoga Asanas and the benefits she has derived from these Yoga Asanas" (Krishnamacharya c. 1941: iii). The allusion suggests an appeal to those sections of Mysore youth who were attracted to the Western-style, Macfadden-inspired fitness programs such as Iyer's and Rao's, as well as an attempt to invest yoga with some of the glitter that it lacked in the popular imagination. The preface largely treats of the "scientific" health benefits of yoga and argues for the superiority of the "Yogic system" over the "ordinary systems of Physical Culture now in vogue" (iv), much in the manner of Sundaram and others examined in chapter 6.

The Maharaja's state-of-the-art *yogaśālā* functioned to a large extent for the promotion of yoga as a respectable form of indigenous exercise that could challenge the prevalent imported gymnastics and the cultural stereotype of the effete Indian (see chapter 5). The regular demonstrations conducted by Krishnamacharya and his troupe at Mysore University were intended to "drum up trade" for yoga (interview, Sharma, September 29, 2005) and to attract students who might otherwise have gone the way of Western-style gymnastics. A significant part of Krishnamacharya's mandate at the palace, indeed, seems to have been to develop a spectacular form of *āsana* practice that could then be showcased by the Maharaja—partly to rescue yoga's tainted reputation and partly for sheer entertainment. As B. K. S. Iyengar has noted,

> It was my guru's duty to provide for the edification and amusement of the Maharaja's entourage by putting his students—of whom I was one of the youngest—through their paces and showing off their ability to stretch and bend their bodies into the most impressive and astonishing postures. (2005: xix)

A rare film clip from 1938 depicts Iyengar himself effortlessly demonstrating several series of advanced postures in linked, flowing sequences reminiscent of, though not identical with, Pattabhi Jois's Ashtanga Vinyasa (Iyengar 1938). It seems reasonable to assume that this is the kind of dynamic performance that Iyengar and his peers were called on to give before the Maharaja and other dignitaries, as well as in the innumerable lecture tours. If we are to believe Iyengar's twenty-first-century reminiscences of this period, one of the rationales for the arduous, spectacular system of *āsana* that emerged from the Jaganmohan Palace was to please the royal patron. In other words, the flowing sequences similar to the ones seen today in Ashtanga yoga were conceived at least in part as performance pieces in a modern Indian court as well as spectacular enticements to draw the people (back?) to yoga.[9] Although this can never be a complete explanation, it is a compelling one and is in accord with Krishnamacharya's oath to his guru to spread the message of yoga, as well as with his previous employment in yoga public relations under the sponsorship of N. S. Subarao.

We should also note here the account given of the lean pre-*śālā* years by Fernando Pagés Ruiz in the pages of *Yoga Journal*, during which Krishnamacharya sought to popularize yoga and "stimulate interest in a dying tradition" by demonstrating extraordinary feats of strength and physiological control, such as suspending his pulse, stopping cars with his hands, performing difficult *āsanas*, and lifting heavy objects with his teeth (Ruiz 2006). As Ruiz comments, "to teach people about yoga, Krishnamacharya felt, he first had to get their attention" (Ruiz 2006). It seems eminently possible that the advanced *āsana* extravaganzas performed in later years by his senior students had a similar function and shared in a common "modern strongman" discourse. As we saw in chapter 5, such feats of strength are common in modern Indian physical culture literature, where they are often (at least nominally) associated with *haṭha* yoga. We recall, for instance, the case of the bodybuilder and physical culture luminary Ramamurthy, who regularly performed stock feats of strength such as Krishnamacharya's. These demonstrations, in other words, were leitmotifs that straddled the worlds of modern bodybuilding and yoga.

Another example of this overlap comes from within the walls of the Jaganmohan Palace itself. The previously mentioned palace physical instruction teacher V. D. S. Naidu—entrusted, like Krishnamacharya himself, with the fitness of the Arasu boys—was a prominent Mysore physical educationalist and strongman. Pattabhi Jois relates that as a boy, he and a group of friends one day attended Naidu's class. Seeing the physical prowess of these youngsters on gymnastic equipment like parallel bars, Naidu asked them how they had gained such bodily control. When they told him they were students at Krishnamacharya's *yogaśālā*, he said "go back there then. Yoga is much better than this kind of exercise." Naidu was renowned for his feats of strength, such as hauling cars, and letting trucks roll over his body. In one fateful demonstration, he had a student jump from a height of eighteen feet onto his chest. However, the boy jumped before Naidu was ready, and he died five days later in hospital from ruptured organs (interview, Pattabhi Jois, September 25, 2005). The same story of Naidu's demise was related to me by Iyer student and Krishnamacharya's bodybuilding neighbor at the Jaganmohan Palace, Ananta Rao (interview September 19, 2005). What is important about this story is that while Naidu acknowledges the superiority of Krishnamacharya's system over his own, it is nevertheless perceived as essentially a *kind of exercise* and thus comparable in form and intent to the Krishnamacharya's regime. We should understand Krishnamacharya's strongman demonstrations in this light. That is to say, Krishnamacharya arrived at the *yogaśālā* with a charge similar to Naidu's: to ensure the physical fitness of the royal youth and to popularize their respective forms of physical culture. What is more, both men were adept at the kind of strength exploits standardized by earlier bodybuilders like Ramamurthy. It is in this sense that the Krishnamacharya of this period must be considered (among other things) as an inheritor of the nineteenth- and twentieth-century physical culture lineages that are the topic of this book's foregoing chapters.

A common refrain among the first- and second-generation students of Krishnamacharya whom I interviewed, as well as others who knew him during his Mysore days, is the association of his teaching with the circus. For example, the bodybuilding and gymnastics teacher Anant Rao, who for several years shared a wing of the Jaganmohan Palace with Krishnamacharya, feels that the latter was "teaching circus tricks and calling it yoga" (interview, September 19, 2005). T. R. S. Sharma considers the yoga he learned at Kaivalyadhama to be "more rounded" than Krishnamacharya's approach, which "was more like circus" (interview, September 29, 2005) but nonetheless feels that it is inappropriate to call the postures "tricks" (personal communication, February 3, 2006, after reading a first draft of this chapter). And Śrīnivāsa Rangācar (one of Krishnamacharya's earliest students, about whom more shortly) similarly deemed the *āsana* forms he learned "circus tricks" (interview, Shankara Narayan Jois, September 26, 2005). A later student of Krishnamacharya, A. V. Balasubramaniam, states in a recent film documentary on the history of yoga:

> In the thirties and forties when he felt that yoga and interest in it was in a low ebb, [Krishnamacharya] wanted to create some enthusiasm and some faith in people, and at that point in time he did a bit of that kind of circus work...to draw people's attention. (Desai and Desai 2004)

The *āsana* systems derived from this early chapter of Krishnamacharya's career dominate the popular practice of yoga in the West today, and yet it is largely overlooked that they stem from a pragmatic program of solicitation that exploits a long theatrical tradition of acrobatics and contortionism. This is not to say, of course, that Krishnamacharya approached his demonstrations like sideshows at a *mela*, but merely that audiences would have recognized the performances as belonging to a well-established topos of *haṭha* yogic fakirism and circus turns (see chapter 3 above). The demonstrations were a "hook" to grab the attention of an audience who might otherwise have had little interest in the arche arcane topic of yoga. Shankar Narayan Jois, a disciple of early *yogaśālā* student Śrīnivāsa Rangācar, summarizes as follows:

> Krishnamacharya had an interest in body-oriented sciences by nature, and because of this interest, he gathered different postures from places (like Northern India) and evolved them.[10] He started teaching like that because it can be taught easily to many, like a drill. Some of the higher yoga techniques are hard to understand and to teach, so he used that as a simple device to commence something. It was a way of bringing people in. (interview, September 29, 2005)

Krishnamacharya was sent all over south India by the Maharaja on what was candidly called "propaganda work" (Sjoman 1996: 50). One such tour to Pune, recorded in the Jaganmohan Palace administrative records, was conducted in the summer of 1938 (n. a. 1931–1947, Year 1938–1939: 9). T. R. S. Sharma, who was one of the four boys chosen to represent the *yogaśālā*, remembers a demonstration in a large hall there, where he and his friends performed *āsana* to thunderous applause. Krishnamacharya would pick the young boy Sharma up while he performed a difficult pose and display him to the audience (interview, September 29, 2005). Sharma also remembers being impressed at the time that Krishnamacharya lectured in fluent Hindi.

Pattabhi Jois also participated in a large number of demonstrations, along with senior Pāṭhaśālā students like Mahadev Bhat and a number of Arasu boys. The *āsanas* were distributed beforehand into primary, intermediate, and advanced categories, with the younger boys performing the easiest poses while Jois and his peers demonstrated the most advanced (interview, Pattabhi Jois, September 25, 2005). These sequences were, according to Jois, virtually identical to the aerobic schema he still teaches today: that is, several distinct "series" within which each main *āsana* is conjoined by a short, repeated, linking series of postures and jumps based on the *sūryanamaskār* model. Although he would never endorse such an interpretation himself, his description suggests that the three sequences of the *Ashtanga* system may well have been devised as a "set list" for public demonstrations: a shared repertoire for student displays.

The need for a coordinated, high-speed showcase might also explain why, in Jois's system, postures are usually held only for five (but up to a maximum of eight) audible "ujjayi" breaths: this would not only allow the models to perfectly synchronize their entry and exit from a pose but would also provide enough time for Krishnamacharya to explain the significance of a posture without taxing the attention of the audience. Significantly, Krishnamacharya's *Yoga*

Makaranda of 1935 advocates long timings for most poses, generally from three to fifteen minutes, suggesting that the relatively rapid-fire *āsana* sequences inherited and developed by Pattabhi Jois represent a very particularized and specific approach within the broader scheme of Krishnamacharya's teaching, even at this time (Narasimhan [trans.] 2005 [1935]). Although this explanation of the five-breath system is speculation on my part (and bound to be contentious insofar as it elides other reasons for this format, such as buildup of heat; see Smith 2008), it *was* independently suggested by Krishnamacharya's Mysore student B. N. S. Iyengar and was considered to be a distinct possibility by T. R. S. Sharma, who does not remember any "five breath" format being taught in the *yogaśālā*. On the contrary, Krishnamacharya taught him that "you should gradually stay in the pose for up to three minutes" (interview, September 29, 2005), a scheme that seems more in line with Krishnamacharya's intention in *Yoga Makaranda*. That said, the Ashtanga practice always concludes with a "finishing sequence" that usually does include longer stays in the shoulderstand (*sarvāṅgāsana*) and its variations, headstand (*śīrṣāsana*) and its variations, a seated "bound" lotus (*baddhapadmāsana* and *yogamudrāsana*), twenty-five deep breaths in lotus pose, and a supine relaxation (*śavāsana*). This part of the sequence is generally conducted in a separate room from the main *vinyāsa* section, thus marking it as a different phase of the practice. This does not, however, help to explain the unique format of the main part of each "series."

Dissent

At the time (even as now) Krishnamacharya's gymnastic Mysore style came in for criticism. One of his earliest students was Śrīnivāsa Rangācar (later known as Śrīrangaguru) who, like Pattabhi Jois and many of the Pāṭhaśālā students, was from a poor village in an outlying district of Mysore. Rangācar was naturally predisposed to *āsana*, quickly mastering the difficult poses and becoming an assistant teacher at the *yogaśālā* (Chanu 1992: 6).[11] However, Rangācar became disgusted with the methods taught there, concluding that "but for Yogic exercises [Krishnamacharya] had no idea of the real inner bases of [yoga]" (18). He had, by 1938, attained his own profound yogic realization but was discouraged and obstructed by Krishnamacharya in his ambitions; according to Chanu, when he expressed the wish to present his *āsanas* to the Maharaja, Krishnamacharya blocked his access (1992: 18). Rangācar then returned to his own village to live a solitary life of contemplation. Three decades later he was to found his own school in Mysore named, pointedly, "Aṣṭāṅga Yoga Vijñāna Mandiram."

Despite the generally hagiographic presentations of the "Krishnamacharya industry" (such as T. K. V. Desikachar 1982 and 1998; Srivatsan 1997; and K. Desikachar 2005 and 2009) it seems difficult to square Rangācar's summary dismissal of his teacher's worth with the genius usually presented. How is it possible that a long-term, dedicated student like Rangācar, a member of the select inner circle of palace yoga students—deemed proficient enough, moreover, to teach in Krishnamacharya's stead—could fail to recognize the profundity of his master's learning or the inner logic of his method? It would be easy to simply dismiss Rangācar's criticism of Krishnamacharya as the petulance of youth, but as we have seen, the evidence from the period, and oral testimony, suggests that in his role at the *yogaśālā* Krishnamacharya did certainly focus almost exclusively on the external, physical exercise component of yoga. T. R. S. Sharma states that Krishnamacharya's nightly teaching at the *śālā* was concerned uniquely with *aṅgalāghava* ("lightness of limb" see the section "Haṭha Yoga" in chapter 1) and that "the spiritual aspects of yoga like *dhyāna*, *dhāranā* and the *samādhi* states were rarely talked about" (interview, August 29, 2005). B. K. S. Iyengar remarks dryly of his *āsana* regime prepared by Krishnamacharya: "If my brother-in-law also had an eye to my deeper spiritual or personal development, he did not say so at the time" (2005: xix).[12]

B. K. S. Iyengar also notes that at the beginning of his royal employ, Krishnamacharya had originally been engaged to teach *mīmāṃsā* at the Pāṭhaśālā, but was reassigned to the *yogaśālā* when the students complained to the Maharaja that the lessons were too difficult (Iyengar 2000: 53). This anecdote once again suggests the ultimate authority of the Maharaja over what and where Krishnamacharya was to teach and the role the Maharaja played in directing the curriculum of the *yogaśālā*. Despite his reputation as a fiercely independent man who did as he pleased and spurned royal largesse (Desikachar 2005: 97), Krishnamacharya remained, in administration if not in spirit, an employee of the Maharaja with a family to feed. After his marriage, indeed, Krishnamacharya had been forced by circumstance to work in a coffee plantation in the Hasan district of Karnataka (Iyengar 2000: 52), a fact that is often eliminated from "official" biographies. During this time (from 1927 until 1931?),[13] he wore "half-pants and half-sleeved shirt, socks and shoes, a hat on his head and a stick in his hand" (52) rather than the dress of the orthodox Brahmin. As Iyengar remarks, "destiny had played its trick on him even" (52). It was only after a lecture on the Upaniṣads in Mysore town hall in 1931 that Krishnamacharya began to attract the attention as a learned scholar that eventually led to his employment at the palace. If Krishnamacharya was to keep his position at the *yogaśālā*, he would have to conform to the Maharaja's mandate. And this mandate seems to have been that he teach *āsana* in keeping both with the strong gymnastic tradition of the palace itself and with the changing face of indigenous physical education programs across the region.

Gymnastics Indian and Foreign: The Derivation of the Mysore Style

> The treatise before us is however confined to that part of [Yoga] that deals with the training of the Body. But this should not be confounded with what is generally known as physical culture or manly games with which it is often compared, though by mistake. The Yogic descriptions of the body chiefly aim at the preservation of health and not at the development of the muscles or of the skill and courage of the field. It has been rightly characterized as "a system of hygienic practices." Modern conditions demand a judicious combination of all these different items.
>
> From V. Subrahmanya Iyer's Preface to *Yoga Makaranda* (Krishnamacharya 1935: iii)

John Rosselli notes that from the 1870s onward, gymnastics taught in Indian government schools "often had a strong element of individual body-building or acrobatics" (1980: 137). The method that Krishnamacharya taught the children at the palace invites comparison to a number of these educational disciplines, particularly several that rose to prominence in Indian education establishments during the second and third decades of the early twentieth century. Although not necessarily conceived within the rubric of yoga, these regimens of pedagogical gymnastics, I contend, create the context for understanding the otherwise anomalous athletic systems of Krishnamacharya's Mysore years. The 1930 physical education report of Mysore's Department of Public Instruction, for example, recommends that school children be instructed in "Gymnastics, Indian or Foreign" (n.a. 1930: 10) and Krishnamacharya's teaching evinces a clear permeability to such trends of physical education in Indian schools. His system can be fruitfully considered *a synthetic revival of indigenous exercise (comprising* yogāsana *alongside other types) within the context of Westernized curricular physical education in late colonial India.*

Norman Sjoman's study of the Mysore yoga tradition points out that there was a long-established tradition of royal gymnastics at the palace and that the Maharaja himself had followed a regimen of gymnastic exercise as a child (Sjoman 1996: 52). He makes the case that Krishnamacharya drew freely on the gymnastic texts that he found there in the elaboration of his own teaching system (Sjoman 1996) and moreover, that he inherited "the old gymnastics hall containing gymnastic apparatus and ropes hanging from the ceiling as his *yogaśālā*" (Sjoman 1996: 53).[14] Indeed, Śrīnivāsa Rangācar related to one of his senior students that during his time as a student-teacher at the *yogaśālā* Krishnamacharya used "all kinds of gymnastic equipment" in his teaching (including rope climbing apparatus) and that in those days, Krishnamacharya's teaching "was considered gymnastics alone" (interview, Shankara Naryan Jois, September 26, 2005). T. R. S. Sharma, who entered the *yogaśālā* after Rangācar departure, does not remember any such equipment, which suggests that it was not a prominent feature of Krishnamcharya's teaching there except in the early years of his tenure (interview, September 29, 2005). It might also be worth noting that with Anant Rao's departure as the principal teacher at K. V. Iyer's Mysore *vyāyamśālā* in 1941, a large quantity of gymnastic equipment was just left "lying around" the wing of the Jaganmohan Palace where Krishnamacharya also taught (interview, Anant Rao, September 29, 2005).

This passage from equipment-based gymnastics to a nonapparatus regime would mirror the more general and pervasive trend in Indian physical culture away from costly installations—like the once-popular Maclaren gymnasiums—and toward more economically accessible routines drawn from European freehand gymnastics and indigenous exercise (see chapter 4). Prior to and during Krishnamacharya's time in Mysore this physical education zeitgeist was being given official form in government school syllabi (as the Mysore Department of Public Instruction report suggests) and by the end of the decade it had been concretized into fairly standard format across the nation.

I wish to consider briefly two examples of physical education regimens that enjoyed widespread popularity in 1930s India: the first drawn from an imported, European system, and the other from a government-endorsed compilation of "homegrown" exercises. These concrete details concerning technique will, I hope, show that Krishnamacharya's "Mysore style" was far from out of step with the dominant forms of physical education in late colonial India and was in fact a variant of standard exercise routines of the time.

Foreign

As we saw have seen, the modern Indian physical culture movement grew up in reaction to foreign, colonial forms of body discipline such as Maclaren and Ling. However, these systems of exercise were generally not rejected wholesale but incorporated into a broad syncretic scheme that eventually gave more weight to revived indigenous practices. The system called Primitive (or "Primary") Gymnastics, developed by the Dane Niels Bukh (1880–1950), was one such European system that came to occupy a central position in the Indian physical education scene. Through the first decades of the twentieth century,

Ling's hitherto dominant system was increasingly deemed insufficient for creating able-bodied men (we remember that K. V. Iyer criticizes it on precisely these grounds), and a more vigorous Danish gymnastics gained popularity. In 1906, Danish gymnastics even became part of the official British army training program (Leonard 1947: 212). Bukh's system, which "emphasized continuity of movement, rhythmic exercise, and intensive stretching to seek elasticity, flexibility, and freedom" (Dixon and McIntosh 1957: 101), attained such exponential popularity from the early 1920s onward that by 1930, YMCA National Physical Director Henry Gray could rank it as second only to Ling in terms of "full national approval or... general recognition" among exercise regimes in India (Gray 1930: 7).

To indicate the extent of overlap between the two systems, let us consider briefly some of the particulars of Bukh's system in comparison with *yogāsana*, as taught by Krishnamacharya in Mysore during the 1930's (see figures below). Bukh's *Primary Gymnastics* (first English edition 1925, completely revised in 1939) offers a complete course of stretching and strengthening exercises—graded, like the Ashtanga Vinyasa system, into six progressive series. The exercises are aerobic in nature and practiced in a "vigorous rhythm" (Bukh 1925: 8) so that heat is generated in the body (8). All movements are accompanied by deep breathing. The same is true for Ashtanga, in which one of the main rationales for the intensely aerobic posture work and the deep *ujjayi* breathing is the heat that it generates in the practitioner.[15] At least *twenty-eight* of the exercises in the first edition of Bukh's manual are strikingly similar (often identical) to yoga postures occurring in Pattabhi Jois's Ashtanga sequence or in Iyengar's *Light on Yoga* (Iyengar 1966). There are several more in the second edition of 1939. Not only do Bukh's positions suggest modern yoga postures but the linking movements between them are reminiscent of the jumping sequences of Ashtanga Vinyasa.

Bukh's American student, Dorothy Sumption, summarizes the underlying principles of the maestro's work as follows: "Advanced work in Fundamental Danish Gymnastics consists of the harmonious combination of exercises into a unified whole.... The main idea in combining is to make the work continuous without distinct pauses, which are superfluous and a waste of time" (1927: 169).

For example, one sequence begins with "Long Sitting," a position comparable to Krishnamacharya's *daṇḍāsana*, from which the student jumps back into a plank-type pose ("prone falling (front hand lying)"), then turns and balances on one hand and one foot ("side falling (side hand lying)"), taking a position reminiscent of *vaśiṣṭāsana*. From there he or she jumps into "Hand Standing" (*adho mukha vṛkṣāsana*) and then lies down (*śavāsana*) (Bukh 1925: 27–29). These linking movements, as well as the positions themselves, strongly suggest Ashtanga Vinyasa's system in which, between poses, the student jumps from

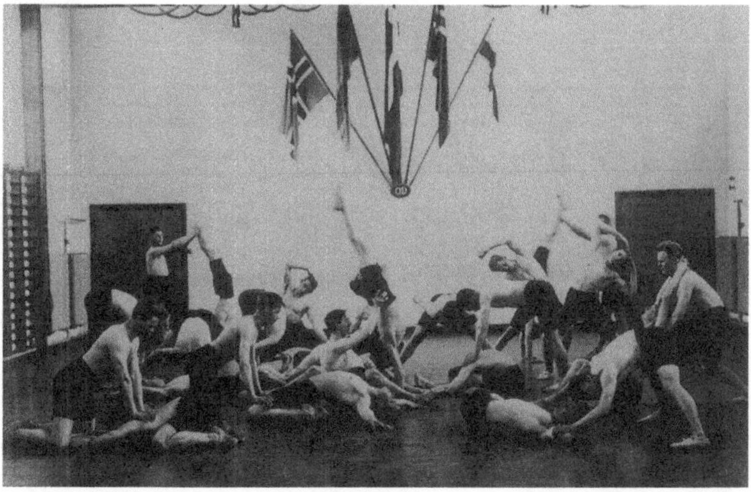

Bukh's gymnasium in Ollerup, Denmark (postcard)

sitting into a push-up position, and then (with some variation) jumps into the next successive pose. Bukh's "athletic" or "serial" gymnastics were performed, like Ashtanga, to a count, with each posture (as in Ashtanga) being called out while the previous sequence was finishing, reflecting a modernist fascination with dynamic movement (Bonde 2000: 107; Sumption 1927: 7). As for many forms of postural modern yoga, including Ashtanga, "the drive-shaft of Bukh's system was suppleness" (Bonde 2006: 33). The functional/descriptive names given to Bukh's exercises are also mirrored in the functional/descriptive names that characterize what Sjoman postulates are late *āsanas* (in contradistinction to the symbolic objects, animals, sages, and deities that gave their name to earlier postures, Sjoman 1996: 49).

I point out these similarities not to suggest that Krishnamacharya borrowed directly from Bukh but to indicate how closely his system matches one of the most prominent modalities of gymnastic culture in India, as well as in Europe. And as we saw in chapter 4, Bukh-influenced gymnastics were, by the mid-1930s, a standard choice for children's physical culture in popular publications like *Health and Strength.* While this notion challenges the narrative of origins commonly rehearsed among Ashtanga practitioners and teachers today, it is really hardly surprising, given the context, to see elements of Danish children's gymnastics emerge in Krishnamacharya's pedagogy in Mysore. Sjoman inquires with regard to Krishnamacharya's system, "are the asanas really part of the yoga system or are they created or enlarged upon in the very recent past in response to modern emphasis on movement?" (1996: 39–40). Given the similarities

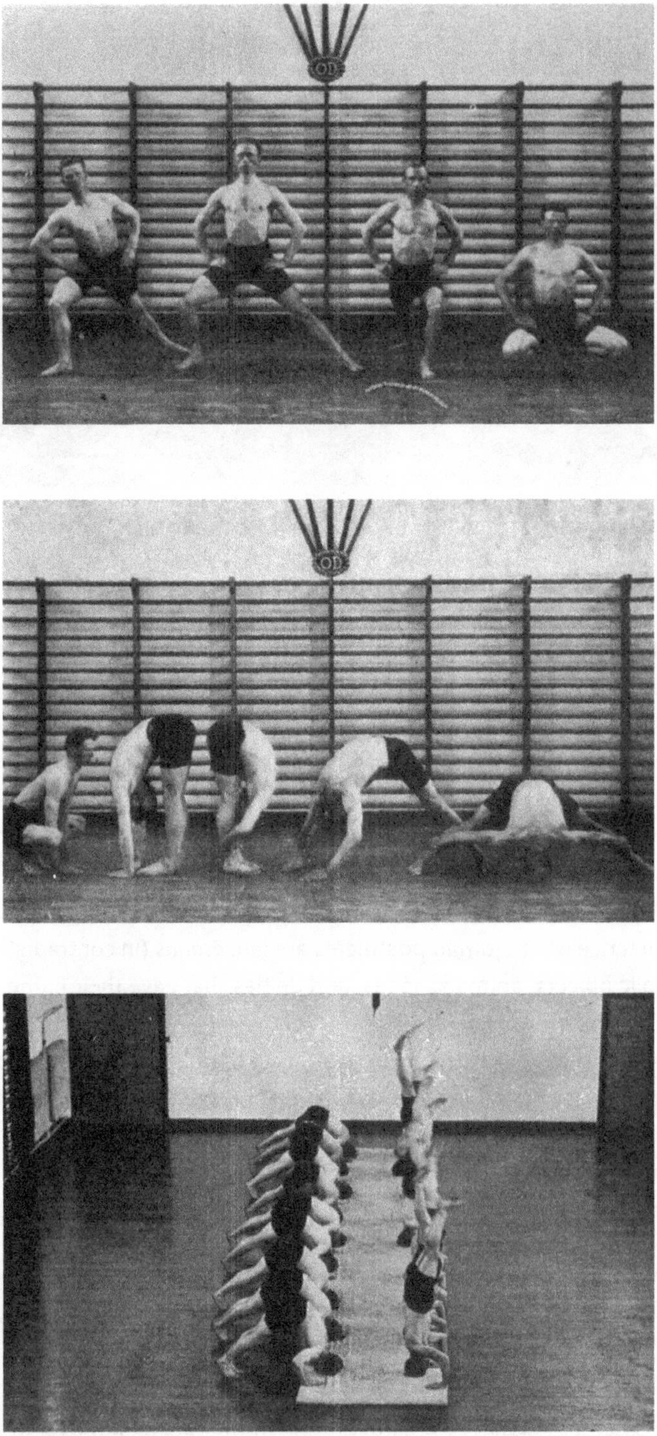

Exercises from Bukh 1925

between Bukh's Primitive Gymnastics and these dynamic yoga sequences, it is the latter scenario that seems more compelling.[16]

Indian

During the first year of his tenure at the palace, Krishnamacharya was sent by the Maharaja to Kuvalayananda's pioneer research institute, Kaivalyadhama, to observe the work carried out there.[17] Gharote and Gharote point out that "one of the ideals of Kaivalyadhama was to evolve a system of physical culture based on Yoga and to take steps to popularise that system" (1999: 37). Many went there to seek advice and assistance "in organising physical culture courses based on Yoga" (37), and Krishnamacharya, we can say with some certainty, was among their number.

From 1927, Kuvalayananda sat on a committee on physical training in the Bombay presidency, the goal of which was to build an ideal of physical education that would "foster those personal and civic virtues in pupils which would make them better citizens" (Gharote and Gharote 1999: 105). By 1933 Kuvalayanda's curricula of "Yogic Physical Education" had been introduced into education establishments across the United Provinces (Gharote and Gharote 1999: 38; Kuvalayananda 1936: ii). By the time of Krishnamacharya's visit, Kuvalayananda's *āsana* regimes were *the* paradigm of pedagogic yoga instruction in India, and it is reasonable to suppose that Krishnamacharya absorbed some of their core elements and applied them to his work with the children in Mysore. Kuvalayananda's syllabi are recorded in his *Yaugik Saṅgh Vyāyam* ("Yogic Group Exercise") of 1936,[18] a book originally written for the Education Commission of the United Provinces (1936: ii). These mass exercises, states Kuvalayananda, are based on the drill techniques (*huku-mo* in Hindi) popularized by his guru Manick Rao (ii; see also Mujumdar 1950: 450), a figure we also previously encountered as the physical culture preceptor of the revolutionary yogin Tiruka (chapter 5).

As we have seen, drill was the standard form of instruction in physical education after the introduction of Ling gymnastics (see chapter 4), and the instruction format does not differ greatly here. First, the posture is named by the instructor, after which the students are counted through the three phases of the *āsana* (entry, posture proper, exit). This is of course precisely the format adopted by Krishnamacharya in his early school teaching and which has been transmitted into postural modern yoga as the "count class" or "led practice" format of Ashtanga Vinyasa. These influences provide a more satisfying explanation of the count sequence of Ashtanga Vinyasa, perhaps, than the "official" version examined above, wherein the exact counts are said to be specified in the five-thousand-year-old lost text, *Yoga Kurunta* of Vamana, or in the Yajur and Ṛg Vedas. While

Kuvalayananda limits himself in *Yaugik Saṅgh Vyāyam* to simple, dynamically performed callisthenic postures and some easy *āsanas* (referring the interested reader to his *āsanas* of 1933), it would seem clear that Krishnamacharya adopted this format and wove in other, sometimes advanced, yoga postures, much as Kuvalayananda himself would do.

In practice, such syntheses, built on this increasingly conventional format, were not unusual. To take an example, the Bombay Physical Education Committee syllabus—based on Kuvalayananda's work, and compulsory in the province's schools from 1937 (Old Students' Association 1940: iii)—shows striking similarities with the system enshrined in postural modern yoga as Ashtanga Vinyasa. The drills often closely match the "*vinyāsas*" of Krishnamacharya's method, such as in the "Calisthenics" section, which contains a drill called "Kukh Kas Ek," close in form and execution to Ashtanga yoga's *utthita trikoṇāsana.*[19]

Many other such suggestive correspondences can be found in this section. However, it is chapter 10, devoted to "Individualistic Exercises, Dands, Baithaks, Namaskars and Asanas,"[20] that makes clear the functional position occupied by *āsanas* in educational programs. Although *āsanas* are presented separately from the other exercises, it is clear that they belong here unequivocally in the category of fitness training and that they are blended with aerobic exercises from outside any known yoga tradition.

At the time, it seems that this was a widespread and perfectly acceptable practice: *āsanas were there to be pragmatically utilized in gymnastic bricolage*. The *āsanas* described in this chapter all originate and finish with the fundamental standing position known as "Husshyar" or "attention" (Old Students' Association 1940: 206), just as the full Ashtanga Vinyasa sequence begins and ends each pose in *samasthiti* (also known as *tadāsana* in some modern postural systems). From here, the student bends forward, places the hands, and jumps back to a "prone support position" before lowering into a push-up (207). He or she then executes one of a number of "dands," whose movements correspond to the central Ashtanga "*vinyāsa*" sequence: *caturaṅga daṇḍāsana, urdhva mukha śvanāsana*, and *adho mukha svanāsana* in Ashtanga nomenclature (see figure on page 182). The dand position corresponding to this last posture (popularly translated as "Downward Facing Dog") and described earlier in the book, appears to describe the use of the *jālandhara* and *uddiyāna* bandhas ("locks") in a manner characteristic of the Ashtanga *āsana* system: "at the same time, take the head in, chin touching the chest, draw the abdomen in" (195).

Once again exactly matching the Ashtanga sequence, the student then *jumps through* his or her arms to a sitting position with the legs stretched out straight in front (207). This commonly occurring movement is known as "Saf-Suf Do" in the dand section and "Baith Jao" in the *āsana* section and corresponds

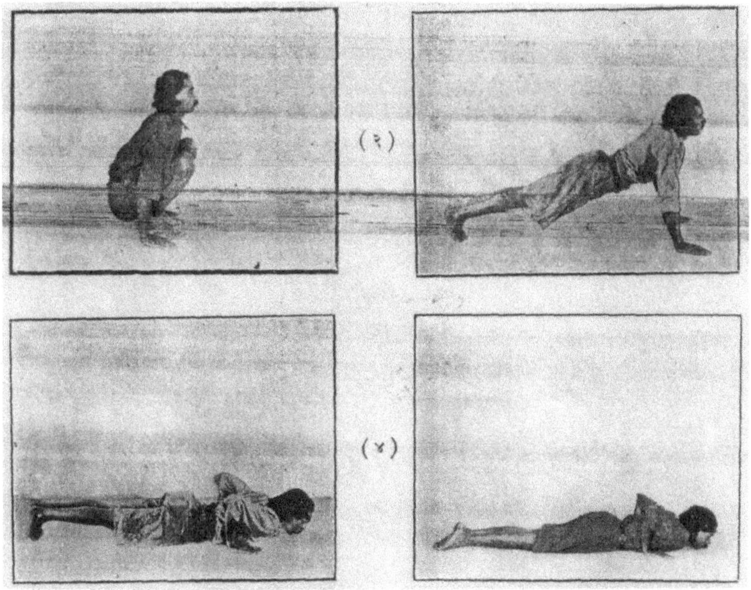

"Jumping back" sequence in Kuvalayananda's *Yaugik Saṅgh Vyāyam*, 1936 (with permission of Kaivalyadhama Institute)

to the "jump through" to *daṇḍāsana* in Ashtanga Vinyasa. From here, the student assumes the *āsana* itself, which is held *for five breaths.* Thereafter he or she lifts the legs through the arms without touching the floor (known as "Khade Ho Jao") to a press-up position and reverses the previous movements to a standing "attention." The form corresponds in every detail to the dynamic aspect of the Ashtanga system, even down to the standardized number of breaths for each posture.

It is significant that the "*sūryanamaskār*" sequence (which is itself nothing more than a particular arrangement of dands) is in this book known as "Ashtang Dand" (205), probably with reference to the position known in certain quarters as "*aṣṭāṅga namaskāra*," in which eight parts of the body (feet, knees, hands, chest, and chin) touch the ground simultaneously. Although this position is replaced in Krishnamacharya's sequence with the "push-up" posture known as *caturāṅga daṇḍāsana*, it is not unreasonable to speculate that the appellation "ashtanga yoga" may indicate the system's foundations in dands (reformulated as *āsana*) rather than any genealogical relationship with Patañjali's eightfold yoga. Mujumdar's *Encyclopedia of Indian Physical Culture* of 1950 states that *sūryanamaskār* is also known as "sashtanga namaskar" (456), with reference to the same central posture. In this view, *sūryanamaskar* is a modern, physical

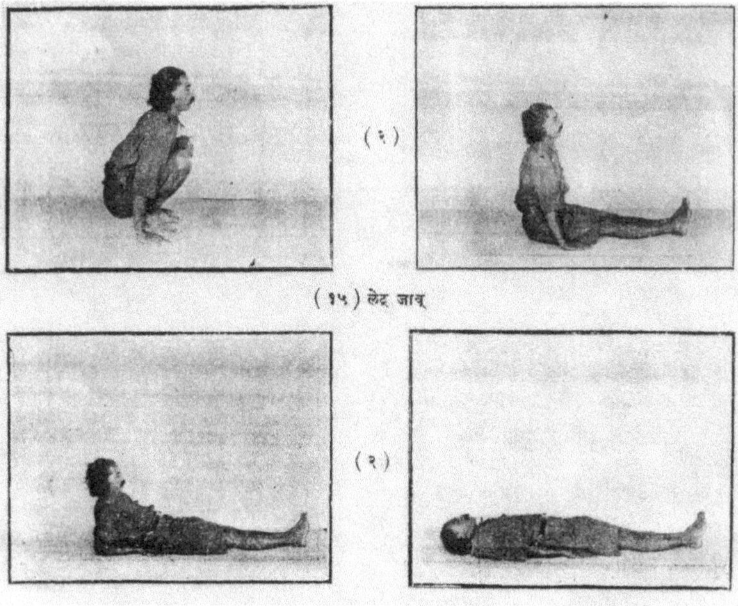

"Jumping through" in Kuvalayananda's *Yaugik Saṅgh Vyāyam*, 1936 (with permission of Kaivalyadhama Institute)

culture–oriented rendition of the far more ancient practice of prostrating to the sun (see also De Maitre, 1936: 134, on *aṣṭāṅga dands* used as prostrations during pilgrimage). And Ashtanga Vinyasa is a powerful synthesis of *āsanas* and *dands*, after the manner of Kuvalayananda's national physical culture programs.

It is clear that these sections of the syllabus represent a fusion of popular "indigenous" aerobic exercises with *āsana* to create a system of athletic yoga mostly unknown in India before the 1920s. This was partly a response to the influence of the rhythmic acrobatics of Western gymnastics. Krishnamacharya's dynamic teaching style in Mysore is of a piece with this trend, and his elaborate innovations in *āsana* represent virtuoso additions to what was, by the time he began teaching in Mysore, becoming a standard exercise format across the nation. Although the evident proficiency of his young troupe was probably unsurpassed at the time, the *mode* of practice was in itself by no means exceptional.

Modernity in Tradition

An attempt to exhaust the possible influences that may have given rise to Krishnamacharya's *āsana* system would be fruitless and dull. It has rather been my intention in this chapter to establish that Krishnamacharya was not working within a historical vacuum and that his teaching represents an admixture of cultural adaptation, radical innovation, and fidelity to tradition. This is *not* a particularly contentious assertion. The attribution of all his learning to the grace of his guru and to the mysteriously vanished *Yoga Kurunta* can be understood as a standard convention in a living (Sanskritic) tradition where conservation and innovation are tandem imperatives. As Pierre-Sylvain Filliozat explains,

> The orthodox pandit is not in the least concerned to restore an ancient state of affairs. If he were to point out the diachronic differences between the base-text and his own epoch, he would have to reveal his own share of innovation and his individuality. He prefers to keep this latter hidden. For him, the important thing is to present the whole of his knowledge—which contains both the ancient heritage and his new vision—as an organized totality. (Filliozat 1992: 92, my trans.)

To point up the influences and unmistakably modern innovations that contribute to Krishnamacharya's Mysore method (and by extrapolation to the current Ashtanga Vinyasa system) is, by this reasoning, not to impute any kind of inauthenticity to it. Krishnamacharya, like legions of pandits before him, adapted his teaching to the cultural temper of the times while remaining within the bounds of orthodoxy. Krishnamacharya's (and K. Pattabhi Jois's) account of Ashtanga Vinyasa's origins legitimated this modernized yoga in traditionally acceptable fashion, with reference to *śāstra* and guru. We should also add to this that, as Joseph Alter puts it, the modern yoga renaissance was "self-consciously concerned with modernity, and the programmatic modernization of tradition" (2006: 762). Although today's "Krishnamacharya industry" tends to foreground the timeless and traditional in his teaching—such as his direct and transhistorical access to the sage Śrī Nāthamūni, and his study of the orthodox *darśanas*—there is no question that Krishnamacharya's time in Mysore was heavily influenced by the same kind of "programmatic modernization" that was occurring all around him.

It would be a mistake to think that the present work's focus on the genesis of Ashtanga as a partial result of modern Indian physical culture implies either a diminution of its value or a denial of the other practical and philosophical elements that so manifestly inform the practice, such as the "classical" procedures of *haṭha* yoga (viz. *mudrā, bandha, dṛṣṭi*, and *prāṇāyāma*) and the orthodox Hindu intellectual tradition in which T. Krishnamcharya was steeped. The modern practice of Ashtanga Vinyasa yoga stands in a complex relationship to history, and the influence of pedagogical gymnastics is just one element in its composition. It is, nevertheless, a major one, and Krishnamacharya's early phase of dynamic yoga teaching, which persists (at least in mode)[21] in the Ashtanga Vinyasa method of Pattabhi Jois, cannot be fully understood without reference to it. That Krishnamacharya drew on a variety of popular physical culture forms and exploited the topos of *haṭha* yogic "circus turns" in his elaboration and promotion of yoga need not in any way invalidate the method. It does, however, provide an invaluable insight into the dynamics of knowledge transmission with regard to one of the twentieth century's most revered yoga teachers and into a far more widespread osmosis between modernity and tradition.

Concluding Reflections

This chapter and those which precede it have outlined some of the ways in which the early modern practice of *āsana* was influenced by various expressions of physical culture. This does not mean that the kind of posture-based yogas that predominate globally today are "mere gymnastics" nor that they are necessarily less "real" or "spiritual" than other forms of yoga. The history of modern physical culture overlaps and intersects with the histories of para-religious, "unchurched" spirituality; Western esotericism; medicine, health, and hygiene; chiropractic, osteopathy, and bodywork; body-centered psychotherapy; the modern revival of Hinduism; and the sociopolitical demands of the emergent modern Indian nation (to name but a few). In turn, each of these histories is intimately linked to the development of modern transnational, anglophone yoga. Historically speaking, then, physical culture encompasses a far broader range of concerns and influences than "mere gymnastics," and in many instances the modes of practice, belief frameworks, and aspirations of its practitioners are coterminous with those of modern, posture-based yoga. They may indeed be at variance with "Classical Yoga," but it does not follow from this that these practices, beliefs, and aspirations (whether conceived as yoga or not) are thereby lacking in seriousness, dignity, or spiritual profundity.

For some, such as best-selling yoga scholar Georg Feuerstein, the modern fascination with postural yoga can only be a perversion of the authentic yoga of tradition. "When traditional yoga reached our Western shores in the late nineteenth century," writes Feuerstein, "it was gradually stripped of its spiritual orientation and remodeled into fitness training" (2003: 27).[22] However, as should be clear by now, several aspects of Feuerstein's assessment are misplaced. First, Vivekananda's system should not be considered "traditional yoga" in any strict sense but rather the first (and possibly most enduring) expression of what I have termed "transnational anglophone yoga." Second, the notion that "fitness" is somehow opposed to the "spiritual" ignores the possibility of physical training as spiritual practice, in India as elsewhere (e.g., Alter 1992a). It also misses the deeply "spiritual" orientation of some modern bodybuilding and of women's fitness training in the harmonial gymnastics tradition (chapters 6 and 7 above). Third, the merger of "traditional yoga" (viz. the modern yoga of Vivekananda) with physical culture did not begin on North American shores, even though its development was, and continues to be, influenced by experiments and innovations there.

As I write this conclusion, winners of regional and national heats are gathering at the Bikram Yoga College of India Headquarters near Hollywood, Los Angeles, to compete in the 2009 Bishnu Charan Ghosh Yoga Asana Championship (named in honor of international bodybuilding champion B. C. Ghosh, brother of Paramahansa Yogananda, and guru of event organizer Bikram Choudhury; see chapter 6). Each contender will have three minutes to perform five compulsory postures plus two additional postures of choice, drawn, as the official entry form specifies, "from the 84 asanas as derived from Patanjali." Competitors will be judged on three main criteria: "a) Proportion of the body, b) Performance regarding steadiness of the posture, c) Dress, style, and grace in asana execution" ("Rules and Regulations," Choudhury 2009). In many respects, Bikram's competition represents a culmination of the historical processes described in this book. Each of its elements can be traced ultimately to the encounter of international physical culture and modern yoga during the early twentieth century: the aesthetic concern for grace, beauty, and sartorial style; the focus on the muscular and structural perfection of the body and the "pose-off" format reminiscent of bodybuilding competitions; and the erroneous but ubiquitous notion that such posture practice derives from Patañjali. A competition like this in the name of yoga would scarcely have been conceivable were it not for the early merger of physical exercise and international yoga and its subsequent normalization as the practical substance of yoga itself in the post–World War II West—and this in spite of Bikram's claim that *āsana* competitions have a two-thousand-year history in India (Daggersfield 2009).

Not satisfied with his own international tournament, however, Bikram is currently negotiating with British Olympic Committee chairman Sebastian Coe to make yoga an event at the London Olympic Games in 2012. Whether the bid is successful or not, it is a sign that global yoga has entered a new phase, one that foregrounds the same Grecian-inspired ideal of psychosomatic fitness that characterized the creation of the modern Games twelve decades ago. The first modern Olympics in Athens and the publication of Vivekananda's *Raja Yoga*, both in 1896, simultaneously brought modern physical culture and modern yoga onto the international stage in unprecedented fashion. Bikram's bid is a powerful symbol of the marriage of these two cultural phenomena and is exemplary of the way in which yoga and physical culture have merged in the modern era.

His guru, as we have seen, was one of the driving forces behind the refashioning of yoga as a democratic health and fitness regime in India during the early to mid-twentieth century. For Bikram (as perhaps for the recently deceased Pattabhi Jois and his yogic heir Sharat Rangaswamy), the lines of influence are clear-cut, and we can pinpoint fairly accurately the historical reasons for the way they practice and teach their yoga. In other cases the vectors may not be so easily traceable. One thing, however, seems evident: yoga as it is practiced in the globalized world today is the result of a new emphasis on physical culture, understood in the various and multiform ways we have examined here. What will become of yoga as it grows and acculturates in the West remains to be seen.

notes

◇◇◇◇◇◇◇

INTRODUCTION

1. In 2004 there were more than 2.5 million practitioners of yoga in Britain alone (statistics from the consumer research company TGI as reported in the London *Times*, Carter 2004). For practitioner numbers in Britain, see also De Michelis (1995) and Newcombe (2007b). A 1994 Roper poll commissioned for the world's most popular yoga magazine, *Yoga Journal*, estimated that over six million Americans (approximately 3.3% of the population) were practicing yoga—1.86 million of them regularly (Cushman 1994: 47–48). Ten years later in 2004, another national poll estimated that 15 million Americans were practicing yoga regularly (Carter 2004), while the proportion "interested in yoga" had also risen substantially. *Yoga Journal* estimated in 2003 that approximately 25.5 million Americans (12%) of the population were "very interested" in yoga. A further 35.3 million people (16%) intended to try yoga within the next year, and 109.7 million (over half the population!) had at least a "casual interest" in yoga (Arnold 2003: 10). The 2008 *Yoga Journal* market study suggests that while the US population practicing yoga has stablized, spending on classes, yoga vacations and products has almost doubled (Yoga Journal 2008).

2. On the initiatives by Bikram Choudhury (1945–) to franchise his yoga technique, see Fish (2006). See Srivastava (2005) for a report on the Indian government's countermeasures to Bikram's strategy.

3. I use the term *yogas*, instead of the singular *yoga*, to emphasize the plurality and variety of experiments and syntheses that sprang up under the name "yoga" during the modern period.

4. Alter's excellent 2006 piece "Yoga at the *Fin de Siècle*" goes a long way toward redressing this, and in fact covers many of the same "moments" in the history of modern yoga as I do here. Unfortunately, the article came to my attention too late for it to be incorporated with any care into the argument, but I nevertheless highly recommend it to interested readers as a sophisticated and insightful counterpart to the material in this book.

5. In this book I will be concerned principally with references to *haṭha* yoga in these early manuals. A fuller account of my early survey of the popular, practical yoga primer genre can be found in Singleton (forthcoming-a).

6. By "popular" here I mean intended for nonscholastic readerships. The word is not meant to say anything about circulation statistics for these books and journals.

7. Burley (2008) is one example of this approach. I might include here some earlier phases of my own writing on modern yoga (for example, Singleton 2005). The "authenticity drive" in contemporary modern yoga scholarship is the subject of Singleton 2008b.

8. In the context of Pattabhi Jois's system, the term *aṣṭāṅga* is popularly transliterated in various ways, including "Astanga," "Ashthanga," and "Ashtanga." Ashtanga seems to be the most common choice and is therefore the one I have adopted here.

CHAPTER 1

1. For a discussion of various systems of "yoga ancillaries" (i.e., *yogāṅgas*), see Vasudeva 2004: 367–436.

2. *mayi sarvāṇi karmāṇi saṃnyasyādhyātmacetasā/ nirāśīr nirmamo bhūtvā yudhyasva vigatajvaraḥ//* "Leaving all actions to me, with your mind intent upon the universal self, be without personal aspirations or concern for possessions, and fight unconcernedly" (25 [3]: 30, trans. van Buitenen 1981).

3. *māṃ hi pārtha vyapāśritya ye 'pi syuḥ pāpayonayaḥ/ striyo vaiśyās tathā śūdrās te 'pi yānti parāṃ gatim//* "Even people of low origins, women, *vaiśyas*, nay *śūdras*, go the highest course if they rely on me, Pārtha" (31[9]: 32).

4. The fullest exposition of the yoga of knowledge appears in 35 [13]. The philosophical underpinning for this yoga is the Sāṃkhya system.

5. Larson 1989 gives a useful survey of the "hybridity" debate as well as a lexical comparison of the YS and Vasubandhu's *Abhidharmakośa*. Bronkhorst (1993) goes so far as to argue that the YS is theoretically dependent on Buddhist sources.

6. Sarbacker (2005: 101) includes Sénart, de la Vallé Poussin, and Oldenburg as scholars who assert this latter.

7. There is no space to go into detail regarding the history and philosophy of Tantra, but the reader is referred to the studies by White (1996, 2000, 2003) and Flood (2006) for introductions to the topic. See Urban 2003 for a study of "modern Tantra."

8. See Briggs (1989 [1938]) chapter 11 on the legend of Gorakṣa, and Bouy 1994 on the difficulty of dating this figure.

9. On the dating of these texts, see Bouy 1994. On the less well-known *Jogapradīpakā*, see Bühnemann 2007a and 2007b.

10. The nine Upaniṣads that show evidence of such assimlation are *Nādabindu* (36th), *Dhyānabindu* (39th), *Yogacūḍāmaṇi* (46th), *Nirvāṇa* (47th), *Maṇḍalabrāhmaṇa* (48th), *Śāṇḍilya* (58th), *Yogaśikhā* (63rd), *Yogakuṇḍalī* (86th), and *Saubhāgyalakṣmī* (105th).

11. In *khecarīmudrā* the tongue is lengthened by gradually cutting the fraenum linguae and stretching the tongue outward until it eventually reaches the space between

the eyebrows. It is then reversed and inserted into the nasopharyngeal cavity. As a result of this practice, the yogin is said to drink the nectar of immortality that drips from a point in the head known as *bindu*. See HYP 3.32–53; GS 3.25–32.

12. GhS I.8: *āmakumbha ivāmbhastho jīryamāṇaḥ sadā ghaṭaḥ/ yogānalena saṃdahya ghaṭaśuddhiṃ samācaret*. ŚS refers to the perfection of *prāṇāyāma* as "*ghaṭāvasthā*," "the state of the pot" (3.55).

13. HYP names seven *mudrās* (III.6). ŚS names the same seven and adds four more (IV). GhS names twenty-five (III). In 2005 I was taught these same twenty-five *haṭha* yoga *mudrās* (with "modifications for householders") by B. N. S. Iyengar in Mysore.

14. For example, Satyananda Yoga (aka Bihar School of Yoga) routinely teaches three of the *ṣaṭkarmāṇi*, namely, "kunjal," a form of *vamanadhauti* (GhS I.39); "śankhaprakṣalāna," a form of *vārisāradhauti* (GhS I.17); and *neti* (GhS I.50). *Haṭha* yoga *prāṇāyāmas* are also taught from the beginning, and some *haṭha* yoga *mudrās* are taught in the later stages of training. The BSY, although the foremost yoga teacher training institution in Northern India, remains relatively unknown in the West, in comparison to the *āsana*-based systems stemming from the teachings of T. Krishnamacharya. This is not to say that BSY teachings are not imbued with the kinds of Western esoteric beliefs that De Michelis identifies as a key feature of post-Vivekanandan "Modern Yoga." See Singleton 2005 for an examination of this as it pertains to yoga relaxation.

15. Paul and Basu's contributions are considered in chapter 2. Kuvalayananda and Yogendra are treated in chapter 6.

16. Significantly, Theos Bernard was advised by his *haṭha* yoga teacher near Ranchi to further his studies of the subject in Tibet, for "what has become mere tradition in India is still living and visible in the ancient monasteries of that isolated land of mysteries" (1950: 11). It is also vitally important that two of the "ur-gurus" of the early twentieth century, Madhavadas-ji and T. Krishnamacharya, are also said to have traveled to Tibet as part of their yogic apprenticeships (although Sjoman 1996 suggests that Krishnamcharya probably studied with his guru Rammohan Brahmacari in southern India). As previously noted, *haṭha* yoga began to decline in India from the eighteenth century onward.

17. Samuel 2008 contains an excellent discussion and critical overview of scholarship regarding the origins of yoga and tantra and their history up to the thirteenth century. For a sound, if slightly dated, treatment of *haṭha* yoga, see Briggs 1989 [1938]. Burley 2000 offers a comprehensive but accessible overview of *haṭha* yoga as interpreted through the "classical triad" of texts (GhS, HYP, ŚS). Regarding *siddha* and *haṭha* traditions, see White 1996 (a more condensed version will be found in White 1984), who considerably expands and deepens the work of Eliade (1969, see especially chapters VI, VII, and VIII). Larson and Bhattacharya's encyclopedia volume on yoga (2008) contains a chapter on *haṭha* yoga as a "satellite" of Pātañjalayoga. For various aspects of tantric yoga, including Jain forms of practice, see Part II of Whicher and Carpenter 2003. Hartzell 1997 treats Śaiva and Buddhist forms of tantric yoga. For treatments of the body in tantra, see Flood 2006, Padoux 2002, and White 2002. About *āsanas*, including a brief survey of the role they play in traditional forms of yoga, see Bühnemann 2007a. For more anthropologically situated accounts, see Mallinson

2005, van der Veer 1989, Gross 1992, Bouiller 1997, and Hausner 2007. Bernard's 1950 participant/observer account still represents an interesting addition to these.

CHAPTER 2

1. Peter Mundy, writing in 1628–1634, similarly describes a group "Jooguees" who carry "greate Chaines of iron about the middle, to which is fastned a broad plate of the same, which is made fast over their privities to take from them the use and the very thought of women" (Mundy 1914: 177). Farquhar suggests that yogins began to carry heavy chains to symbolize their shame at being enslaved by the Muslim invaders (1925b: 440). The handstand position is a common feature of modern *āsana* (*adhomukha vṛkṣāsana* in Iyengar's 1966 nomenclature).

2. Also worthy of note here are Mundy's descriptions of "Fackeeres" and "Joogues" from vol. 2 of his travels during 1628–1634 (in Mundy 1914: 176–77); vol. 6 of the illustrated *Cérémonies et Coutumes religieuses des peuples idolatres*, edited by J. F. Bernard (1723); and Bishop of Calcutta Reginald Heber's short account of fakirs in his *Narrative of a Journey through the Upper Provinces of India* (Heber 1828). These accounts do not differ greatly in substance to those already described.

3. See Pinch 2006: 61–70 for a more extensive review of "Old World Encounters" with yogins, and Smith 2003: 65–85 for a general overview of the "European discovery of Hinduism," which includes a lengthier consideration of Bernier.

4. Bhalla 1944; Ghurye 1953: 112; van der Veer 1987: 693; Pinch 2006: 18, 84–86, 195–96.

5. See Dalmia 1995 on the British-facilitated construction of Vaiṣṇavism and the *bhakti mārga* (path of devotion) as "the only real religion of the Hindus." Also Pinch 2003, and Urban 2003: 69–70.

6. See also his description of how "the popular Yoga parts from philosophical Yoga" in his "Yoga Techniques in the Great Epic" (1901: 337).

7. I am grateful to Dagmar Wujastyk for help with this translation.

8. Although referred to on the title page as Rai Bahadur Śrīśa Chandra Vidyārṇava, the preface names the author as "Babu Srish Chandra Bose," that is, S. C. Vasu (Vidyārṇava 1919: i).

9. Note that GhS III.45–48, gives a rather unclear description of a posture called *vajrolī* in which the body is raised from the ground by the hands. This is distinct from the practice of *vajrolīmudrā* under discussion here.

10. This enthusiasm to modernize and render scientifically respectable is encapsulated in Vasu's attitude toward the alteration of consciousness by chemical means. "The practice of some class of inferior Yogis of stimulating psychic development by opium, *bhang*, *charas*, and *ganja*," he warns, "are to be strongly denounced by every sane and reasonable creature" (1895: xv). On the other hand, certain medical substances "which may be termed scientific"—chloroform, ether, and nitrous oxide—are subject to no such condemnation and are instead presented as a rapid means of attaining the state of *pratyāhāra*, or withdrawal of the senses (lvi). While Vasu is not recommending that the reader experiment with anaesthetics, it is clear that he considers them to be of a different order from the opium and cannabis derivatives favored by the *haṭha* yogis.

11. For a modern revisiting of this question, see Ken Wilber, "Are the Chakras Real?" (1979). Wilber, one of the leading lights of the Transpersonal Psychology movement, is widely read in New Age modern yoga circles.

12. These machines are called the AMI (Apparatus for Measuring the Functional Conditions of Meridians and their Corresponding Internal Organs) and the Chakra Instrument. The latter "was designed to detect the energy generated in the body and then emitted from it in terms of various physical variables" and "to detect minute energy changes (electric magnetic, optical) in the immediate environment of the subject" (1981: 257–58).

13. Note also Basu's contribution to the cataloguing of an Indian *materia medica* in his beautifully illustrated *Indian Medicinal Plants* of 1918 (with K. R. Kirtikar).

CHAPTER 3

1. The spelling is an anglicization of Baba Lakṣmaṇḍas.

2. For a description of Joseph Clark, see Ackroyd 2000: 148. The picaresque seventh book of Wordsworth's "The Prelude" (1805) depicts Posture Masters "perform[ing] their feats" at a Sadler's Wells saturnalia. See also the advertisement in the London *Spectator* of April 10, 1712, for performances of "postures as never was seen" by an unnamed "famous Posture-Master of Europe" and the advertisement in *Mist's Weekly Journal* of August 24, 1723, for Fawkes's show at London's Bartholomew Fair.

3. The *siddhis* in modern yoga will be the subject of Singleton (forthcoming-c).

4. At the time of publication I have as yet been unable to make a thorough survey of this genre but hope to do so in the near future. Significant titles include *Rêve de Pariah, aka Dream of a Hindu Beggar* (dir. George Melies, 1902); *The Yogi* (George Loane Tucker, 1913); *Beggars and Fakirs of India* (1920); *Raja Yogi, aka Prince Ascetic* (Manilal Joshi 1925); *Mystic India* (1927); and *Yogi Vemana* (1947).

5. Dane's book was, like Theos Bernard's seminal "report" on *haṭha* yoga of 1950, and B. K. S. Iyengar's "bible" of postural yoga, *Light on Yoga* (1966), one of a series of books on yoga by actual (or claimed) practitioners of yoga published by Rider Press.

6. Unlike live burials, the rope trick is not normally associated with *haṭha* yogins per se but rather with performing magicians styling themselves "yogis." However, as Eliade notes, "it has long been considered the prototype of yogic powers" and may reflect the close relationship that obtains between yoga and "fakiric miracles" (Eliade 1969: 321).

7. Compare this with a remark by Blavatsky in 1887 that *haṭha* yogis "converse with the devil" (1982e: 51, my trans. from the French). See section "Fakir's Avenue," this chapter.

8. It seems, however, that Vivekananda's American disciple, Swami Kripananda (also known as Leon Landsberg) was in fact teaching *āsana* as early as 1898, as evidenced by an article in the *New York Herald* of Sunday March 27 (fifth section) entitled, "If you want to be a yogi and have heavenly dreams, study these postures." One can only speculate as to whether Vivekananda taught these directly to his disciple or whether Kripananda learned them on his own initiative. The former option seems unlikely, given what we have seen of Vivekananda's attitude to *āsana*, but it is not unthinkable. I thank Eric Shaw for drawing my attention to this article.

9. See also Blavatsky 1982a: 462–64; 1982e: 113; 1982d: 604, 615; and Neff 1937: 96.

10. See Bouiller (1997: 51) on the *kāpālikas* and their relationship to modern day *haṭha* yogis; and Urban (2003: 147–64) on Vivekananda's hostility toward tantra more generally.

CHAPTER 4

1. Elsewhere Roth writes, "The ultimate aim of rational Gymnastics is the harmonious development of the physical and psychical life of man" (1852: 1).

2. The British army also adopted the practice of Indian Clubs (*jori*) in the nineteenth century, combining them with callisthenics and Swedish gymnastics (Todd 2003: 73). Indian Clubs, indeed, gained widespread popularity in the physical culture movement as a whole, speaking to the fact that the vectors of exchange were never unilaterally from West to East.

3. See also Alter 2005: 126–27, on the differentiation of the Pātañjalan notion of *kāya saṃpat*—perfection of the body—from modern medicalized yoga. See De Michelis 2004: 211–17 on specific therapeutic correspondences in Iyengar.

4. For examples of yoga compared to gymnastics, see Yogananda 1925b: 10; Yogendra 1989 [1928]: 83; Jambunathan (1933: xi); McLaurin 1933: 10; Sivananda 1935: 22.

5. Gulick's "clarion call 'that Christ's Kingdom should include the athletic world' provided a philosophical rationale for operating sports in society" (Ladd and Mathison 1999: 63).

6. Note, however, that it was the Hanuman Vyayam Prasarak Mandal of Amaravati that "had the honour of organising the first successful demonstration of Indian Physical Culture at the Berlin Olympic gathering in 1936" (Gharote and Gharote 1999: 108). Buck's early efforts did much to launch India on the worldwide physiological nationalist scene.

7. See Alter 2004c on the marginalization of yoga and individualistic physical culture (such as Swedish drill) as team sports gained precedence at the turn of the century. Conversely, McDonald (1999) points out that sport is discouraged in the Hindu cultural supremacist organization the RSS because it encourages competition and individualism, whereas "physical culture" (including *yogāsana* drill) promotes solidarity and selflessness (356n.1).

CHAPTER 5

1. Ramamurthy appears on the title page of his book as "The Indian Hercules" (1923). See also Nadkarni 1927. Ghose confers the same title on one Asananda Dhenki (1925: 15).

2. Budd points out that physical culture publications of the time often sustained "a hysterical rhetoric of biological degeneration" alongside "the more euphoric positivism of their own methods" (1997: 82). See also Pick 1989 on the anxiety of biological decline ("dégénérescence") as specifically "European disorder."

3. "Callisthenics" (American spelling, "calisthenics") refers to the system of gymnastics invented by Phokion Heinrich Clias (1782–1854), a native of Boston who helped train the Swiss army early in the nineteenth century and later became superintendent of physical training in the royal military and naval academies of England. His major work is *An Elementary Course of Gymnastic Exercises, Intended to Develop and Improve the Physical Powers of Man* of 1823. In later years, the term *callisthenics* came to refer more generally to free-standing gymnastics regimes, particularly those aimed at women (Todd 1998).

4. *My System* was published in a Danish edition in 1904, was translated the following year, and continued to enjoy an astounding success for the next five decades. Here, and in chapter 6, I use the first authorized English edition of *My System* from 1905, which is based on the fifth Danish edition. Remarkably, by the time of its appearance in English, 20,000 copies had already been issued in Swedish, and 70,000 in German (1905: xi). The English edition was reprinted very regularly until at least 1957.

5. A 1916 textbook written for the Central Hindu College in Benares, entitled *Sanātana Dharma*, conveniently summarizes the enduring tenets of this creed. As well as the injunction to "avoid all doctrines which are the subject of controversy between schools recognised as orthodox" (Central Hindu College 1916: v) three principles are listed as the essence of the college's pedagogical message: (1) the instruction must be acceptable to *all* Hindus, (2) it must "include the special teachings which mark Hinduism out from other religions," and (3) it "must not include the distinctive views of any special school or sect" (vi). Unlike Bankim's religion, however, the book is not overtly nationalistic in tone, aiming rather to shape the students into "pious, moral, loyal and useful citizens of their Motherland and Empire" (viii). See Halbfass 1988: 345 on the spread of "sanatana-dharma-text-books" in India.

6. Pinch notes, "After her marriage in 1905, she was referred to as 'Debi Chaudhurani' in an explicit appeal to the sense of male patriotic duty evoked in Bankim's work by the same name (*Debi Chaudhurani*, 1884, featuring another married woman warrior-patriot" (2006: 242). See also Lise McKean's description of Debi's dramatic stage production of *Ānandamaṭh* as part of an "annual festival of heroes" that she instituted in 1903 (1996: 252–53).

7. *nāyam ātmā pravacanena labhyo na medhayā na bahunā śrutena/ yam evaiṣa vṛṇute tena labhyas tasyaiṣa ātmā vivṛṇute tanūṃ svām*. Olivelle (1996) translates this as "This self cannot be grasped/ by teachings or by intelligence,/ or even by great learning./ Only the man he chooses can grasp him,/ whose body this self chooses as his own."

8. Nivedita was closely involved in the nationalist extremist group, the *Anuśīlam Samitī* (Guha-Thakurta 1992: 171).

9. Included are "the combat techniques of lathi, kati, spear, patta, sword, bandesh, daggerfighting, Jujuitsu and wrestling as well as techniques of physical culture such as dand, baithak, karel, jodi, mallakambha, spring dumb-bells, weight-dumb bells, weight lifting, roman rings, techniques of sport such as lejhim, dumb bells, bala-kavayat, boxing, Sarvang sundara-vyayama etc." (Tiruka 1977: v).

10. See also Ruiz 2006, and chapter 9 below, on T. Krishnamacharya's performances of yogic feats of strength.

CHAPTER 6

1. See Alter 2004a on Kuvalayananda's "medicalisation" of *haṭha* yoga, and Singleton 2006 for my review of this book; Alter 2007 for an analysis of his contributions to physical culture; and Singleton 2007g for a concise summary of his life and work.

2. For example, in another incident later in life, Yogendra's son Jayadeva is cured of chronic eczema by a wandering fakir. Both Yogendra and his father are by nature "distrustful of *sadhus* and *fakirs*" but cannot deny the efficacy of the remedy. The noble fakir, moreover, will not accept remuneration for his cure (Rodrigues 1997: 149). This episode points again to the ambivalence surrounding the yogī which Joseph Alter (2005) diagnoses within certain practical modern formulations: although purged of all things mystical and magical, modern medical yoga derives an element of potency from association with yoga's "other history" of sex, magic, and alchemy. See also Briggs 1938: 128 on the reputation of certain yogis for curing sick children.

3. The following from the Institute's newsletter of 1962 is a good example of the later official change in outlook: "In modern times, Hatha Yoga, at best, has been regarded as a system of physical culture. This is absolute nonsense. Hatha Yoga unfolds a way of life and its ideals dove-tail into the ideals of other Indian cultural disciplines like polity, sociology, education art, etc." (Sondhi 1962: 80). *Haṭha* yoga, the same passage insists, is neither "perverted or magical," nor "only... philosophical scholarship" (80). Note also that I had hoped at this point in the discussion to include several images from Yogendra's 1928 manual *Yoga Āsanas Simplified* but was refused permission by Shri Yogendra's son, Dr. Jayadeva Yogendra, who now runs the Yoga Institute.

4. This book is a collection of writings by Yogendra that originally appeared in the Yoga Institute's periodical during the 1930s.

5. Regrettably, the edition I am working from is a 1989 reprint of the 1928 original and contains some additions and modifications that are not flagged as such in the text. I have not been able to track down the original edition. Even Yogendra's own Yoga Institute seems not to own a copy.

6. Yogendra was by no means alone in his fascination with eugenics and human engineering; many others contributed to the wider percolation of social Darwinist ideas into popular modern yoga: see Singleton 2007p. One further example will suffice here: Kuvalayananda's collaboration (at his research institute Kaivalyadhamma) with the aforementioned evolutionary biologist and eugenicist J. B. S. Haldane would doubtlessly make for an interesting appendix to Alter's case study of the Swami in his *Yoga in Modern India, the Body Between Science and Philosophy* (2006). Haldane, whose eugenic science fiction *Daedalus* of 1924 foresaw the predominance of designer test-tube babies by the late twentieth century, had a fascination with Hinduism and yoga and even lived in India between 1958 and 1963 (Dronaraju 1985). He occasionally referred to himself as a "Hindu agnostic" (Dronaraju 1985, 171) and was increasingly influenced by Hinduism's "contributions to discussions on human evolution" (98).

7. My information on Iyer's life derives mainly from interviews with his only child, K. V. Karna (September 17, 2005), and his chief student, now 100 years old, Anant Rao (September 19, 2005), who ran a physical culture school during the early 1930s in the same wing of Mysore's Jaganmohan Palace as the postural modern yoga guru,

T. Krishnamacharya (see chapter 9 and Goldberg forthcoming). Elliott Goldberg also helped me greatly with details of Iyer's life. It is to be hoped that Goldberg's forthcoming work will complement and expand the sketch of Iyer that I present here. Also note that a photograph of this original "Hercules Gymnasium" can be found in *Vyāyam, the Bodybuilder* of August 1927 (vol. 1, issue 8).

8. This book, as well as Iyer's *Perfect Physique* (1936), *Physique and Figure* (1940), and a short biopic of Iyer, can be found on Roger Fillary's Sandow Web site, www.sandowplus.co.uk/sandowindex.htm.

9. Thanks to Elliott Goldberg for drawing my attention to this quotation.

10. The following section is a partial reworking of Singleton 2007 (with permission of Brill). For further treatment of the history of Mind Cure and New Thought see Meyer (1965), Parker (1973), Jackson (1975), and Fuller (1982, 1989, 2001). Catherine Albanese's masterful cultural history of American metaphysical religion, *A Republic of Mind and Spirit* (2007), has much to say on New Thought and goes into more far more detail than is possible here below on the topic of Yogi Ramacharaka.

11. For example, in 2004 alone, *Hatha Yoga, or the Yogi Philosophy of Physical Well-Being* (discussed below) was published in New Delhi by Cosmo Publications and by Indigo Publications. In the same year it was published in London by L. N. Fowler and Co. Ramacharaka's books continue to be published in the United States by the Yoga Publications Society (Homewood, Illinois).

12. Consider also the following assessment by the prominent modern postural yoga teacher Goswami of his training in *haṭha* yoga with his (significantly named) guru Balaka Bharati: "My muscles increased in size and strength and finally I controlled them completely" (1959: 15).

13. *Haṭha Yoga Pradīpikā* 2.33–34, and *Gheraṇda Saṃhita* 1.52, where the same process is named *lauliki* and classed as a *śodhanam*, or "purification" (as opposed to *kriyā*, or *action*, in HYP).

14. It is of course Vishnudevananda, author of *The Complete Illustrated Book of Yoga* (1960), who is generally credited as the *āsana* pioneer within Sivananda-inspired yoga. See on this topic Strauss 2005: 97–100. Strauss herself is not aware of any involvement of Sivananda with Ghosh but considers Sanchez's scenario far from unlikely given that "the circles of contact were really quite small" within modern yoga (Sarah Strauss, personal communication, October 11, 2006).

15. See also the example of Ghamande's proto-correspondence course in chapter 8 below.

16. See bibliography for a list of Gherwal's later work, including the quarterly journal *India's Message* (from 1932), published out of Santa Barbara, CA.

17. Out of this group of yogis in America, Hari Rama is the one most concerned about food. His book is a curious juxtaposition of modern Hinduism and nutrition with, for example, "Extracts from Rama Tirtha" sandwiched between recipes for an "Egg Drink" and "French Dressing" (1926: 84).

18. Roland Robertson's (1992) term *glocalization* "refers to the provision within global marketing for the marketing of difference according to local taste" (Beckerlegge 2004: 309).

CHAPTER 7

1. See Singleton 2005 for an extended consideration of yogic relaxation in terms of harmonial religion.

2. See Shawn (n.d.) for an early summary of Delsarte's life and work, and his influence on contemporary American dance. See Ruyter 2005 for a more recent, scholarly consideration of Delsarte.

3. It was from Ling preceptor George H. Taylor that Stebbins learned "the therapeutic value of different forms of exercise" (Stebbins 1893: vi). See Taylor 1860 and 1885. As Jan Todd notes, Taylor experimented with partner work to increase the range of motion in various postures (1998: 147).

4. See also in this regard Bharati's now famous analysis of the "pizza effect" in transnational Hinduism (1970).

5. Stebbins's term *rhythmic breathing* quickly became a synonym for *prāṇāyāma*. Ramacharaka's *Hatha Yoga* refers to "Rhythmic Breathing" as "the keynote to much of the Hatha Yoga practices" (1904: 159). Yogendra also claims a "unique" system of "rhythmic breathing" which has common features with Stebbins (1928). See also Pratinidhi (1938) on the place of "rhythmic breathing" in *sūryanamaskār* practice.

6. Another fruitful avenue of research within the "esoteric gymnastic" tradition would be the emphasis on pelvic floor exercises prevalent not only in Stebbins but also in works by medical gymnastic luminaries Austin, Buchanan, Kellogg, and Taylor (see Ruyter 1999: 108). This emphasis, I would speculate, may have facilitated (via Pilates) the prevalent contemporary understanding of the *haṭha* yoga "locks" known as *mūlabhandha* and *uddiyānabandha* as exercises for "pelvic floor stability" and "core strength."

7. Choisy also founded the psychoanalytic movement "Psyché" (in which Jacques Lacan began his career) and was an important figure in the ongoing dialogue between yoga and psychoanalysis (see Choisy 1949 and Ceccomori 2001). See also her *Exercises du Yoga* of 1963.

8. Apparently one in a series of books that included *Mind Control Postures* and *Breath Culture* (Ali 1928 : 7). I have not, however, been able to track down these other titles.

9. My information regarding Stack's life is taken from her daughter Prunella Stack's 1988 biography, *Zest for Life*.

10. The postures correspond (from left to right and in Iyengar's 1966 nomenclature) to *salambhasarvāṅgāsana, eka pāda sarvāṅgāsana*, supported *setubandhāsana* (a common prop-assisted pose in Iyengar yoga), *śalabhāsana, daṇḍāsana, halāsana*, and *paścimottanāsana*.

11. Consider the following from Stack: "I believe...that a new civilisation is dawning, which will materialise around the year A.D. 2000 as a result of the foundations which are beginning to be laid by the enlightened women and men of today" (1931: 3). We might indeed wonder if Stack's prediction was a glimpse of the yoga boom of the late 1990s!

12. "Vegetotherapy has nothing to do with any kind of calisthenics or breathing exercises such as yoga. If anything it is diametrically opposed to these methods" (1952

interview in Reich 1967: 77). In his seminal *Bioenergetics* of 1975, Lowen attempts a "reconciliation" of Reichian therapy and yoga (71).

13. The review is found in the "Book Corner" section of *Yoga and Health*, a short-running independent magazine not to be confused with today's popular glossy of the same name. Thanks to Suzanne Newcombe for this reference.

14. Another figure worthy of study in relation to medical and remedial postural yoga is Bess Mensendieck (1861–1957), whose system of bodily alignment and awareness has had a profound influence on physical therapy today. See Mensendieck 1906, 1918, 1937, 1954. Such a study would situate her work within a wider history of postural correction in relation to yoga. Mrozek 1992 writes, "During the first half of the twentieth century, a highly orchestrated movement to improve the posture of America's young people developed, also linking concerns for the individual with care for the society at large" (289).

15. The League emerged from a surge of enthusiasm for the building and disciplining of the body in the early twentieth century. This "working-class and lower-middle-class organisation" went from 13,000 members in 1911 to 125,000 members by 1935 (Mosse 1996: 137).

16. Hariharananda Aranya, for example, glosses Patañjali's sūtra 3.24 (*baleṣu hastibalādīni*) thus: "All physical culturists know that by consciously applying the will-power on particular muscles, their strength can be developed. Saṃyama on strength is only the highest form of the same process" (1983: 296)

17. Indeed, we might note that "Modern Yoga" in the person of Vivekananda (according to De Michelis's 2004 thesis), and American women's first involvement with purposive exercise both "began in New England" (Todd 1998: 301). See also Park 1978.

CHAPTER 8

1. I am grateful to Aparna Lalingkar for translating portions of this text for me.

CHAPTER 9

1. Although Jois has certainly added to and amended sequences, my informants for this chapter (as well as an early publication by Krishnamacharya himself) corroborate the view that an aerobic "jumping" system similar to that now known as Ashtanga yoga was indeed sometimes taught by Krishnamacharya during this period (alongside other, nondynamic modes of *āsana* practice).

2. Srivatsan names this preceptor as Gaṅgānātha Jhā (1997: 23), the renowned Sanskrit scholar of Benares and Allahabad. See Jhā 1907.

3. This 1919 initiative coincided with the arrival in India of H. C. Buck, the dynamic American YMCA physical educationalist who was to have such an impact on physical culture in the succeeding years (see chapter 4), and with the establishment of Sri Yogendra's Yoga Institute at Santa Cruz. The equally influential Kaivalyadhama yoga center of Swami Kuvalayananda would open two years later.

4. Jois states that the *Aruṇa Mantra* from the *Yajur Veda* delineates the nine postures of *sūryanamaskār* "A" and that a section of the *Ṛg Veda* delineates the eighteen

postures of "B" (interview September 25, 2005). The verses that he recited to me at this time as being a delineation of *sūryanamaskār* "A" were in fact from an oft-used Śanti mantra employed at the commencement of a range of ritual invocations, and which begins, "Oṃ bhadraṃ karṇebhiḥ śṛṇuyāma devāḥ/ Bhadraṃ paśyemākṣarabhir jajatrāḥ..." ("O Gods! Let us hear auspicious words through our ears./ Let us see auspicious things through our eyes in the sacrifices..."). The mantra that he recited to me as being a delineation of *sūryanamaskār* "B" was from Ṛgveda 1.50.11cd (repeated elsewhere in the Vedic literature, e.g., Taittirīya Brāhmaṇa, Fourth Part): "hṛdrogaṃ mama sūrya harimāṇaṃ ca nāśaya" ("O Sūrya, please destroy my heart (hṛd) disease (rogam) and jaundice (harimāṇam—yellowness)"). This mantra has been used widely in the last few decades by Indians who say it can help cure heart disease. It is hard to see how either of these verses pertain in any way to *sūryanamaskār*, let alone delineate the individual movements. I am grateful to Frederick M. Smith for his help in tracking down and translating these verses.

5. Yogendra's "authority" here is cited as *Haṭhayogapradīpikā*, with *Jyotsnā*, 1.51. However, this verse and commentary are a straightforward description and gloss on the technique of *siṃhāsana* and do not mention *sūryanamaskāra*. Yogendra's point probably still obtains in spite of this confusing reference.

6. Sjoman, however, refers to "complaints of lack of interest" in the *yogaśālā* from 1945 (1996: 51). From October 1942 onward, the records note an annual "Yogasala Day."

7. Krishnamacharya lists his sources in the dedication/preface, which is dated October 10, 1934. They are 1. Haṭhayogapradīpikā, 2. Rājayogaratnākara, 3. Yogatārāvali, 4. Yogaphalapradīpikā, 5. Rāvaṇanāḍi, 6. Bhairavakalpa, 7. Śrītattvanidhi, 8. Yogaratnakaraṇḍa, 9. Mahānārāyaṇīya, 10. Rudrayāmala, 11. Brahmayāmala, 12. Atharvaṇarahasya, 13. Pātañjalayogadarśana, 14. Kapilasūtra, 15. Yogayājñavalkya, 16. Gheraṇḍasaṃhitā, 17. Nāradapañcarātrasaṃhitā, 18. Sattvasaṃhitā, 19. Sūtasaṃhitā, 20. Dhyānabindūpaniṣad, 21. Śāṇḍilyopaniṣad, 22. Yogaśikhopaniṣad, 23. Yogakuṇḍalyupaniṣad, 24. Ahirbudhnyasaṃhitā, 25. Nādabindūpaniṣad, 26. Amṛtabindūpaniṣad, 27. Garbhopaniṣad. Sjoman gives a similar list (with a couple of variant spellings) in *The Yoga Tradition of the Mysore Palace*, along with the observation that this is "a padded academic bibliography with works referred to that have nothing to do with the tradition that [Krishanamachariar] is teaching in" (1996:66, fn.69).

8. Haldane, whose eugenic science fiction *Daedalus* of 1924 foresaw the predominance of designer test-tube babies by the late twentieth century, had a fascination with Hinduism and yoga and even lived in India between 1958 and 1963 (Dronamraju 1985). He occasionally referred to himself as a "Hindu agnostic" (171) and was increasingly influenced by Hinduism's "contributions to discussions on human evolution" (98). According to Alter, experiments conducted by Kuvalayananda in 1934 disproved the eminent physiologist J. S. Haldane's conclusions regarding "the so-called alveolar air plateau" (2004a: 93). This refers to J. B. S.'s father. See also Singleton 2005.

9. In *Yoga Makaranda* of 1935, Krishnamcharya himself states, "In *haṭha* yoga prominence is given to the technique of *āsana*, and strange kinds of practices, which are only to enthrall the audience, are also over-emphasised" (Narasimhan [trans.] 2005

[1935]: 34). Here, he acknowledges the spectacular applications of *āsana* but appears to judge them unfavorably. Might this indicate a degree of discomfiture regarding his public performance duties at the time?

10. This is corroborated by V. Subrahmanya Iyer's English foreword to Krishnamacharya's *Yoga Makaranda* in which it is stated that the book is "based upon the vast technical knowledge that the learned author, Sriman Krishnamacharya, has gathered from his extensive travels all over India, wherever the *Asanas* are specially practiced" (1935: iv).

11. The Maharaja offered poor children like these a stipend to attend the Sanskrit college. As T. R. S. Sharma points out, the Pāṭhaśālā and yoga teaching offered them a glimmer of hope in what was otherwise a desperate economic situation (interview with Sharma, September 29, 2005). Pattabhi Jois insists that Śrīnivāsa Rangācar did not teach at the *śālā* (interview with Jois, September 25, 2005). It is possible that Rangācar was already persona non grata there by the time Jois arrived.

12. Elsewhere, however, Iyengar has noted that the small coterie of students from the Pāṭhaśālā would sometimes go to Krishnamacharya's house for theory lessons (2000: 53).

13. Pattabhi Jois, who lived in a village four miles from Hasan, met Krishnamacharya for the first time in 1927 after a lecture at Hasan town hall. He says that Krishnamacharya stayed in the town for four years (interview with Jois, September 25, 2005), which would indicate that Krishnamacharya took up this job at the plantation in late 1927.

14. I should remark that Sjoman's otherwise insightful study of Krishnamacharya's yoga tends not to dwell on the physical culture education context that I describe here.

15. Of course, this is not to ignore the yogic principle of *tapas* (heat) which is used to explain the vigorous physical practices of Ashtanga Vinyasa (see Smith 2008).

16. We might note, finally, that Krishnamacharya's guru, Rāmmohan Brahmācari is referred to in the preface of the first edition of *Yoga Makaranda* as "sjt.," that is, "sergeant" (see Sjoman 1996: 51). As an ex-military man, it is even possible that the "*vinyāsa*" system that he taught to Krishnamacharya was informed by the dynamic army training regimes, such as Bukh's, which dominated physical culture in India at the time (see chapters 4 and 5).

17. V. Subrahmanya Iyer mentions this "special visit with his pupils" in his preface to *Yoga Makaranda*, which is dated September 1, 1934 [Krishnamacharya 1935: i]. Krishnamacharya began work at the *yogaśālā* in late August 1933 (Krishnamacharya 1935: v). The visit must therefore have occurred within the first year of his work at the *yogaśālā*.

18. I am grateful to Mahima Natrajan for partially translating this text for me. Joseph Alter's otherwise excellent examination of Kuvalayananda's yogic physical culture programs in relation to Muscular Christianity (Alter 2007) does not take into account this seminal publication.

19. "Jumping feet astride and stretching arms sideward. One. Bending trunk to the left and touching the left ankle with left hand. Two. Returning to position one. Returning to original position" (n.a. 1940: 91). See also Miele n.d.: 23.

20. They are called "Individualist Exercises" in contradistinction to the group games to which much of the rest of the book is devoted. For a description of dands, baithaks, and namaskars, see Alter 1992a: 98–105.

21. Ashtanga represents a particular "way" of practicing yoga that was evolved and transmitted by Krishnamacharya. The details of the sequencing and of individual poses seem to have been subject to some modification over the decades by Pattabhi Jois.

22. It could well be, of course, that Feuerstein's thinking on this matter has altered somewhat since 2003, especially given the wealth of historical material that has emerged since then on modern yoga, with which he is no doubt familiar.

bibliography

Abhedananda, S. 1902. *Vedânta Philosophy, How to Be a Yogi*. New York: Vedanta Society.
Abraham, N. 1933. Posture. *Vyayam* 4(4): 22–27.
Ackroyd, P. 2000. *London: The Biography*. London: Chatto & Windus.
Ahlstrom, S. 1972. *A Religious History of the American People*. New Haven: Yale University Press.
Ahmed, S. T. 1988. *The Mysore Palace*. Mysore: Academy Publishers.
Alain, P. 1957. *Yoga for Perfect Health*. London: Thorsons.
Albanese, C. L. 1992. *America, Religions and Religion*. Belmont, Calif.: Wadsworth.
———. 2007. *A Republic of Mind and Spirit : a Cultural History of American Metaphysical Religion*, New Haven, Conn.: Yale University Press.
Alexander, M. F. 1969. *The Resurrection of the Body, the Writings of F. Matthias Alexander*. New York: University Books.
Ali, C. 1928. *Divine Posture Influence upon Endocrine Glands*. New York: Cajzoran Ali.
Allen, A. L. 1914. *The Message of New Thought*. London: Harrap.
Allen, M. H. 1997. Rewriting the Script for South Indian Dance. *Drama Review* 41(3): 63–100.
———. 1998. Tales Tunes Tell: Deepening the Dialogue between "Classical" and "Non-Classical" in the Music of India. *Yearbook for Traditional Music* 30: 22–52.
Alter, J. S. 1992a. The "Sannyasi" and the Indian Wrestler: The Anatomy of a Relationship. *American Ethnologist* 19(2): 317–36.
———. 1992b. *The Wrestler's Body: Identity and Ideology in North India*. Berkeley: University of California Press.
———. 1994. Somatic Nationalism: Indian Wrestling and Militant Hinduism. *Modern Asian Studies* 28(3): 557–88.
———. 2000. *Gandhi's Body: Sex, Diet, and the Politics of Nationalism*. Philadelphia: University of Philadelphia Press.
———. 2004a. *Yoga in Modern India: The Body between Science and Philosophy*. Princeton, N.J.: Princeton University Press.

———. 2004b. Body, Text, Nation: Writing the Physically Fit Body in Post-Colonial India. In J. H. Mills and S. Sen (eds.), *Confronting the Body*. London: Anthem, pp. 16–39.

———. 2004c. Indian Clubs and Colonialism: Hindu Masculinity and Muscular Christianity. *Comparative Studies in Society and History* 46(3): 497–534.

———. 2005. Modern Medical Yoga: Struggling with a History of Magic, Alchemy and Sex. *Asian Medicine, Tradition and Modernity* 1(1): 119–46.

———. 2006. Yoga at the *Fin de Siècle*: Muscular Christianity with a "Hindu" Twist. *International Journal of the History of Sport* 23(5): 759–76.

———. 2007. Yoga and Physical Education: Swami Kuvalayananda's Nationalist Project. *Asian Medicine, Tradition and Modernity* 3(1): 20–36.

———. 2008. Yoga Shivir: Performativity and the Study of Modern Yoga. In M. Singleton and J. Byrne (eds.), *Yoga in the Modern World: Contemporary Perspectives*. London: Routledge Hindu Studies Series.

Ames, R. T., W. Dissanayake, et al. (eds.). 1994. *Self as Person in Asian Theory and Practice*. New York: State University of New York Press.

Anzieu, D. 1989. *The Skin Ego*. New Haven: Yale University Press.

Aranya, H. 1983. *Yoga Philosophy of Patañjali, containing his Yoga aphorisms with Vyāsa's commentary in Sanskrit and a translation with annotations including suggestions for the practice of Yoga*. Albany: State University of New York Press.

Archer, W. 1918. *India and the Future*. New York: Alfred A. Knopf.

Arnold, K. 2003. We're Listening. *Yoga Journal* 174: 10.

Asad, T. 1993. *Genealogies of Religion: Discipline and Reasons of Power in Christianity and Islam*. Baltimore: Johns Hopkins University Press.

———. 2003. *Formations of the Secular: Christianity, Islam, Modernity*. Stanford, Calif.: Stanford University Press.

Ash, B. 1934. Mainly for the Ladies: Building the Body Beautiful. S-T-R-E-T-C-H Your Way to Figure Perfection. *Health and Strength*, August 4, p. 170.

———. 1935. Preparing the Pupils' Programme. *Health and Strength*, December 21, p. 767.

Asturel, F., H. Price, et al. 1912. *Wunder indischer Fakire*. Berlin: C. Georgi.

Atkinson, W. W. 1911. *The Message of the New Thought*. London: L. N. Fowler.

Atkinson, W. W. and E. E. Beals. 1922. *Personal Power or Your Master Self*. London: L. N. Fowler.

Ayangar, C. R. S. 1893. *The Hatha Yoga Pradipika*. Bombay: Tookaram Tatya on behalf of the Bombay Theosophical Publication Fund.

Ayangar, C. R. S., and N. Iyer, 1893. *Occult Physiology. Notes on Hata Yoga*. London: Theosophical Publication Society.

B.K.S.Iyengar.com. 2006. *Inauguration of the WORLD's FIRST "Sage Patanjali" Temple at Bellur, Karnataka, India*. Available at http://www.bksiyengar.com/modules/Institut/Yogini/temple.htm. Accessed July 12, 2006.

Baier, K. 1998. *Yoga auf dem Weg nach Westen*. Würzburg: Beiträge zur Rezeptionsgeschichte.

Balfour, H. 1897. Life History of an Aghori Fakir. *Journal of the Anthropological Institute* 26: 340–57.

Ballantyne, J. R. 1852. *The Aphorisms of the Yoga Philosophy of Patanjali with Illustrative Extracts from the Commentary by Bhoja Raja*. Allahabad: Presbyterian Mission Press.

Balsekar, R. 1940. *Streamlines*. Bombay: Sindhula.

Banerjee, B. N. 1894. *Practical Yoga Philosophy or Siva-Sanhita in English; the Masterpiece of Occult Philosophy and Esoteric Yoga Science with Copious Explanatory Notes*. Calcutta: R. C. Bhattacharya, People's Press.

Bannister, R. C. 1979. *Social Darwinism, Science and Myth in Anglo-American Social Thought*. Philadelphia: Temple University Press.

Barthes, R., and R. Howard 1981. *Camera Lucida: Reflections on Photography*. New York: Hill and Wang.

Basu, B. D., and K. R. Kirtikar. 1918. *Indian Medicinal Plants*. Bahadurganj: Sudhindra Nath Basu, Panini Office.

Basu, S. 1893. *The Esoteric Science and Philosophy of the Tantras, Shiva Sanhita*. Calcutta: Heeralal Dhole.

Bayly, S. 1995. Caste and "Race" in the Colonial Ethnography of India. In P. Robb (ed.), *The Concept of Race in South Asia*. Delhi: Oxford University Press, pp. 165–218.

———. 1998. Hindu Modernisers and the "Public" Arena: Indigenous Critiques of Caste in Colonial India. In W. Radice (ed.), *Swami Vivekananda and the Modernization of Hinduism*. Delhi: Oxford University Press, pp. 93–137.

Beckerlegge, G. 2004. The Early Spread of Vedanta Societies: An Example of "Imported Localism." *Numen* 51(3): 296–320.

Bender Birch, B. 1995. *Power Yoga, the Total Strength and Flexibility Workout*. New York: Simon & Schuster.

Bernard, J. F. (ed.). 1733–36. *Cérémonies des peuples des Indes occidentales. Des Indiens orientaux. Vol. 6: Cérémonies et coutumes religieuses des peuples idolatres*, 9 vols. Amsterdam: J. F. Bernard.

Bernard, T. 1950. *Hatha Yoga: The Report of a Personal Experience*. London: Rider.

Bernier, F. 1688. Mémoire de Mr. Bernier sur le Quiétisme des Indes. *Histoire des Ouvrages des Sçavants* (September), art. V: 47–52.

———. 1968 [1670]. *Travels in the Mogul Empire, a.d. 1656–1668*, 2nd ed. Delhi: S. Chand.

Besant, A. 1908/1959. *An Introduction to Yoga*. Madras: Theosophical Publishing House.

Bhakta Vishita, S. 1918. *A Course of Lessons in Practical Yoga*. Chicago: Advanced Thought Publications.

Bhalla, P. N. 1944. The Gosain Brothers. *Journal of Indian History* 23, Part 2 (68): 128–36.

Bharati, A. 1976. *The Light at the Center, Context and Pretext of Modern Mysticism*. Santa Barbara: Ross-Erikson.

———. 1970. The Hindu Renaissance and Its Apologetic Patterns. *Journal of Asian Studies* 29(2): 267–88.

Bhashyacharya, P. N. 1905. *The Age of Patanjali*. Madras: Theosophist Office.

Bhonsle, R. K. R. 1933. Indian Sports in Olden Days in Madras. Some Games Described. *Vyayam* 4(4): 18–21.

Bhopatkar, L. B. 1928. *Physical Culture*. Poona: S. V. Damle.

Bickerdike, P. 1934. The Importance of Correct Posture. *Health and Strength*, December 8, p. 5.

Bishop, E. M. 1892. *Americanized Delsarte Culture*. Washington, D.C.: Emily M. Bishop.

Blavatsky, H. P. 1982a. *Collected Writings, Vol. II: 1879–1880*. Wheaton, Ill.: Theosophical Publishing House.

———. 1982b. *Collected Writings, Vol. III: 1881–1882*. Wheaton Ill.: Theosophical Publishing House.

———. 1982c. *Collected Writings, Vol. IV: 1882–3*. Wheaton, Ill.: Theosophical Publishing House.

———. 1982d. *Collected Writings, Vol. VI: 1883–1885*. Wheaton, Ill.: Theosophical Publishing House.

———. 1982e. *Collected Writings, Vol. VIII: 1887*. Wheaton, Ill.: Theosophical Publishing House.

———. 1982f. *Collected Writings, Vol. XII: 1889–1890*. Wheaton, Ill.: Theosophical Publishing House.

Bodas, R. J. R. M. S. 1892. *Patañjalasūtrāṇi with the Scholium of Vyāsa and the Commentary of Vāchaspati*. Bombay: Department of Public Instruction and Government Central Book Depot.

Bohlman, P. V., and B. Nettl. 1991. *Comparative Musicology and Anthropology of Music: Essays on the History of Ethnomusicology: Conference Entitled "Ideas, Concepts, and Personalities in the History of Ethnomusicology": Papers*. Chicago: University of Chicago Press.

Bonde, H. 2000. The Iconic Symbolism of Niels Bukh: Aryan Body Culture, Danish Gymnastics and Nordic Tradition. In J. A. Mangan (ed.), *Superman Supreme, Fascist Body as Political Icon—Global Fascism*. London: Frank Cass, pp. 103–18.

———. 2001. *Niels Bukh, en Politisk-Ideologisk Biografi*. Copenhagen: Museum Tusculanums Forlag.

———. 2006. *Gymnastics and Politics, Niels Bukh and Male Aesthetics*. Copenhagen: Museum Tusculanum Press, University of Copenhagen.

Bosc, E. 1913. *Yoghisme et Fakirisme Hindous (Introduction au Yoga)*. Paris: G. A. Mann.

Bose, R. C. 1884a. *Brahmoism, or History of Reformed Hinduism from Its Origin in 1830 under Rajah Mohun Roy to the Present Time, with a Particular Account of Babu Keshub Chunder Sen's Connection with the Movement*. London: Funk and Wagnalls.

———. 1884b. *Hindu Philosophy Popularly Explained, the Orthodox Systems*. New York: Funk and Wagnalls.

Bouiller, V. 1997. *Ascètes et Rois, un Monastère de Kanphata Yogis au Népal*. Paris: CNRS Editions.

Bouillier, V., and Tarabout, G. (eds.). 2002. *Images du Corps dans le Monde Hindou*. Paris: CNRS Editions.

Bourdieu, P. 1977. *Outline of a Theory of Practice*. Cambridge: Cambridge University Press.

———. 1978. Sport and Social Class. *Social Science Information* 17(6): 819–840.

———. 1984. *Distinction: A Social Critique of the Judgement of Taste*. London: Routledge.

Bouy, C. 1994. *Les Nātha Yogin et Les Upaniṣads, Étude d'histoire de la littérature Hindoue*. Collège de France, Publications de l'Institut de Civilisation Indienne. Paris: Édition-Diffusion de Bocard.

Branting, L. G. 1882. *Delar af L. G. Brantings efterlemnade handskrifter*. Upsala: R. Almqvist & J. Wiksell.
Briggs, G. W. 1989 [1938]. *Gorakhnāth and the Kānphaṭa Yogīs*. Delhi: Motilal Banarsidass.
Brink, B. D. 1916. *The Bodybuilder, Robert J. Roberts*. New York: Association Press.
Brockington, J. L. 1996. *The Sacred Thread, Hinduism in Its Continuity and Diversity*. Edinburgh: Edinburgh University Press.
Bronkhorst, J. 1981. Yoga and Seśvara Sāṃkhya. *Journal of Indian Philosophy* 9: 309–20.
———. 1985. Patañjali and the Yoga Sūtras. *Studien zur Indologie und Iranistik* 10: 191–212.
———. 1993. *The Two Traditions of Meditation in Ancient India*. Delhi: Motilal Banarsidass.
———. 2005. The Reliability of Tradition. In F. Squarcini (ed.), *Boundaries, Dynamics and Construction of Traditions in South Asia*. Delhi: Firenze University Press and Munshiram Manoharlal, pp. 63–76.
Brooks, D. R. 1992. Encountering the Hindu "Other": Tantrism and the Brahmans of South India. *Journal of the American Academy of Religion* 60(3): 405–36.
Broom, H. 1934a. Age-Old Physical Culture of the East. Even Modern Physical Culturists Can Learn Not a Little from the Yogis. *Health and Strength*, June 30, p. 738.
———. 1934b. The Gentle Art of Doing Nothing. *Health and Strength*, August 18, p. 224.
Bruce, K. 1931. *The Fakir's Curse*. London: H. Jenkins.
Bryant, E. 2005. Was the Author of the *Yogasūtras* a Vaiṣṇava? *Journal of Vaiṣṇava Studies* 14(1): 7–28.
Buchanan, J. 1932. Brief Notes on Physical Education in Bengal. *Vyayam* 4(2): 20–24.
Buck, H. C. 1929. The Coming of "Vyayam." *Vyayam* 1(1): 5–6.
———. 1930. *Syllabus of Physical Activities for Secondary Schools and Manual of Instructions for Teachers*. Madras: Government Press.
———. 1936. Physical Education—Its Place and Value in Modern Life. *Vyayam* 7(3): 80–83.
———. 1939. The Place of Indigenous Activities in the Physical Education Programme. *Vyayam* 10(3): 75–78.
Buckley, N. 1932. Will Nudism Be Nationalised? *The Superman* 3: 22–23.
Budd, M. A. 1997. *The Sculpture Machine: Physical Culture and Body Politics in the Age of Empire*. Basingstoke: Macmillan.
Bühnemann, G. 2007a. *Eighty-Four Āsanas in Yoga: A Survey of Traditions*. New Delhi: D. K. Printworld.
———. 2007b. The Identification of an Illustrated Haṭhayoga Manuscript and Its Significance for Traditions of 84 Āsanas in Yoga. *Asian Medicine, Tradition and Modernity* 3(1): 156–76.
Bukh, N. 1925. *Primary Gymnastics, the Basis of Rational Physical Development*. Translated and adapted by F. N. Punchard and J. Johansson. London: Methuen.
———. 1939. *Primary Gymnastics, the Basis of Rational Physical Development*. Translated and adapted by F. N. Punchard and J. Johansson. London: Methuen.
Burger, M. 2003. *Yoga Transmission in the Situations of Encounter*. Delhi: IHAR.
Burgin, V. 1982. *Thinking Photography*. London: Macmillan.

Burley, M. 2000. *Haṭha Yoga: Its Context, Theory and Practice*. Delhi: Motilal Banarsidass.

———. 2008. From Fusion to Confusion: A Consideration of Sex and Sexuality in Traditional and Contemporary Yoga. In M. Singleton and J. Byrne (eds.), *Yoga in the Modern World: Contemporary Perspectives*. London: Routledge Hindu Studies Series.

Bynum, C. W. 1995. *The Resurrection of the Body in Western Christianity, 200–1336*. New York: Columbia University Press.

Call, A. P. 1891. *Power through Repose*. London: S. Low, Marston.

Caplan, L. 1995. Martial Gurkhas: The Persistence of British Military Discourse on "Race." In P. Robb (ed.), *The Concept of Race in South Asia*. Delhi: Oxford University Press, pp. 571–607.

Carnac, L. 1897. The King of Contortionists. *Pearson's Magazine* III.iv:74.

Carpenter, E. 1911. *A Visit to a Gnani, or Wise Man of the East*. London: George Allen.

Carrette, J. 2000. *Foucault and Religion, Spiritual Corporality and Political Spirituality*. London: Routledge.

Carrette, J., and R. King 2005. *Selling Spirituality, the Silent Takeover of Religion*. London: Routledge.

Carrington, H. 1909. *Hindu Magic*. London: Annals of Psychical Science.

Carrington, H., and H. Price. 1913. *Hindu Magic: An Expose of the Tricks of the Yogis and Fakirs of India*. Kansas City, Mo.: The Sphinx.

Carter, M. 2004. New Poses for Macho Men. *The Times Body & Soul Supplement*, Saturday, May 22. Available at http://www.newsint-archive.co.uk. Accessed October 15, 2007.

Caton, A. R. 1936. *Activity and Rest: The Life and Work of Mrs. William Archer*. London: P. Allan.

Ceccomori, S. 2001. *Cent Ans de Yoga en France*. Paris: Edidit.

Chakraborty, C. 2007. The Hindu Ascetic as Fitness Instructor: Reviving Faith in Yoga. *Journal of the History of Sport* 24(9): 1172–1186.

Chambers, R. (ed.). 1862–1864. *The Book of Days: A Miscellany of Popular Antiquities in Connection with the Calendar, including Anecdote, Biography and History, Curiosities of Literature and Oddities of Human Life and Character*. Edinburgh: W. & R. Chambers, vol. 2.

Chanu, D. S. V. 1992. *Sriranga Sadguru, a Short Biography*. Mysore: Astanga Vijnana Mandiram.

Chaoul, M. A. 2007. Magical Movement (*'Phrul 'Khor*): Ancient Tibetan Yogic Practices from the Bön Religion and their Migration into Contemporary Medical Settings. *Asian Medicine, Tradition and Modernity* 3(1): 130–155

Chapelle, P. 1989. La Traversée d"une siècle. *Viniyoga*, December 24, pp. 27–32.

Charpentier, J. 1934. Haṭha-Yoga-Pradīpikā of Swātmārāma Swāmin by Yogī Śrīnivāsa Iyangār. *Bulletin of the School of Oriental Studies, University of London* 7(4): 959–60.

Chatterjee, B. C., and J. Lipner (eds.). 2005. *Ānandamaṭh, or the Sacred Brotherhood*. Oxford: Oxford University Press.

Choisy, M. 1949. *Yoga et Psychanalyse*. Geneva: Éditions du Mont-Blanc.

———. 1963. *Exercises de Yoga*. Geneva: Éditions du Mont Blanc.

Choudhury, B. 2009. Rules and Regulations, Bishnu Charan Ghosh Yoga Asana Championship. Available at www.bikramyoga.com/YogaExpo/5rulesnregs.pdf. Accessed March 2009.

Chowdhury-Sengupta, I. 1996. Reconstructing Spiritual Heroism: The Evolution of the Swadeshi Sannyasi in Bengal. In J. Leslie (ed.), *Myth and Mythmaking*. London: Curzon, pp. 124–43.

Christy, A. 1932. *The Orient in American Transcendentalism: A Study of Emerson, Thoreau, and Alcott*. New York: Columbia University Press.

Chvaicer, M. T. 2002. The Criminalization of Capoeira in Nineteenth-Century Brazil. *Hispanic American Historical Review* 82(3): 525–47.

C.I.A. 2008. The World Factbook. South Asia: Nepal. Available at https://www.cia.gov/library/publications/the-world-factbook/geos/np.html. Accessed May 2009.

Claeys, G. 2000. The "Survival of the Fittest" and the Origins of Social Darwinism. *Journal of the History of Ideas* 61(2): 223–40.

Clarke, J. J. 1997. *Oriental Enlightenment: The Encounter between Asian and Western Thought*. London: Routledge.

Clark, M. 2006. *Śaṅkarācārya and the Founding of the Four Monasteries*. Leiden: Brill.

Clayton, L. D. O. 1930. Eve's Ideal Path to Grace, Health and Fitness. *Health and Strength*, March 22, p. 314. Central Hindu College. 1916. *Sanâtana Dharma, an Elementary Text-Book of Hindu Religion and Ethics*. Benares: Board of Trustees, Central Hindu College.

Collingham, E. M. 2001. *Imperial Bodies, the Physical Experience of the Raj c.1800–1947*. Cambridge: Polity.

Connolly, P. 2007. *A Student's Guide to the History and Philosophy of Yoga*. London: Equinox.

Coomaraswamy, A. K. 1948. *The Dance of Shiva: Fourteen Indian Essays*. Bombay: Published for Asia Publishing House by P. S. Jayasinghe.

Coué, E. 1923. *My Method, including American Impressions*. London: W. Heinemann.

———. 1924. *Conscious Auto-suggestion*. London: T. F. Unwin.

Crisp, T. 1970. *Yoga and Relaxation*. London: Collins.

Crossley, N. 2005. Mapping Reflexive Body Techniques: On Body Modification and Maintenance. *Body and Society* 11(1): 1–35.

Crowley, A., and M. d'Este Sturges (under the pseudonyms Frater Perdurabo and Soror Virakam). 1911. *Book Four*. London: Wieland.

Crowley, A., (under the pseudonym Mahatma Guru Sri Paramahaṃsa Shivaji). 1939. *Eight Lectures on Yoga*. London: O.T.O.

Cushman, A. 1994. Guess Who's Coming to Yoga? *Yoga Journal* 118 (September/October): 47–48.

Daggersfield, A. 2009. Experts Train to Sweat It Out at the British Championships. Available at http://news.bbc.co.uk/2/hi/uk_news/magazine/7844691.stm. Accessed February 20, 2009.

Dalen, V. 1953. *A World History of Physical Education: Cultural. Philosophical. Comparative*. Englewood Cliffs, N.J.: Prentice Hall.

Dalmia, V. 1995. The Only Real Religion of the Hindus: Vaiṣṇava Self-representation in the Late Nineteenth Century. In V. Dalmia and H. V. Stietencron (eds.), *Representing Hinduism, the Construction of Religious Traditions and National Identity*. Thousand Oaks, Calif.: Sage, pp. 176–209.

Dane, V. 1933. *Naked Ascetic*. London: Rider.

———. 1934. *Modern Fitness, or the Five Minute Plan*. London: Thorsons.

———. 1937. *The Gateway to Prosperity, Leading to Health, Happiness and Success*. London: Master Key.

Danielson, A. J. 1934. *Health and Physical Education for Schools in India*. Calcutta: YMCA Publishing House.

Dars, S. 1989. Au Pied de la Montagne. *Viniyoga*, December 24, pp. 4–14.

Das, B. 1930. *Eugenics, Ethics and Metaphysics*. Adyar, Madras: Theosophical Publishing House.

Dasgupta, A. K. 1992. *The Fakir and Sannyasi Uprisings*. Calcutta: K. P. Bagchi.

David, M. D. 1992. *The YMCA and the Making of Modern India (a Centenary History)*. New Delhi: National Council of YMCAs of India.

David-Neel, A. 1954. *L'Inde, Hier, Aujourd'hui, Demain*. Paris: Plon.

Day, H. 1971. *Yoga Illustrated Dictionary*. Delhi: Jaico.

Deleuze, G. 1983. *Nietzsche and Philosophy*. London: Athlone Press.

Demaître, E. 1936. *Fakirs et Yogis des Indes*. Paris: Hachette.

De Michelis, E. 2004. *A History of Modern Yoga: Patañjali and Western Esotericism*. London: Continuum.

———. 2005. The Role of the Hindu Renaissance and New Age Ideas in the Development of Modern Haṭha Yoga. Unpublished paper.

———. 2007. A Preliminary Survey of Modern Yoga Studies. *Asian Medicine, Tradition and Modernity, Special Yoga Issue* 3: 1–19.

Desai, G., and M. Desai 2004. Yoga Unveiled, the Evolution and Essence of a Spiritual Tradition. DVD. Connecticut, New England: Yoga Unveiled.

Descamps, M.-A. 2004. *Histoire du Yoga en Occident*. Available at http://europsy.org/marc-alain/histyog.html. Accessed May 2005.

Deshpande, S. H. 1992. *Physical Education in Ancient India*. Delhi: Bharatiya Vidya Pakashan.

Desikachar, K. 2005. *The Yoga of the Yogi: The Legacy of T. Krishnamacharya*. Chennai: Krishnamcharya Yoga Mandiram.

———. 2009. *Masters in Focus*. Chennai: Krishnamcharya Healing and Yoga Foundation.

Desikachar, T. K. V. 1982. *The Yoga of T. Krishnamacharya*. Madras: Krishnamacharya Yoga Mandiram.

———. 1993. Introduction to the Yoga Makaranda. *Krishnamacharya Yoga Mandiram Darśanam* 2(3): 3–5.

———. 1995. Yoga Makaranda, for the Attention of the Readers. *Krishnamacharya Yoga Mandiram Darśanam* 3(4): 4.

———. 1998. *Health, Healing and Beyond, Yoga and the Living Tradition of Krishnamacharya*. New York: Aperture.

Dew, N. 2009. *Orientalism in Louis XIV's France.* Oxford Historical Monographs. Oxford: Oxford University Press.

Dimeo, P. 2004. "A Parcel of Dummies"? Sport and the Body in Indian History. In J. H. Mills and S. Sen (eds.), *Confronting the Body, the Politics of Physicality in Colonial and Post-Colonial India.* London: Anthem.

Disciples East and West. 1979. *The Life of Swami Vivekananda.* Calcutta: Advaita Ashrama.

Dixon, J. G. and P. C. McIntosh 1957. *Landmarks in the History of Physical Education*: Routledge and Kegan Paul.

Dodson, M. S. 2002. Re-Presented for the Pandits: James Ballantyne, "Useful Knowledge," and Sanskrit Scholarship in Benares College during the Mid-Nineteenth Century. *Modern Asian Studies* 36(2): 257–98.

Douglas, M. 1970. *Natural Symbols, Explorations in Cosmology.* London: Barrie and Jenkins.

Dresser, H. W. 1917. *Handbook of the New Thought.* New York: G. P. Putnam's Sons.

———. n.d. *A History of the New Thought Movement.* London: Harrap.

Dronamraju, K. R. 1985. *Haldane, The Life and Work of J.B.S. Haldane with special reference to India.* Aberdeen: Aberdeen University Press.

Duff, A. 1988 [1840]. *India and Indian Missions: Including Sketches of the Gigantic System of Hinduism both in Theory and in Practice.* Delhi: Swati.

Dukes, P. 1950. *The Unending Quest: Autobiographical Sketches.* London: Cassell.

Dutt, R. C. 1975. *Isvar Chandra Vidyasagar, a Story of His Life and Work.* New Delhi: Ashish.

Dutton, K. R. 1995. The Perfectible Body: The Western Ideal of Physical Development. London: Cassell.

Dvivedi, M. N. 1885. *Raja Yoga, or the Practical Metaphysics of the Vedanta.* Bombay: Sobhodha-Prakasha Press.

———. 1890. *The Yoga-Sutra of Patanjali.* Bombay: Tookaram Tatya for the Bombay Theosophical Publication Fund.

Dwight, T. 1889. The Anatomy of the Contortionist. *Scribner's Magazine*, April 5, pp. 493–504.

Eeman, L. E. 1929. *Self and Superman, the Technique of Conscious Evolution.* London: Christophers.

Eliade, M. 1963. *Patanjali et le Yoga.* Paris: Seuil.

———. 1969. *Yoga, Immortality and Freedom.* London: Routledge and Kegan Paul.

Elkins, J. 1999. *Pictures of the Body: Pain and Metamorphosis.* Stanford, Calif.: Stanford University Press.

Erdman, J. L. 1987. Performance as Translation, Uday Shankar in the West. *Drama Review* 31(1): 64–88.

Eubanks, L. E. 1934. Mind and Muscle. *Health and Strength*, April 7, p. 393.

Ewing, A. H. 1901. The Hindu Conception of the Functions of Breath. A Study in Early Hindu Psycho-Physics. *Journal of the American Oriental Society* 22: 249–308.

Farquhar, J. N. 1912. *A Primer of Hinduism.* London: Oxford University Press.

———. 1915. *Modern Religious Movements in India.* New York: Macmillan.

———. 1925a. The Organization of the Sannyasis of the Vedanta. *Journal of the Royal Asiatic Society of Great Britain and Ireland* 45(3): 479–86.

———. 1925b. The Fighting Ascetics of India. *Bulletin of the John Rylands Library* 9(2): 431–52.

Featherstone, M. 1991. The Body in Consumer Culture. In B. S. Turner (ed.), *The Body, Social Process and Cultural Theory*. London: Sage, pp. 170–96.

Feuerstein, G. 1989. *The Yoga-Sūtra of Patañjali*. Rochester, Vermont: Inner Traditions.

———. 2003. The Lost Teachings of Yoga. *Common Ground* 140: 4, 16, 27.

Filliozat, P.-S. 1992. *Le Sanskrit*. Paris: Presses Universitaires de France.

Fish, A. 2006. The Commodification and Exchange of Knowledge in the Case of Transnational Commercial Yoga. *International Journal of Cultural Property*, 13: 189–206.

Fitzgerald, W. G. 1897a. Side Shows 1. *The Strand Magazine, An Illustrated Monthly*, vol 13, January-June: 320–328.

———. 1897b. Side Shows 5. *The Strand Magazine, An Illustrated Monthly*, vol. 14 (79) July: 91–97.

Flagg, W. J. 1898. *Yoga or Transformation, a Comparative Statement of the Various Religious Dogmas concerning the Soul and Its Destiny, and of Akkadian, Hindu, Taoist, Egyptian, Hebrew, Greek, Christian, Mohammedan, Japanese and Other Magic*. New York: J.W. Bouton.

Flood, G. 1998. *An Introduction to Hinduism*. Cambridge: Cambridge University Press.

———. 1999. *Beyond Phenomenology. Rethinking the Study of Religion*. London: Cassell.

———. 2006. *The Tantric Body, the Secret Tradition of Hindu Religion*. London: I. B. Tauris.

Foucault, M. 1975. *Surveiller et punir: naissance de la prison*. Paris: Gallimard.

———. 1979. *The History of Sexuality*. London: Allen Lane.

———. 1997a. Subjectivity and Truth. In P. Rabinow (ed.), *The Essential Works*. London: Allen Lane, vol. 1, pp. 87–92.

———. 1997b. The Hermeneutic of the Subject. In P. Rabinow (ed.), *The Essential Works*. London: Allen Lane, vol. 1, pp. 93–106.

———. 1997c. Technologies of the Self. In P. Rabinow (ed.), *The Essential Works*. London: Allen Lane, vol. 1, pp. 223–51.

———. 1997d. The Ethics of the Concern for Self as a Practice of Freedom. In P. Rabinow (ed.), *The Essential Works*. London: Allen Lane, vol. 1, pp. 281–301.

French, H. W. 1974. *The Swan's Wide Waters: Ramakrishna and Western Culture*. Port Washington: Kennikat Press [Distributed by Bailey and Swinfen].

Freud, S., and P. Gay 1995. *The Freud Reader*. London: Vintage.

Fryer, J. 1967 [1698]. *A New Account of East India and Persia, Being Nine Years' Travels, 1672–1681*. Nendeln/Lichtenstein: Hakluyt Society.

Frykenberg, R. E. 2000. The Construction of Hinduism as a "Public" Religion: Looking Again at the Religious Roots of Company Raj in South India. In K. E. Yandell and J. J. Paul (eds.), *Religion and Public Culture. Encounters and Identities in Modern South India*. Richmond, Surrey: Curzon.

Fuchs, C. 1990. *Yoga in Deutschland: Rezeption-Organisation-Typologie*. Stuttgart: Kohlhammer Verlag.

Fuller, R. C. 1982. *Mesmerism and the American Cure of Souls.* Philadelphia: University of Pennsylvania Press.

———. 1986. *Americans and the Unconscious.* New York: Oxford University Press.

———. 1989. *Alternative Medicine and American Religious Life.* New York: Oxford University Press.

———. 2001. *Spiritual but Not Religious: Understanding Unchurched America.* Oxford: Oxford University Press.

Gervis, P. 1956. *Naked They Pray.* London: Cassell.

Ghamande, Y. 1905. *Yogasopāna Pūrvacatuṣka.* Bombay: Janardan Mahadev Gurjar, Niranayasagar Press.

Ghanekar, V. B. 1954. Suryanamaskar. *Vyayam*, June, pp. 2–5.

Gharote, M. L., and M. M. Gharote. 1999. *Swami Kuvalayananda—A Pioneer of Scientific Yoga and Indian Physical Education.* Lonavla: Lonavla Yoga Institute.

Gherwal, Y. R. S. 1923. *Practical Hatha Yoga, Science of Health. How to Keep Well and Cure Diseases by Hindu Yogic Practice.* Tacoma, Wash.: L. J. Storms.

———. 1927. *Great Masters of the Himalayas, Their Lives and Temple Teaching.* Santa Barbara, Calif.: R. S. Gherwal.

———. 1930. *Kundalini, the Mother of the Universe, the Mystery of Piercing the Six Chakras.* Santa Barbara, Calif.: R. S. Gherwal.

———. 1931. *Lexicon of Hindu Terms of Yoga and Vedanta Philosophies.* Santa Barbara, Calif.: R. S. Gherwal.

———. 1932. *India's Message* (Quarterly Journal). Santa Barbara, Calif.: R. S. Gherwal.

———. 1935. *Patanjali's Raja Yoga: A Revelation of the Science of Yoga.* Santa Barbara, Calif.: R. S. Gherwal.

———. 1939. *Lives and Teachings of the Yogis of India.* Santa Barbara, Calif.: R. S. Gherwal.

———. 1941. *World Prophecies: Dictators and Taxation Foretold in Ancient Hindu Philosophy.* Santa Barbara, Calif.: R. S. Gherwal.

Ghose, P. K. 1925. *Sad Neglect of Physical Culture among the Indians.* Calcutta: Ghosh.

Ghosh, B. C., and K. C. Sen Gupta. 1930. *Muscle Control and Barbell Exercise.* Calcutta: College of Physical Education.

Ghosh, J. M. 1930. *Sannyasi and Fakir Raiders in Bengal.* Calcutta: Bengali Secretariat Book Depot.

Ghosh, S. L. 1980. *Mejda, the Family and Early Life of Paramahansa Yogananda.* Los Angeles: Self- Realization Fellowship.

Ghurye, G. S. 1953. *Indian Sadhus.* Bombay: Popular Prakashan.

Girardot, N. J. 2002. Max Muller's "Sacred Books" and the Nineteenth-Century Production of the Comparative Science of Religions. *History of Religions* 41(3): 213–50.

Glucklich, A. 2001. *Sacred Pain: Hurting the Body for the Sake of the Soul.* Oxford: Oxford University Press.

Godwin, J. 1994. *The Theosophical Enlightenment.* Albany: State University of New York Press.

Godwin, J., C. Chanel, and J.P. Deveney (eds.). 1995. *The Hermetic Brotherhood of Luxor: initiatic and historical documents of an order of practical occultism.* York Beach, ME.: S. Weiser.

Gold, D. 1999. Nath Yogis as Established Alternatives: Householders and Ascetics Today. In K. Ishwaran (ed.), *Ascetic Culture, Renunciation and Wordly Engagement*. Leiden: Brill, pp. 68–89.

Goldberg, E. 2006. *Worshiping the Sun Indoors: The Beginnings of Modern Surya Namaskar in Muscle Cult*. Paper presented at a workshop organized at the Faculty of Divinity, University of Cambridge, Cambridge, April 22–23.

———. Forthcoming. *Radiant Bodies: The Formation of Modern Hatha Yoga*.

Gombrich, R., and G. Obeyesekere 1988. *Buddhism Transformed, Religious Change in Sri Lanka*. Princeton, N.J.: Princeton University Press.

Gonda, J. 1965. *Les Religions de l'Inde, Vol. II: L'Hindouisme Récent*. Paris: Payot.

Goswami, S. S. 1959. *Hatha-Yoga: An Advanced Method of Physical Education and Concentration*. London: Fowler.

Govindarajulu, L. K. (ed.). 1949. *Buck Commemoration Volume: Being a Memorial, Dedicated to Harry Crowe Buck*. Saidapet, Madras: Buck Commemoration Volume Committee of the Alumni Association of the YMCA College of Physical Education.

Gray, J. H. 1930. India's Physical Education What Shall It Be. *Vyayam* 1(4): 5–9.

———. 1931. Physical Culture: Physical Training: Physical Education. *Vyayam* 2(3): 15–16.

Green, N. 2008. Breathing in India, c. 1890. *Modern Asian Studies* 42(2-3 [Double Issue]): 283-315.

Griffith, R. M. 2001. Body Salvation: New Thought, Father Divine, and the Feast of Material Pleasures. *Religion and American Culture* 11(2): 119–53.

Grinshpon, Y. 2002. *Silence Unheard: Deathly Otherness in Pātañjala-yoga*. Albany: State University of New York Press.

Gross, R. L. 1992. *The Sadhus of India: A Study of Indian Asceticism*. Jaipur: Rawat Publications.

Guha-Thakurta, T. 1992. *The Making of a New "Indian" Art, Artists, Aesthetics and Nationalism in Bengal, c.1850–1920*. Cambridge: Cambridge University Press.

Gupta, C. P. K. 1925. *My System of Physical Culture*. Calcutta: P. K. Gupta.

Gupta, K. R. L. 1986. *Hindu Anatomy, Physiology, Therapeutics, History of Medicine and Practice of Physic*. New Delhi: Sri Satguru.

Gyanee, B. S. 1931. *Yogi Exercises*. Tacoma, Wash.: Bhagwan S. Gyanee.

Gymnast 1934. Amateur Acrobatics for "Bounding" Health. *Health and Strength*, February 10, p. 147.

Haanel, C. F., V. S. Perera, et al. 1937. *The Amazing Secrets of the Yogi, Followed by the Gateway to Prosperity*. London: Master Key.

Haddock, F. C. 1909. *The Power of Will*. Meriden, Conn.: Pelton and L. N. Fowler.

Halbfass, W. 1988. *India and Europe: An Essay in Understanding*. Albany: State University of New York Press.

Haldane, J. B. S., and A. Lunn. 1935. *Science and the Supernatural*. London: Eyre and Spottiswoode.

Hamilton, D. 1986. *The Monkey Gland Affair*. London: Chatto & Windus.

Hamilton, G. 1827. *The Elements of Gymnastics for Boys and of Calisthenics for Young Ladies*. London: Poole and Edwards.

Hanegraaff, W. J. 1998. *New Age Religion and Western Culture*. New York: State University of New York Press.

Hannah, C. 1933a. Health Wisdom of the East 1. Introductory. *Health and Strength*, July 29, p. 153.

———. 1933b. Health Wisdom of the East 2. Breathe "Prana" for Vitality and Strength. *Health and Strength*, August 5, p. 180.

———. 1933c. Health Wisdom of the East 3. Step-by-Step to Perfect Health. *Health and Strength*, August 12, p. 208.

———. 1933d. Health Wisdom of the East 4. Body and Mind in Perfect Partnership. The Full Fitness that Safeguards You against Debility or Disease. *Health and Strength*, August 19, p. 239.

———. 1933e. Health Wisdom of the East 5. The Yogi Way to "Sexual Balance." *Health and Strength*, August 26, p. 269.

Hara, O. H. 1906. *Practical Yoga, with a Chapter Devoted to Persian Magic*. London: L. N. Fowler.

Hargreaves, J. (ed.). 1982. *Sport, Culture and Ideology*. London: Routledge and Kegan Paul.

Hargreaves, J. 1986. *Sport, Power and Culture. A Social and Historical Analysis of Popular Sports in Britain*. Cambridge: Polity.

Hari Rama, Y. 1926. *Yoga System of Study. Philosophy, Breathing, Food and Exercises*. N.p.: H. Mohan.

———. 1927. *Super Yoga Science*. N.p.: H. Mohan.

Hartog, P. J. 1929. The Indian Universities. *Annals of the American Academy of Political and Social Science* 145(2): 138–50.

Hartzell, J. F. 1997. Tantric Yoga: A Study of the Vedic Precursors, Historical Evolution, Literatures, Cultures, Doctrines, and Practices of the 11th Century Kashmiri Saivite and Buddhist Unexcelled Tantric Yogas. Unpublished Diss., Columbia University, New York.

Hasselle-Newcombe, S. 2002. Yoga in Contemporary Britain: A Preliminary Sociological Exploration. M.A. Diss., Department of Sociology, London School of Economics and Political Science.

Hastam. 1989. Le Jeune Homme et le Rajah. *Viniyoga*, December 24, pp. 14–20.

Hatcher, B. A. 1999. *Eclecticism and Modern Hindu Discourse*. New York: Oxford University Press.

Hausner, S. L. 2007. *Wandering with Sadhus: Ascetics in the Hindu Himalayas*. Bloomington.: Indiana University Press.

Hay, S. N. 1988. *Sources of Indian Tradition: Vol. 2: Modern India and Pakistan*. New York: Columbia University Press.

Heber, Rev. R. 1828. *Narrative of a Journey through the Upper Provinces of India, from Calcutta to Bombay, 1824–1825 (with notes upon Ceylon), an Account of a Journey to Madras and the Southern Provinces, 1826, and Letters Written in India*, 2nd ed., 3 vols. London: John Murray.

Heehs, P. 1994. Foreign Influences on Bengali Revolutionary Terrorism 1902–1908. *Modern Asian Studies* 28(3): 533–56.

Hobsbawm, E. J., and T. O. Ranger. 1983. *The Invention of Tradition*. Cambridge: Cambridge University Press.

Holland, C. (ed.). 1998. *Strange Feats and Clever Turns, Remarkable Speciality Acts in Variety, Vaudeville and Sideshows at the Turn of the Twentieth Century as Seen by their Contemporaries*. London: Holland and Palmer.

Honigberger, J. M. 1852. *Thirty-five Years in the East*. London: H. Bailliere.

Hopkins, E. W. 1901. Yoga Technique in the Great Epic. *Journal of the American Oriental Society* 22: 333–79.

———. 1970 [1885]. *The Religions of India*. New Delhi: Munshiram Manoharlal.

Inden, R. 1986. Orientalist Constructions of India. *Modern Asian Studies* 20: 401–46.

———. 1992. *Imagining India*. Oxford: Basil Blackwell.

Ishwaran, K. 1999. *Ascetic Culture: Renunciation and Worldly Engagement*. Leiden: Brill.

Iyengar, B. K. S. 1938. 1938 Demonstration. DVD. London, Iyengar Yoga Institute.

———. 1966. *Light on Yoga*. London: Allen & Unwin.

———. 1987 [1978]. *Iyengar, His Life and Work*. Porthill, Idaho: Timeless Books.

———. 1993a. *Light on the Yoga Sūtras of Patañjali*. London: Aquarian/Thorsons.

———. 1993b. The Yogi on Yoga, an Interview with B. K. S. Iyengar. *Krishnamacharya Yoga Mandiram Darśana* 2(3): 36–38.

———. 2000. *Aṣṭādala Yogamālā*. New Delhi: Allied Publishers., vol. 1.

———. 2005. *Light on Life*. London: Rodale.

Iyer, K. V. 1927. The Beauties of a Symmetrical Body. *Vyayam, the Bodybuilder* 1(6): 163–66.

———. 1927. A Message to the Youth of My Country. *Vyayam, the Bodybuilder* 1(12): 245–48.

———. 1930. *Muscle Cult. A Pro-Em to My System*. Bangalore: Hercules Gymnasium and Correspondence School of Physical Culture.

———. 1936. *Perfect Physique*. Bangalore: Hercules Gymnasium and Correspondence School of Physical Culture.

———. 1937. *Suryanamaskar*. Bangalore: Bangalore Press.

———. 1940. *Physique and Figure*. Bangalore: Hercules Gymnasium and Correspondence School of Physical Culture.

Jackson, C. T. 1975. The New Thought Movement and the Nineteenth Century Discovery of Oriental Philosophy. *Journal of Popular Culture* 9: 523–48.

———. 1981. *The Oriental Religions and American Thought: Nineteenth-Century Explorations*. Westport, Conn.: Greenwood.

Jacobsen, A., and R. V. S. Sundaram (trans.) 2006 [c.1941]. *Yogāsanagalu by Vidvān T. Krishnamacharya*. Unpublished translation based on the 2nd Edition, Mysore: University of Mysore, 1973.

Jacolliot, L. and W. L. Felt 1884. *Occult Science in India and among the Ancients: With an Account of Their Mystic Initiations, and the History of Spiritism*. New York: J.W. Lovell.

Jacques, D. H. 1861. *Hints towards Physical Perfection: or, the Philosophy of Human Beauty; Showing How to Acquire and Retain Bodily Symmetry, Health, and Vigor, Secure Long Life, and Avoid The Infirmities of Age*. New York: Fowler and Wells.

Jambunathan, M. R. 1933. *Yoga Asanas. Illustrated. Being an Exposition of Yoga Poses*. Madras: Jambunathan Book Shop.

James, E. 1861. *The Yogi. A Tale*. London: Whittaker.
James, W. 1907. The Energies of Man. *Science* 25(635): 321–32.
Jensen, A. 1920. *Massage and Exercise Combined; A Permanent Physical Culture Course for Men Women and Children; Health-Giving, Vitalizing, Prophylatic* [sic], *Beautifying; A New System of the Characteristic Essentials of Gymastic and Indian Yogis Concentration Exercises Combined with Scientific Massage Movements; with 86 Illustrations and Deep Breathing Exercises*. New York: Albrecht Jensen.
Jhā, Gnt. 1907. *The Yoga-Darśana, the Sutras of Patañjali with the Bhāṣya of Vyāsa*. Bombay: Rajaram Tukaram Tatya for the Bombay Theosophical Publication Fund.
Johnson, E. L. 1979. *The History of YMCA Physical Education*. Chicago: Association Press.
Jois, S. K. P. 1999. *Yoga Mala*. New York: Eddie Stern.
Jordens, J. T. F. 1998. A Fake Autobiography. *Dayananda Sarasvati: Essays on His Life and Ideas*. Delhi: Oxford University Press.
K. P. L. 1944. Hatha Yoga. The Report of a Personal Experience. *Journal of Philosophy* 41(19): 530.
Kamath, S. 1933. Indigenous Activities. *Vyayam* 4(3): 22–28.
Kapferer, B. 1986. Performance and the Structuring of Meaning and Experience. In V. W. Turner and E. M. Bruner (eds.), *The Anthropology of Experience*. Urbana: University of Illinois Press, pp. 188–203.
Kasulis, T. P., R. T. Ames, et al. (eds.). 1993. *Self as Body in Asian Theory and Practice*. New York: State University of New York Press.
Katdare, D. M. 1927a. Rules for the Guidance of Subscribers and Contributors. *Vyāyam, the Bodybuilder* 1(1). No page number.
———. 1927b. Virile Humanity Is the Real Basis of Nationalism. *Vyāyam, the Bodybuilder* 1(4): 89–90.
Keat, R. 1986. The Human Body in Social Theory: Reich, Foucault and the Repressive Hypothesis. *Radical Philosophy* 42: 24–32.
Kern, S. 1975. *Anatomy and Destiny: A Cultural History of the Human Body*. Indianapolis Bobbs-Merrill.
Kersenboom, S. 1987. *Nityasumangali: Devadasi Tradition in South India*. Delhi: Motilal Banarsidass.
Ketkar, G. V. 1927. Tilak's Example and Precept on Physical Development. *Vyayam*, November 11, pp. 230–33.
Kevles, D. J. 1995. *In the Name of Eugenics, Genetics and the Use of Human Heredity*. Cambridge, Mass.: Harvard University Press.
Killingley, D. 1990. Yoga-Sūtra IV, 2–3 and Vivekānanda's Interpretation of Evolution. *Journal of Indian Philosophy* 18(2): 151–80.
———. 1995. Hinduism, Darwinism and Evolution in Late-Nineteenth-Century India. In D. Amigoni and J. Wallace (eds.), *Charles Darwin's* The Origin of Species, *New Interdisciplinary Essays*. Manchester: Manchester University Press, pp. 174–202.
King, R. 1999. *Orientalism and Religion: Post-Colonial Theory, India, and the Mystic East*. London: Routledge.
Kirkland, W. 1941. Speaking of Pictures, This Is Real Yoga. *Life*, February 24, pp. 10–12.

Koller, J. M. 1993. Human Embodiment: Indian Perspectives. In T. P. Kasulis, R. T. Ames, and W. Dissanayake (eds.), *Self as Body in Asian Theory and Practice.* New York: State University of New York Press, pp. 45–58.

Kopf, D. 1975. An Historiographical Essay on the Goddess Kāli. In T. K. Stewart (ed.), *Shaping Bengali Worlds: Public and Private.* East Lansing: Asian Studies Center, University of Michigan.

Kothiwale, D. B. 1935. Mass Physical Training. *Vyayam* 6(3): 4–9.

Kripal, J. J. 1995. Kali's Child: The Mystical and the Erotic in the Life and Teachings of Ramakrishna. Chicago: University of Chicago Press.

———. 2007. *Esalen: America and the Religion of No Religion.* Chicago: University of Chicago Press.

Krishnamacharya, T. 1935. *Yoga Makaranda.* Bangalore: Bangalore Press.

———. c. 1941. *Yogāsanagalu.* Mysore: University of Mysore.

———. 2004. *Yoga Rahasya.* Chennai: Krishnamacharya Yoga Mandiram.

Kumar, R. 1993. *The History of Doing, an Illustrated Account of Movements for Women's Rights and Feminism in India 1800–1990.* London: Verso.

Kuvalayananda, S. (ed.). 1924–. *Yoga-Mīmāṁsā.* Lonavla: Kaivalyadhama.

———. 1933. *Popular Yoga: Āsanas.* Bombay: Popular Prakashan.

———. 1935. *Popular Yoga: Prāṇāyāma.* Lonavla: Kaivalyadhama.

———. 1936. *Yaugik Saṅgh Vyāyam.* Lonavla: Kaivalyadhama.

———. 1972 [1931]. *Popular Yoga: Āsanas.* Hemel Hempstead: C. E. Tuttle.

Ladd, T., and J. A. Mathisen. 1999. *Muscular Christianity, Evangelical Protestants and the Development of American Sport.* Grand Rapids, Mich.: Baker Books.

Laidlaw, J. 2002. For an Anthropology of Ethics and Freedom. *Journal of the Royal Anthropological Institute* 8(2): 311–32.

Lamsley, A. T. 1930. Build a Better Race. *Health and Strength,* February 8, p. 144.

Lanman, C. R. 1917. Hindu Ascetics and Their Powers. *Transactions and Proceedings of the American Philological Association* 48: 133–51.

Larson, G., and Bhattacharya, R. S. (eds.). 2008. *Yoga: India's Philosophy of Meditation.* Delhi: Motilal Banarsidass.

Larson, J. G. 1989. An Old Problem Revisited: The Relation between Sāṃkhya, Yoga and Buddhism. *Studien zur Indologie und Iranistik* 15: 129–46.

———. 1999. "Classical Yoga as Neo-Sāṃkhya: A Chapter in the History of Indian Philosophy," *Asiatische Studien* 53(3): 723–32.

Leadbeater, C. W. 1927. *The Chakras.* Adyar: Theosophical Publishing House.

Lee, M. 1983. *A History of Physical Education and Sport in the U.S.A.* New York: Wiley, c1983.

Lee, M. M. A. 2005. *Turn Stress into Bliss: The Proven Phoenix Rising Yoga Therapy Programme for Relaxation and Stress-relief.* Gloucester, Mass.: Fair Winds.

Leonard, F. E. 1947. *A Guide to the History of Physical Education.* London: Henry Kimpton.

Levin, D. M. 1985. *The Body's Recollection of Being: Phenomenological Psychology and the Deconstruction of Nihilism.* London: Routledge and Kegan Paul.

Liberman, K. 2008. The Reflexivity of the Authenticity of Yoga. In M. Singleton and J. Byrne (eds.), *Yoga in the Modern World: Contemporary Perspectives.* London: Routledge Hindu Studies Series.

Lorenzen, D. N. 1978. Warrior Ascetics in Indian History. *Journal of the American Oriental Society* 98(1): 61–75.
Lorenzen, D. N. 1999. Who Invented Hinduism? *Comparative Studies in Society and History* 41(4): 630–59.
Losty, J. P. 1985. The Thousand Petals of Bliss: The Yoga Force. *Kos, Franco Maria Ricci (FMR) (American Edition)* 4(17): 91–194.
Lowen, A. 1975. *Bioenergetics*. New York: Coward, McCann & Geoghegan.
Lowen, A., and L. Lowen 1977. *The Way to Vibrant Health: A Manual of Bioenergetic Eexercises*. New York: Harper Colophon Books.
Macfadden, B. 1900. *The Virile Power of Superb Manhood*. New York: Physical Culture Publishing.
———. 1904a. *Building of Vital Power*. New York: Physical Culture Publishing.
———. 1904b. *How Success Is Won*. New York: Physical Culture Publishing.
———. 1912. *Macfadden's Encyclopedia of Physical Culture*. New York: Physical Culture Publishing.
———. 1926. *The Book of Health*. New York: Macfadden Publications.
Maclaren, A. 1866. *Training in Theory and Practice*. London: Macmillan.
———. 1869. *A System of Physical Education, Theoretical and Practical*. Oxford: Clarendon Press.
MacMunn, G. 1931. *The Religions and Hidden Cults of India*. London: Sampson Low, Marston.
Madhava and I. Vidyasagara. 1858. *Sarvadarsana Sangraha, or, An Epitome of the Different Systems of Indian Philosophy*. Calcutta: Asiatic Society of Bengal.
Madhavacharya. 1914. *The Sarva-Darśana-Saṃgraha, or Review of the Different Systems of Hindu Philosophy*. London: Kegan Paul, Trench, Trubner.
———. 2002. *Sarva-Darśana-Saṃgraha*. Delhi: Chaukhamba Sanskrit Pratishthan.
Maehle, G. 2006. *Ashtanga Yoga: Practice and Philosophy*. Innaloo City: Kaivalya Publications.
Mallinson, J. 2005. Rāmānandī Tyāgīs and Haṭha Yoga. *Journal of Vaishnava Studies* 14(1): 107–21.
———. 2007. The Khecarīvidyā of Ādinātha: A Critical Edition and Annotated Translation of an Early Text of Haṭhayoga. London: Routledge.
Mangan, J. A. 1999. *Shaping the Superman: Fascist Body as Political Icon: Aryan Fascism*. London: Frank Cass.
———. 2000. *Superman Supreme: Fascist Body as Political Icon: Global Fascism*. London: Frank Cass.
Manor, J. 1977. *Political Change in an Indian State: Mysore, 1917–1955*. New Delhi: Manohar.
Maranto, G. 1996. *Quest for Perfection, The Drive to Breed Better Human Beings*. New York: Lisa Drew/Scribner.
Marshall, P. J. (ed.). *The British Discovery of Hinduism in the Eighteenth Century*. Cambridge: Cambridge University Press.

Mathews, B. 1937. *Flaming Milestones, Being an Interpretation and the Official Report of the Twenty-First World's Conference of the World's Alliance of Y.M.C.A.'s, Held in January 1937, in Mysore, South India*. Geneva: World Committee of Y.M.C.A.s.

Matilal, B. K. 1994. The Perception of Self in Indian Tradition. In R. T. Ames (ed.), *Self as Person in Asian Theory and Practice*. New York: State University of New York Press, pp. 279–95.

Mauss, M. 1979. Body Techniques. In *Sociology and Psychology*. London: Routledge and Kegan Paul, pp. 95–123.

Maxick. 1913. *Muscle Control; or, Body Development by Will-power*. London: Ewart, Seymour.

———. 1914. *Great Strength by Muscle-Control.... With 54 Full-page Illustrations*. London: Ewart, Seymour.

Mayo, K. 1927. *Mother India*. London: Butler and Tanner.

———. 1928. *The Face of Mother India*. London: Hamish Hamilton.

McCrone, K. E. 1988. *Playing the Game: Sport and the Physical Emancipation of English Women, 1870–1914*. Lexington: University Press of Kentucky.

McDonald, I. 1999. "Physiological Patriots"? The Politics of Physical Culture and Hindu Nationalism in India. *International Review for the Sociology of Sport* 34(4): 343–57.

McEvilley, T. 1981. An Archaeology of Yoga. *Res* 1: 44–78.

McKean, L. 1996. *Divine Enterprise: Gurus and the Hindu Nationalist Movement*. Chicago: University of Chicago Press.

McLaurin, H. 1933. *Eastern Philosophy for Western Minds: An Approach to the Principles and Modern Practice of Yoga*. Boston, Mass: Stratford.

McLuhan, H. M. 1962. *The Gutenberg Galaxy: The Making of Typographic Man*. London: Routledge & Kegan Paul.

McLuhan, M., Q. Fiore, et al. 1967. *The Medium Is the Massage*. New York: Bantam.

Medin, A. 2004. Yoga for the Twenty-first Century: Krishnamacharya and the Modern Developments of Yoga, with Reference to the Schools of Aṣṭāṅga Yoga, Iyengar Yoga and Desikachar Yoga. *Indian Religions*. London, School of Oriental and African Studies, p. 108.

———. Forthcoming. *The Three Gurus*.

Mehta, N. D. 1919. *Hindu Eugenics*. Bandra: N.D. Mehta.

Melton, J. G. 1990. *New Age Encyclopedia*. Detroit: Gale Research Institute.

Mensendieck, B. 1918. *Standards of Female Beauty, Based on Conscious Muscle Education. [With Illustrations.]*. New York: Mensendieck.

———. 1906. *Körperkultur des Weibes : praktisch hygienische und praktisch ästhetische Winkel*. München: F. Bruckmann.

———. 1937. *The Mensendieck System of Functional Exercises*. Portland, Maine: Southworth- Anthoensen Press.

———. 1954. *Look Better, Feel Better: The World-renowned Mensendieck System of Functional Movements—for a Youthful Body and Vibrant Health*. New York: Harper.

Meyer, D. 1965. *The Positive Thinkers*. New York: Doubleday.

Midgley. 1985. *Evolution as Religion, Strange Hopes and Stranger Fears*. London: Methuen.

Miles, F. 1937. The Truth about Suppleness. *Health and Strength* 17: 572.

Mills, J. H., and S. Sen 2004. *Confronting the Body: The Politics of Physicality in Colonial and Post-colonial India*. London: Anthem.

Mitchell, S. 1977. Women's Participation in the Olympic Games 1900–1926. *Journal of Sport History* 4(2): 208–28.

Mitra, D. 2003. *Asanas, 608 Yoga Poses*. Novato, Calif.: New World Library.

Mitra, R. 1883. *The Yoga Aphorisms of Patanjali with the Commentary of Bhoja Raja and and English Translation*. Calcutta: Asiatic Society of Bengal.

Mitter, P. 1994. *Art and Nationalism in Colonial India, 1850–1922*. Cambridge: Cambridge University Press.

Monier-Williams, M. 1879. *Modern India and the Indians, Being a Series of Impressions, Notes and Essays*. London: Trubner.

———. 1891. *Brāhmanism and Hinduism or, Religious Thought and Life in India as Based on the Veda and Other Sacred Books of the Hindus*. London: John Murray.

Moore, S. D. 1996. *God's Gym: Divine Male Bodies of the Bible*. New York: Routledge.

Morgan, L. 1936. Surya Namaskars. A Rajah's 10-point Way to Health and Youth. *New Chronicle* (London), p. 5.

Morley, J. 2001. Inspiration and Expiration: Yoga Practice through Merleau-Ponty's Phenomenology of the Body. *Philosophy East and West* 51(1): 73–82.

Mosse, G. L. 1996. *The Image of Man: The Creation of Modern Masculinity*. New York: Oxford University Press.

Mosso, A. 1904. *Les Exercises Physiques et le Développement Intellectuel*. Paris: Felix Alcan.

Motoyama, H. 1981. *Theories of the Chakras, Bridge to Higher Consciousness*. Wheaton, Ill.: Quest Books (The Theosophical Publishing House).

Mrozek, D. J. 1992. The Scientific Quest for Physical Culture and the Persistent Appeal of Quackery. In J. W. Berryman and R. J. Park (eds.), *Sport and Exercise Science, Essays in the History of Sports Medicine*. Urbana: University of Illinois Press, pp. 283–96.

Mujumdar, D. C. 1950. *Encyclopedia of Indian Physical Culture*. Baroda: Good Companions.

Mujumdar, S. A. 1927. Presidential Address to the Maharashtra Physical Culture Conference. *Vyāyam, the Bodybuilder* 1(7): 182–95.

Müller, J. P. 1905. *My System, Fifteen Minutes' Work a Day for Health's Sake*. London: Anglo-Danish Publishing. Müller, M. 1881, *Selected Essays on Language, Mythology and Religion*, 2 vols. London: Longmans, Green.

———. 1899. *The Six Systems of Indian Philosophy*. London: Longmans, Green.

———. 1974 [1898]. *Ramakrishna, His Life and Sayings (with a Review of the Book by Swami Vivekananda)*. Calcutta: S. Gupta.

Muller-Ortega, P. E. 2005. "Tarko Yogāṅgam Uttamam": On Subtle Knowledge and the Refinement of Thought in Abhinavagupta's Liberative Tantric Method. In K. A. Jacobsen, *Theory and Practice of Yoga, Essays in Honour of Gerald James Larson*. Leiden: Brill, pp. 181–212.

Mundy, P. 1914. *The Travels of Peter Mundy in Europe and Asia 1608–1667. Vol. II: Travels in Asia, 1628–1634*. London: Hakluyt Society.

Muzumdar, S. 1937a. "Sarvangasana"—the Greatest of Yogic Exercises. The Health Wisdom of the East Contained in One Simple Movement. *Health and Strength*, June 12, pp. 861, 863.

———. 1937b. Gama—the King of Indian Super Wrestlers. *Health and Strength*, September 18, pp. 430–31.

———. 1937c. The Eastern Way to Health. *Health and Strength*, October 30, pp. 648–49.

———. 1949. *Yogic Exercises for the Fit and the Ailing*. Bombay: Orient Longmans.

Myss, C. 1996. *Anatomy of the Spirit: The Seven Stages of Power and Healing*. London: Bantam.

n.a. 1877. *The Saddarshana-Chintanikâ, or Studies in Indian Philosophy. A Monthly Publication Stating and Explaining the Aphorisms of the Six Schools of Indian Philosophy, with Their Translation into Marathi and English*. Poona: Dnyan Prakash Press.

n.a. 1927. Athletic and Gymnastic Exercises. *Vyayam* 1(5): 146.

n.a. 1930. Physical Training in Secondary Schools in Mysore. *Vyayam* 2(2): 10–12.

n.a. 1931. Curriculum of Studies in the Y.M.C.A. School of Physical Education, Madras. *Vyayam* 3(2): 28–31.

n.a. 1931–1947. *Jaganmohan Palace Administrative Records*. Mysore: Jaganmohan Palace Administration.

n.a. 1933. The Amazing Maxick Invades England. *Health and Strength*, July 22, p. 124.

n.a. 1936. The "Yogi" Sensation of the Season at Simla: A Lioness as Visitor at the Viceregal Lodge. *Illustrated London News*, June 27, p. 1163.

n.a. 1938. A New Health Era in the Orient. *Health and Strength*, April 9, p. 525.

n.a. 1970. Book Corner. *Yoga and Health*, 3:48.

Nadkarni, M. M. 1927. Prof. Rammurti, the Indian Hercules. *Vyayam* 1(4): 104–8.

Narasimhan, M. A. (trans.) 2005 [1935]. *The Yoga Makaranda of T. Krishnamacharya*. Unpublished translation.

———. (trans.) 2005 [c.1941]. *The Yogāsanagalu of T. Krishnamacharya*. Unpublished translation.

Narayan, K. 1989. *Storytellers, Saints and Scoundrels, Folk Narrative in Hindu Religious Teaching*. Delhi: Motilal Banarsidass.

———. 1993. Refractions of the Field at Home: American Representations of Hindu Holy Men in the Nineteenth and Twentieth Centuries. *Cultural Anthropology* 8(4): 476–509.

Narayanan, S. 1930. Recent Interesting Developments in Physical Education in India. *Vyayam* 2(2): 9–10.

Nathamuni, S. 1998. *Śrī Nāthamuni's Yogarahasya*. Chennai: Krishnamacharya Yoga Mandiram.

Neff, M. K., and H. P. Blavatsky 1937. *Personal Memoirs*. London: Rider.

Nevrin, K. 2005. Modern Yoga and Śrī Vaishnavism. *Journal of Vaishnava Studies* 14(1): 65–93.

———. Forthcoming. Taming Forces: Empowerment and Authenticity in Modern Hathayoga. Diss., Department of Ethnology, History of Religions, and Gender Studies, Stockholm University, Sweden.

Newcombe, S. 2007a. "A Social History of Yoga and Ayurveda in Britain, 1950–1995. Diss., Faculty of History, University of Cambridge.

———. 2007b. Stretching for Health and Well-Being: Yoga and Women in Britain, 1960–1980. *Asian Medicine, Tradition and Modernity (Special Yoga Issue)* 3: 37–63.

Nikhilananda, S. 1953. *Vivekananda: A Biography*. New York: Ramakrishna Center.

Nivedita, S. 1967. *The Complete Works of Sister Nivedita*. Calcutta: Ramakrishna Sarada Mission.

Noll, R. 1996. *The Jung Cult, the Origins of a Charismatic Movement*. London: Fontana Press.

Old Students'Association. 1940. *Our Physical Activities*. Kandivli: Training Institute for Physical Education.

Old, W. G. 1915. *The Yoga of Yama, What Death Said*. London: William Rider and Son.

Olivelle, P. 1996. *Upaniṣads*. Oxford World's Classics. Oxford: Oxford University Press.

O'Malley, L. S. S. 1935. *Popular Hinduism, the Religion of the Masses*. Cambridge: Cambridge University Press.

Oman, J. C. 1903. *The Mystics, Ascetics and Saints of India: A Study of Sadhuism, with an Account of the Yogis, Sanyasis, Bairagis, and Other Strange Hindu Sectarians*. London: T. Fisher Unwin.

Openshaw, J. 2002. *Seeking the Bauls of Bengal*. Cambridge: Cambridge University Press.

Ovington, J. 1696. *A Voyage to Suratt in the Year 1689*. London: Jacob Tonson.

Padoux, A. 2002. Corps et cosmos: l'image du corps du yogin tantrique. In V. Bouiller and G. Tarabout (eds.), *Images du Corps dans le Monde Hindou*. Paris: CNRS Editions, pp. 163–87.

Pahlajrai, P. 2004. Doxographies—Why Six *Darśanas*? Which Six? Available at www.students.washington.edu/prem/Colloquium04-Doxographies.pdf. Accessed 10 August 2005.

Park, R. J. 1978. "Embodied Selves": The Rise and Development of Concern for Physical Education, Active Games and Recreation for American Women, 1776–1865. *Journal of Sports History* 5: 5–41.

———. 1992. Physiologists, Physicians, and Physical Educators: Nineteenth-Century Biology and Exercise. In J. W. Berryman and R. J. Park (eds.), *Sport and Exercise Science, Essays in the History of Sports Medicine*. Urbana: University of Illinois Press, pp. 138–81.

Parker, G. T. 1973. *The History of Mind Cure in New England*. Hanover, N.H.: University Press of New England.

Parsley, W. L. 1930. Wrestlers of the Rajahs. *Health and Strength* March 20, pp. 400–01.

Partington, T. B. 1924. What Sterilisation Really Means. *Health and Strength*, March 31, p. 359.

———. 1933. Why Girls Become Sex-Morbid. *Health and Strength*, September 2, p. 301.

Patra, B. 1924. *The Mysteries of Nature*. Calcutta: S.C. Kavirata.

Pattabhiram, N. 1988. The Trinity of Bharatanatyam: Bala, Rukmini Devi and Kamala. *Sruti* 48: 23–24.

Paul, N. C. 1888 [1850]. *A Treatise on the Yoga Philosophy*. Bombay: Tukaram Tatya for the Bombay Theosophical Fund.

Payot, J. 1893/1909. *The Education of the Will, the Theory and Practice of Self-Culture*. New York: Funk and Wagnalls.

Phillips, K. 2001. *The Spirit of Yoga*. London: Cassell.

Physician. 1933. The Tibetan Legend, Recent Confirmations and a Dawn of Hope. *Health and Strength*, June 3, p. 640.

Pick, D. 1989. *Faces of Degeneration, a European Disorder, c.1848–1918*. Cambridge: Cambridge University Press.

Pinch, V. 2003. *Bhakti* and the British Empire. *Past and Present* 179(1): 159–96.

———. 2006. Warrior Ascetics and Indian Empires, 1500–2000. Cambridge: Cambridge University Press.

Pinney, C. 1997. *Camera Indica: The Social Life of Indian Photographs*. London: Reaktion.

———. 2003. *Photos of the Gods: The Printed Image and Political Struggle in India*. London: Reaktion.

Pollock, S. 1993. Deep Orientalism? Notes on Sanskrit and Power beyond the Raj. In C. A. Breckenridge and P. van der Veer (eds.), *Orientalism and the Postcolonial Predicament, Perspectives on South Asia*. Philadelphia: University of Pennsylvania Press, pp. 76–133.

Pound, E. 1934. *Make It New: Essays*. London: n.p.

Prasad, R. 1890. *The Science of Breath and the Philosophy of the Tatwas (translated from the Sanskrit), with Fifteen Introductory and Explanatory Essays on Nature's Finer Forces*. London: Theosophical Publishing Society.

———. 1907. *Self-Culture or the Yoga of Patanjali*. Madras: Theosophical Office.

———. 2003 [1912]. *Pātañjali's Yoga Sūtras*. New Delhi: Munshiram Manoharlal.

Pratinidhi, P. and L. Morgan 1938. *The Ten-Point Way to Health. Surya namaskars... Edited with an Introduction by Louise Morgan, etc.* London: J. M. Dent.

Pultz, J. 1995. *Photography and the Body*. London: George Weidenfeld and Nicolson.

Qureshi, R. 1991. Whose Music? Sources and Contexts in Indic Musicology. V. Bohlman Philip and B. Nettl (eds.), *Comparative Musicology and Anthropology of Music: Essays on the History of Ethnomusicology: Conference Entitled "Ideas, Concepts, and Personalities in the History of Ethnomusicology": Papers*. Chicago: University of Chicago Press, pp. 152–68.

Radhakrishnan, S. 1922. The Hindu Dharma. *International Journal of Ethics* 33(1): 1–22.

Radice, W. (ed.). 1998. *Swami Vivekananda and the Modernization of Hinduism*. Delhi: Oxford University Press.

Raghavan, V. 1958. *The Indian Heritage: An Anthology of Sanskrit Literature*. Bangalore, India: Indian Institute of Culture.

Rai, L. 1967. *A History of the Arya Samaj*. Bombay: Orient Longmans.

Raina, D., and S. I. Habib. 1996. The Moral Legitimation of Modern Science: Bhadralok Reflections on Theories of Evolution. *Social Studies of Science* 26(1): 9–42.

Ram Sukul, S. D. (ed.). 1927. *Practical Yoga*. Chicago: Hindu Yoga Society.

Ramacharaka, Y. 1903. *The Hindu-Yogi Science of Breath: A Complete Manual of the Oriental Breathing Philosophy of Physical, Mental, Psychic and Spiritual Development*. Chicago, Ill.: Yogi Publication Society.

———. 1904. *Hatha Yoga or the Yogi Philosophy of Physical Well-Being*. London: L. N. Fowler.

———. 1908. *The Inner Teachings of the Philosophies and Religions of India*. Chicago: Yogi Publication Society.

Ramamurthy, P. K. 1923. *Physical Culture, Being a Scheme Prepared for the Indian Universities*. Ahmedabad: Dharma Vyaya Press.

Ramaswami, S. 2000. *Yoga for the Three Stages of Life*. Rochester, Vt.: Inner Traditions.

Ramayandas, S. D. 1926. *First Steps in Yoga*. London: L. N. Fowler.

Rao, D. S. R. 1913. *In Tune with Nature. Health, Strength and Longevity in Modern India*. Madras: G. C. Loganadham Bros.

Rathbone, J. L. 1931. Some Aspects of Posture Education. *Vyayam* 3(1): 10–14.

Rea, S. 2006. *Yoga Trance Dance*. DVD. Silver Spring, Maryland: Acorn Media Publishing.

Reed, S. A. 1998. The Politics and Poetics of Dance. *Annual Review of Anthropology* 27: 503–32.

Reich, W., and K. R. Eissler. 1967. *Reich Speaks of Freud : Wilhelm Reich Discusses His Work and His Relationship with Sigmund Freud*. New York: Farrar, Straus and Giroux.

Rele, V. G. 1927. *The Mysterious Kundalini: The Physical Basis of the Kundalini (Hatha) Yoga according to Our Present Knowledge of Western Anatomy and Physiology*. Bombay: D. B. Taraporevala.

Rieker, H-U. 1989. *TheYoga of Light: Hatha Yoga Pradipika*, trans. E. Becherer. London: Unwin.

Robertson, R. 1992. *Globalization: Social Theory and Global Culture*. London: Sage.

Rodrigues, S. 1997. *The Householder Yogi: The Life of Shri Yogendra*. Bombay: Yogendra Publications Fund, the Yoga Institute.

Rose, H. A. 1911. *A Glossary of the Tribes and Castes of the Punjab and North-West Frontier Provinces*. Lahore: Civil and Military Gazette Press.

Ross, C. 2005. *Naked Germany: Health, Race and the Nation*. Oxford: Berg.

Rosselli 1980. The Self-Image of Effeteness: Physical Education and Nationalism in Nineteenth-Century Bengal. *Past and Present* 86: 121–48.

Roth, M. 1852. *Movements or Exercises according to Ling's System for the Development and Strengthening of the Human Body in Childhood and in Youth*. London: Groombridge and Sons.

———. 1856. *Gymnastic Exercises without Apparatus*. London: A. N. Myers.

Rothstein, H. 1853. *The Gymnastic Free Exercises of P. H. Ling*. London: Groombridge Bailliere.

Ruiz, F. P. 2006. Krishnamacharya's Legacy. Available at http://www.yogajournal.com/wisdom/465_4.cfm. Accessed March 6, 2006.

Ruyter, N. L. C. 1988. The Intellectual World of Genevieve Stebbins. *Dance Chronicle* 11(3): 381–97.

———. 1996. The Delsarte Heritage. *Journal of the Society for Dance Research* 14(1): 62–74.

———. 1999. *The Cultivation of Body and Mind in Nineteenth-Century American Delsartism*. Westport, Conn.: Greenwood Press.

Ruyter, N. L. C., and T. Leabhart. 2005. *Essays on François Delsarte*. Claremont, Calif.: Pomona College Theater Department for the Claremont Colleges.

Sadananda, Y., and G. A. Jacob. 1881. *A Manual of Hindu Pantheism: The Vedântasâra*. London: Trubner.

Samuel, G. 2006. Tibetan Medicine and Biomedicine: Epistemological Conflicts, Practical Solutions. *Asian Medicine, Tradition and Modernity* 2(1): 72–86.

———. 2007. Endpiece. *Asian Medicine, Tradition and Modernity (Special Yoga Issue)*. 3.1: 177–88.

———. 2008. *Origins of Yoga and Tantra: Indic Religions to the Thirteenth Century*. Cambridge: Cambridge University Press.

Sanchez, T. 2004. Origins of Yoga. Available at http://www.usyoga.org/html/origins.htm. Accessed March 20, 2005.

Sarbacker, S. R. 2005. *Samadhi: Numinous and Cessative in Indo-Tibetan Yoga*. Albany: State University of New York Press.

Sarkar, J. 1958. *A History of Dasnami Naga Sanyasis*. Daraganj: Sri Panchayati Akhara.

Sarkar, K. L. 1902. *The Hindu System of Self-Culture, or the Patanjala Yoga Shastra*. Calcutta: Sarasi Lal Sarkar.

Sarkar, S. 1973. *The Swadeshi Movement in Bengal, 1903–1908*. New Delhi: People's Publishing House.

Schmidt, A. M. 1960. *John Calvin and the Calvinistic Tradition*. New York: Harper.

Schmidt, R. 1908. *Fakire und Fakirtum im alten und modernen Indien : Yoga-Lehre und Yoga-Praxis nach den indischen Originalquellen*. Berlin: Hermann Barsdorf.

Schreiner, P. 2003. *Textualising Yoga: Patanjali's Yogasutras in Tradition and Modernity*. IAHR, Delhi: (Unpublished).

Sédir, P. 1906. *Le Fakirisme Hindou*. Paris: Librairie generale des sciences occultes.

Segel, H. B. 1998. *Body Ascendant: Modernism and the Physical Imperative*. Baltimore: Johns Hopkins University Press.

Self-Realization Fellowship. 2004. The Early Years in America (1920–1928). *The Life of Paramahansa Yogananda*. DVD. Los Angeles, Calif.: Self-Realization Fellowship.

Sen, S. 2004. Schools, Athletes and Confrontation: The Student Body in Colonial India. In J. H. Mills and S. Sen (eds.), *Confronting the Body, the Politics of Physicality in Colonial and Post-Colonial India*. London: Anthem.

Sen, S. P. 1974. *Dictionary of National Biography*. Calcutta: Institute of Historical Studies, vol. III.

Shastrideva, G., and J. Ballantyne. 1885. *The Yoga Philosophy, Being the Text of Patanjali with Bhoja Raja's Commentary; with Their Translations in English by Dr. Ballantyne and Govind Shastri Deva, and Introduction by Col. Olcott and an Appendix*. Bombay: Tookaram Tatya for the Bombay Theosophical Fund.

Shawn, T. n.d. *Every Little Movement: A Book about Francois Delsarte, the Man and His philosophy, His Science and Applied Aesthetics, the Application of This Science to the Art of the Dance, the Influence of Delsarte on American Dance*. Brooklyn: Dance Horizons.

Siegel, L. 1991. *Net of Magic, Wonders and Deceptions in India*. Chicago: University of Chicago Press.

Silvestri, M. 2000. "The Sinn Fein of India": Irish Nationalism and the Policing of Revolutionary Terrorism in Bengal. *Journal of British Studies* 39(4): 454–86.

Sinh, P. 1915. *The Hatha Yoga Pradipika*. Allahabad: Pāṇini Office.

Singh, J. 1979. *Vijñānabhairava or Divine Consciousness, a Treasure of 112 Types of Yoga.* Delhi: Motilal Banarsidass.

Singh, P. 2004. *Indian Cultural Nationalism.* New Delhi: India First Foundation.

Singleton, M. 2005. Salvation through Relaxation: Proprioceptive Therapy in Relation to Yoga. *Journal of Contemporary Religion* 20(3): 289–304.

———. 2006. Review of Joseph Alter's *Yoga in Modern India*, in *Asian Medicine, Tradition and Modernity* 2(1): 91–93.

———. 2007a. British Wheel of Yoga. In D. Cush, C. Robinson, and M. York (eds.), *Encyclopedia of Hinduism*, London: Curzon-Routledge, pp. 123–23.

———. 2007b. Choudhury, Bikram (b. 1946). In D. Cush, C. Robinson, and M. York (eds.), *Encyclopedia of Hinduism.* London: Curzon-Routledge, p. 142.

———. 2007c. Desikachar, T. K. V. and Viniyoga. In D. Cush, C. Robinson, and M. York (eds.), *Encyclopedia of Hinduism.* London: Curzon-Routledge, p. 178.

———. 2007d. Indra Devi (1900–2002). In D. Cush, C. Robinson, and M. York (eds.), *Encyclopedia of Hinduism.* London: Curzon-Routledge, pp. 369–70.

———. 2007e. Iyengar, B. K. S. and Iyengar Yoga (b. 1918). In D. Cush, C. Robinson, and M. York (eds.), *Encyclopedia of Hinduism.* London: Curzon-Routledge, pp. 380–81.

———. 2007f. Krishnamacharya, T. (1888–1989). In D. Cush, C. Robinson, and M. York (eds.), *Encyclopedia of Hinduism.* London: Curzon-Routledge, p. 424.

———. 2007g. Kuvalayananda, Swami (1883–1966) and Kaivalyadhama. In D. Cush, C. Robinson, and M. York (eds.), *Encyclopedia of Hinduism.* London: Curzon-Routledge, pp. 441–42.

———. 2007h. Jois, K. Pattabhi and Ashtanga Vinyasa Yoga. In D. Cush, C. Robinson, and M. York (eds.), *Encyclopedia of Hinduism.* London: Curzon-Routledge, p. 393.

———. 2007i. Satchidananda, Swami and Integral Yoga. In D. Cush, C. Robinson, and M. York (eds.), *Encyclopedia of Hinduism.* London: Curzon-Routledge, p. 769.

———. 2007j. Satyananda, Swami (b. 1923) and the Bihar School of Yoga. In D. Cush, C. Robinson, and M. York (eds.), *Encyclopedia of Hinduism.* London: Curzon-Routledge, p. 776.

———. 2007k. Vishnudevananda (1927–93) and Sivananda Yoga. In D. Cush, C. Robinson, and M. York (eds.), *Encyclopedia of Hinduism.* London: Curzon-Routledge, pp. 960–61.

———. 2007l. Yogendra, Shri (1897–1989) and the Yoga Institute, Santa Cruz. In D. Cush, C. Robinson, and M. York (eds.), *Encyclopedia of Hinduism.* London: Curzon-Routledge, pp. 1041–42.

———. 2007m. Yoga, Modern. In D. Cush, C. Robinson, and M. York (eds.), *Encyclopedia of Hinduism.* London: Curzon-Routledge, pp. 1033–38.

———. (ed.). 2007n. *Asian Medicine, Tradition and Modernity* (3)1 (Leiden: Brill).

———. 2007o. Suggestive Therapeutics: New Thought's Relationship to Modern Yoga. In *Asian Medicine, Tradition and Modernity* 3: 64–84.

———. 2007p. Yoga, Eugenics and Spiritual Darwinism in the Early Twentieth Century. *International Journal of Hindu Studies*, 11(2): 125–46.

———. 2008a. The Classical Reveries of Modern Yoga: Patañjali and Constructive Orientalism In M. Singleton and J. Byrne (eds), *Yoga in the Modern World, Contemporary Perspectives*. London: Routledge Hindu Studies Series.

———. 2008b. Introduction: Putting the Modern in Modern Yoga. In M. Singleton and J. Byrne (eds.), *Yoga in the Modern World: Contemporary Perspectives*. London: Routledge Hindu Studies Series.

———. Forthcoming-a. The American Dream of Yoga. *Nāmarūpa*.

———. Forthcoming-b. Modern Yoga. In K.A. Jacobsen (ed.), *Encyclopedia of Hinduism*. Leiden: Brill.

———. Forthcoming-c. The Siddhis in Modern Yoga, in K.A. Jacobsen (ed.), *The Siddhis of Yoga*. Leiden: Brill.

———. Forthcoming-d. *Yoga Makaranda* of T. Krishnamacharya. In D.G. White (ed.), *Yoga in Practice*. Princeton, N.J.: Princeton University Press.

Singleton, M. and J. Byrne (eds.). 2008. *Yoga in the Modern World: Contemporary Perspectives*. London: Routledge Hindu Studies Series.

Sinh, P. 1915. *The Hatha Yoga Pradipika*. Allahabad: Panini Office.

Sinha, M. 1995. *Colonial Masculinity: The "Manly Englishman" and the "Effeminate Bengali" in the Late Nineteenth Century*. Manchester: Manchester University Press.

Sivananda, S. 1929. *Practice of Yoga, etc.* Madras: Ganesh.

———. 1935. *Yoga Asanas*. Madras: P. K. Vinayagam.

Sjoman, N. E. 1996. *The Yoga Tradition of the Mysore Palace*. New Delhi: Abhinav.

Sklar, D. 1977. *Gods and Beasts: The Nazis and the Occult*. New York: T. Y. Crowell.

Smith, D. 2003. *Hinduism and Modernity*. Oxford: Blackwell.

———. 2004. Nietzsche's Hinduism, Nietzsche's India: Another Look. *Journal of Nietzsche Studies* 28: 37–56.

———. 2005. Orientalism and Hinduism. In G. Flood (ed.), *The Blackwell Companion to Hinduism*. Oxford: Blackwell Publishing.

Smith, B. 2008. With Heat Even Iron Will Bend: Discipline and Authority in Ashtanga Yoga. In M. Singleton and J. Byrne (eds.), *Yoga in the Modern World: Contemporary Perspectives*. London: Routledge Hindu Studies Series.

Sondhi, Krishnan Lal. 1962. Yoga and Indian Culture. *Journal of the Yoga Institute [Santa Cruz]* 7(4): 60–66.

Southard, B. 1993. Colonial Politics and Women's Rights: Woman Suffrage Campaigns in Bengal, British India in the 1920s. *Modern Asian Studies* 27(2): 397–439.

Srinivasan, D. 1984. Unhinging Siva from the Indus Civilization. *Journal of the Royal Asiatic Society of Great Britain and Ireland* 1: 77–89.

Srinivasan, P. 2003. Dancing Modern, Dancing Indian in America. *Pulse*, Autumn, pp. 11–13.

———. 2004. Dancing Modern/Dancing Indian/Dancing... in America. The Myths of Cultural"Purity." *Ballet-Dance Magazine* (April). Available at http://www.ballet-dance.com/200404/articles/asiandance.html. Accessed June 2006.

Srivastava, S. 2005. What happens when spirit meets wallet? It's patently obvious. *Asia Times Online*, July 2. Available at http://www.atimes.com/atimes/South_Asia/GG02Df02.html. Accessed October 2007.

Srivatsan, M. 1997. *Sri Krishnamacharya, the Purnacarya*. Chennai: Krishnamacharya Yoga Mandiram.

Staal, F. 1993. Indian Bodies. In T. P. Kasulis, R. T. Ames, and W. Dissanayake (eds.), *Self as Body in Asian Theory and Practice*. Albany: State University of New York Press, pp. 59–102.

Stack, M. B. 1931. *Building the Body Beautiful, the Bagot Stack Stretch-and-Swing System*. London: Chapman and Hall.

Stack, P. 1988. *Zest for Life, Mary Bagot Stack and the League of Health and Beauty*. London: Peter Owen.

Standwell, T. W. 1934. That Hole in the Brain Discovered by the Super Yogis and So Profitably Exploited by Them. *Health and Strength*, July 14, p. 42.

Stanley, B. 1937. Try Stretching for Strength. *Health and Strength*, February 27, p. 307.

Stebbins, G. 1892. *Dynamic Breathing and Harmonic Gymnastics: A Complete System of Psychical Aesthetic and Physical Culture*. New York: E.S. Werner.

———. 1898. *The Genevieve Stebbins System of Physical Training*. New York: E.S. Werner.

Steelcroft, F. 1896. Some Peculiar Entertainments I. *The Strand Magazine, An Illustrated Monthly*, vol. 11, January-June: 328–35.

———. 1897. A Living Idol. *The Strand Magazine, An Illustrated Monthly*, vol. 13, January-June: 176–80.

Stephen, D. R. 1914. *Patanjali for Western Readers, the Yoga Aphorisms of Patanjali Paraphrased and Modernised from Various English Translations and Recensions*. London: Theosophical Publishing Society.

Sterne, E. 2005. The Yoga of Krishnamacharya. *Journal of Vaishnava Studies* 14(1): 95–106.

Stocker, R. D. 1906. *Yoga Methods. How to Prosper in Mind, Body, and Estate*: London: L. N. Fowler and Co.

———. 1913. *The Time Spirit: A Survey of Contemporary Spiritual Tendencies*. London: Erskine Macdonald.

Stoddart, B. 1988. Sport, Cultural Imperialism, and Colonial Response in the British Empire. *Comparative Studies in Society and History* 30(4): 649–73.

Stone, D. 2002. *Breeding Superman, Nietzsche, Race and Eugenics in Edwardian and Interwar Britain*. Liverpool: Liverpool University Press.

Strauss, S. 2005. *Positioning Yoga: Balancing Acts across Cultures*. Oxford: Berg.

Studdert-Kennedy, G. 1991. *British Christians, Indian Nationalists and the Raj*. Delhi: Oxford University Press.

Sumption, D. 1927. *Fundamental Danish Gymnastics for Women*. New York: A. S. Barnes.

Sundaram, S. 1989 [1928]. *Yogic Physical Culture or the Secret of Happiness*. Bangalore: Brahmacharya Publishing.

Syman, S. 2003. Boston Brahma: How a Group of Turn-of-the-century Cambridge Women Made America Safe for Yoga. *Boston Globe*, August 24. Available at www.boston.com/news/globe/ideas/articles/2003/08/24/boston_brahma?mode=PF Accessed July 2004.

Tavernier, J-B. 1925 [1676]. *Travels in India*. London: Oxford University Press.

Taylor, G. H. 1860. *An Exposition of the Swedish Movement Cure*. New York: Fowler and Wells.

———. 1885. *Pelvic and Hernial Therapeutics. Principles and Methods for Remedying Chronic Affections of the Lower Part of the Trunk, including Processes for Self-Cure.* New York: John B. Alden.

———. 1893. *Mechanical Aids in the Treatment of Chronic Forms of Disease.* New York: G. W. Rogers.

Taylor, K. 2001. *Sir John Woodroffe, Tantra and Bengal: "An Indian Soul in a European Body"?* Richmond: Curzon.

Thevenot, J. de. 1684. *Troisième Partie des Voyages de M. de Thevenot, contenant la relation de l'Indostan, des nouveaux Mogols & des autres Peuples & Pays des Indes.* Paris: Claude Barbin. Available at http://gallica.bnf.fr/ark:/12148/bpt6k86648q.notice. Accessed March 2006.

Thomas, H., and J. Ahmed (eds.). 2004. *Cultural Bodies, Ethnography and Theory.* Oxford: Blackwell.

Thrift, N. 2004. Bare Life. In H. Thomas and J. Ahmed (eds.), *Cultural Bodies, Ethnography and Theory.* Oxford: Blackwell, pp. 145–69.

Tiruka (Sri Raghavendra Swami). 1971. *Suryanamaskara* (Kannada edition). Malladhihalli: Sarvodaya Mudranalaya, Anathasevashrama Trust.

———. 1977. *Suryanamaskara.* Malladhihalli: Sarvodaya Mudranalaya, Anathasevashrama Trust.

———. 1983. *Pranayama for Body and Soul.* Malladihalli: Sarvodaya Mudranalaya, Anathasevashrama Trust.

Tissot, C. J. 1780. *Gymnastique Medicinale et Chirurgicale.* Paris: Bastien.

Todd, J. 1998. *Physical Culture and the Body Beautiful: Purposive Exercise in the Lives of American Women, 1800–1870.* Macon, Ga.: Mercer University Press.

———. 2003. The Strength Builders: A History of Barbells, Dumbbells and Indian Clubs. *The International Journal of the History of Sport* 20(1): 65–90.

Trine, R. W. 1913. *The New Alinement of Life, concerning the Mental Laws of a Greater Personal and Public Power.* London: G. Bell and Sons.

Tripathi, A. 1974. *Vidyasagar: The Traditional Moderniser.* New Delhi: Oriental Longmans.

Turner, B. S. 1991. Recent Developments in the Theory of the Body. In M. Featherstone, M. Hepworth, and B. S. Turner (eds.), *The Body, Social Process and Cultural Theory.* London: Sage, pp. 1–35.

Uberoi, P. 2006. *Body, State and Cosmos: Mao Zedong's "Study of Physical Education"* (1917). Available at http://ignca.nic.in/ks_41018.htm. Accessed March 2006.

Urban, Hugh B. 2003. *Tantra: Sex, Secrecy, Politics, and Power in the Study of Religion.* Berkeley, Calif.: University of California Press.

———. 2006. *Magia Sexualis. Sex, Magic, and Liberation in Modern Western Esotericism.* Berkeley, Calif.: University of California Press.

Valentino, R. 1923. *How You Can Keep Fit.* New York: Macfadden.

van Buitenen, J.A.B. (trans.) 1981. *The Bhagavadgītā in the Mahābhārata.* London: University of Chicago Press.

Van Dalen, D. B., and Bruce L. Bennett, 1953. *A World History of Physical Education, Cultural, Philosophical, Comparative.* Englewood Cliffs, N.J.: Prentice Hall.

van der Veer, P. 1987. Taming the Ascetic: Devotionalism in a Hindu Monastic Order. *Man* 22(4): 680–95.

———. 1989. The Power of Detachment: Disciplines of Body and Mind in the Ramanandi Order. *American Ethnologist* 16(3): 458–70.

———. 1994. *Religious Nationalism, Hindus and Muslims in India*. London: University of California Press.

Vasu, S. C. 1895. *The Gheranda Sanhita, a Treatise on Hatha Yoga*. Bombay: Bombay Theosophical Publication Fund.

——— (ed.). 1913. *The Sacred Laws of the Aryas as Taught in the Schools of Yajnavalkya and Explained by Vijnanesvara in His Well-known Commentary Named the Mitaksara... The Prayaschitta Adhyaya*. Trans. Samarao Narasimha Naraharayya. Allahabad: Pāṇini Office.

———. 1915. *The Yoga Sastra, Consisting of an Introduction to Yoga Philosophy, Sanskrit Text with English Translation of 1. The Siva Samhitâ and of 2. The Gheraṇḍa Samhitâ*. Bahadurganj: Suhindra Nath Vasu (The Pâṇini Office, Bhuvaneśwarī Âśrama).

———. 1996a. *The Gheranda Samhita*. New Delhi: Munshiram Manoharlal.

———. 1996b. *The Siva Samhita*. New Delhi: Munshiram Manoharlal.

———. 2005. *The Siva Samhita*. New Delhi, India: Sri Satguru.

Vasu, S. C., and Y. S. Sabhapaty. 1895. *Om, the Philosophy and Science of Vedanta and Raja Yoga*. Lahore: R. C. Bary and Sons.

Vasudeva, S. 2004. *The Yoga of the Malinivijayottaratantra*. Pondicherry: Institut Francais de Pondichery, Ecole Francaise D" Extreme-Orient, chapters 1–4, 7–11, 11–17.

Versluis, A. 1993. *American Transcendentalism and Asian Religions*. New York: Oxford University Press.

Vidyārṇava, S. C. 1919. *A Catechism of Hindu Dharma*. Allahabad: Sudhindra Natha Vasu, The Pāṇini Office.

Vidyasagara, P. J. 1874. *The Patanjala Darshana, or the Aphorisms of Theistic Philosophy, with the Commentary of Maharshi Vedavyasa and the Gloss of Vachaspati Misra*. Calcutta: Satya Press.

Vijayadev, S. 1962. Genesis of Modern Yoga, The Unbroken Tradition. *Journal of the Yoga Institute* 7(3): 27–30.

Vishnudevananda, S. 1960. *The Complete Book of Yoga*. London: Souvenir Press.

———. 1999. *Hatha Yoga Pradipika: The Classic Guide for the Advanced Practice of Hatha Yoga (Kundalini Yoga): As Written Down in the Seventeenth Century from Ancient Sources by Yogi Swatmarama, Containing the Commentary Jyotsna of Brahmananda. Practical Commentary by Swami Vishnudevananda*. Delhi: Motilal Banarsidass.

Viswanathan, G. 2005. Colonialism and the Construction of Hinduism. In G. Flood (ed.), *The Blackwell Companion to Hinduism*. Oxford: Blackwell Publishing.

Vithaldas, Y. 1939. *The Yoga System of Health*. London: Faber and Faber.

Vivekananda, S. 2001 [1896]. *Raja Yoga, or Conquering the Internal Nature. The Complete Works of Swami Vivekananda*. Calcutta: Advaita Ashrama.

———. 1992 [1894]. Miracles. *The Complete Works of Swami Vivekananda*. Calcutta: Advaita Ashram, vol. 2, pp. 183–85.

———. 1992 [1895]. Epistle LXII. *The Complete Works of Swami Vivekananda*. Calcutta: Advaita Ashram, vol. 8, pp. 361–63.

———. 1992 [1897]. Conversations and Dialogues VIII. *The Complete Works of Swami Vivekananda*. Calcutta: Advaita Ashram, vol. 7, pp. 151–57.

———. 1992 [1900]. Concentration. *The Complete Works of Swami Vivekananda*. Calcutta: Advaita Ashrama, vol. 4, pp. 218–26.

———. 1992 [1902]. Conversations and Dialogues XXIII. *The Complete Works of Swami Vivekananda*. Calcutta: Advaita Ashram, vol. 7, pp. 239–44.

Voronoff, S. 1926. *Étude sur la vieillesse et la rajeunissement par la greffe*. Paris: G. Doin.

Wadia, A. R. 1951. Obituary: Rajasevasakta V. Subrahmanya Iyer, of Mysore, India. *Philosophy* 26: 96.

Wainwright, S. P., and B. S. Turner 2004. Narratives of Embodiment: Body, Aging, and Career in Royal Ballet Dancers. In H. Thomas and J. Ahmed (eds.), *Cultural Bodies, Ethnography and Theory*. Oxford: Blackwell, pp. 98–120.

Wakankar, M. 1995. Body, Crowd, Identity: Genealogy of a Hindu Nationalist Ascetic. *Social Text* 45: 45–73.

Walker, D., H. T. Alken, et al. 1834. *British Manly Exercises: In Which Rowing and Sailing Are Now First Described: and Riding and Driving Are for the First Time Given in a Work of This Kind: As Well as the Usual Subjects of Walking, Balancing, Wrestling, Running, Scating, Boxing, Leaping, Climbing, Training, Vaulting, Swimming, &c. &c. &c.: With Fifty Engravings*. London: T. Hurst.

Walter, H. 1893, *Svâtmârâma's Haṭhayogapradîpikâ (Die Leuchte des Haṭhayoga) aus dem Sanscrit übersetzt*. München: Universität München.

Ward Crampton, C. 1924. *Physical Exercise for Daily Use*. New York: G. P. Putnam's Sons.

Wase, C. 1921. *The Inner Teaching and Yoga*. London: W. Rider.

Wassan, H. Y. 1924. *The Hindu System of Health Development, the Hindu System of Health Koonmb and Ancient Philosophy*. Olympia, Wash.: Yogi Wassan.

———. 1925. *Soroda System of Yoga Philosophy, Applied by Yogi Wassan through Individual Analysis of Body and Mind*. N.p.: Yogi Wassan.

———. 1921. *Secret Key of the Yoga Philosophy, Ida, Pingla, Sukhmuna*. Seattle: Washington Printing.

———. 1922. *Secret Key to Health and Prana*. [Seattle?].

———. 1927. *Secrets of the Himalaya Mountain Masters and Ladder to Cosmic Consciousness*. [Philadelphia].

———. 1934. *Book of Nirvana, Super Cosmic Wisdom, Rajah Yoga System of Yoga Philosophy*. Chicago: Daws Letter Shop.

Watt, C. A. 1997. Education for National Efficiency: Constructive Nationalism in North India, 1909–1916. *Modern Asian Studies* 31(2): 339–74.

Weber, M. 1958 [1909]. *The Religion of India*. Glencoe, Ill.: Free Press.

Werner, K. (ed.). 1989. *The Yogi and the Mystic, Studies in Comparative Indian Mysticism*. London: Curzon Press.

Whalan, M. 2003. "Taking Myself in Hand": Jean Toomer and Physical Culture. *MODERNISM/Modernity* 10(4): 597–616.

Whicher, I. 1998. *The Integrity of the Yoga Darśana: A Reconsideration of Classical Yoga.* Albany, N.Y.: SUNY.

Whicher, I., and D. Carpenter. 2003. *Yoga: The Indian Tradition.* London Routledge/Curzon.

White, D. G. 1984. Why Gurus Are Heavy. *Numen* 31: 40–73.

———. 1996. *The Alchemical Body, Siddha Traditions in Medieval India.* Chicago: University of Chicago Press.

———. 2000. *Tantra in Practice.* Princeton, NJ: Princeton University Press.

———. 2002. Le monde dans le corps du siddha: microcosmologie dans les traditions médiévales indiennes. In V. Bouiller and G. Tarabout (eds.), *Images du Coprs dans le Monde Hindou.* Paris: CNRS Editions, pp. 189–212.

———. 2003. *Kiss of the Yogini: "Tantric Sex" in Its South Asian Contexts.* Chicago: University of Chicago Press.

———. 2004. Early Understandings of Yoga in the Light of Three Aphorisms from the Yoga Sutras of Patañjali. In E. Ciurtin (ed.), *Du corps humain, au Carrefour de plusieurs saviors en Inde. Mélanges offerts à Arion Rosu par ses collègues et ses amis à l'occasion de son 80e anniversaire.* Paris: De Boccard, pp. 611–27.

———. 2006. "Open" and "Closed" Models of the Human Body in Indian Medical and Yogic Traditions. *Asian Medicine, Tradition and Modernity* 2(1): 1–13.

Wilber, K. 1979. Are the Chakras Real? In J. White (ed.), *Kundalini, Evolution and Enlightenment.* Garden City, N.Y.: Anchor, pp. 120–32.

Wile, D. 1996. *Lost T'ai-Chi Classics from the Lat Ch'ing Dynasty.* Albany: State University of New York Press.

Wilke, M. 1926. *Hatha-Yoga. Die indische Fakir-Lehre zur Entwicklung magischer Gewalten im Menschen. 42. bis 49. Tausend.* Dresden: Rudolph.

Wilkins, W. J. 1887. *Modern Hinduism, Being an Account of the Religion and Life of the Hindus in Northern India.* New York: Scribner, Welford.

Williams, J. 2004. The Delsarte System of Expression—Lost in History. Available at http://www.delsarteproject.com/history.htm. Accessed May 10, 2005.

Will, P. J. 1996. Swami Vivekananda and Cultural Stereotyping. In N. Smart and B. S. Murthy (eds.), *East-West Encounters in Philosophy and Religion.* Mumbai: Popular Prakashan, pp. 377–87.

Woodroofe, Sir J. 1924. *The Serpent Power: Being the Shat-chakra-nirûpana and Pâdukâ-panchaka.* Madras: Ganesh.

Wordsworth, W., and W. J. B. Owen. 1985. *The Fourteen-book Prelude.* Ithaca: Cornell University Press.

Wujastyk, D. 2002. Interpréter l'image du corps humain dans l'Inde pré-moderne. In V. Bouiller and G. Tarabout (eds.), *Images du corps dans le monde hindou.* Paris: CNRS Editions.

Yadav, K. C. 2003 [1976]. *The Autobiography of Dayanand Saraswati.* Gugaon: Hope.

Yoga Institute of India. 1936. Editorial Notes. *Yoga, International Journal on the Science of Yoga* 4(26–28): 1–3.

Yoga Journal. 2008. Yoga Journal Releases 2008 "Yoga in America" Market Study. Press Release. Available at http://www.yogajournal.com/advertise/press_releases/10. Accessed January 2009.

Yogananda, P. 1925a. *General Principles and Merits of Yogoda or Tissue-Will System of Body and Mind Perfection, Originated and Taught by Swami Yogananda*. Los Angeles: Sat-Sanga & Yogoda Headquarters.

———. 1925b. *Psychological Chart*. Los Angeles: Yogoda and Sat-Sanga Headquarters.

———. 1946. *Autobiography of a Yogi*. New York: Philosophical Library.

Yogendra, S. 1988 [1928]. *Yoga Asanas Simplified*. Santa Cruz: Yoga Institute.

———. 1931. *Yoga Personal Hygiene*. Santa Cruz: Yoga Institute.

———. 1975. *Facts about Yoga*. Santa Cruz: Yoga Institute.

———. 1976. *Why Yoga*. Santa Cruz: Yoga Institute.

———. 1978. *Yoga Essays*. Santa Cruz: Yoga Institute.

Younger, P. 1995. *The Home of the Dancing Śivan, the Traditions of the Hindu Temple in Citamparam*. New York: Oxford University Press.

Zarrilli, P. B. 1998. *When the Body Becomes All Eyes: Paradigms, Discourses and Practices of Power in Kalarippayatu, a South Indian Martial Art*. Delhi: Oxford University Press.

Zolberg, A. 2006. *A Nation by Design: Immigration Policy in the Fashioning of America*. Cambridge, Mass: Harvard University Press.

index